# Critical Care of the Pediatric Patient

*Editor*

DEREK S. WHEELER

# PEDIATRIC CLINICS OF NORTH AMERICA

www.pediatric.theclinics.com

June 2013 • Volume 60 • Number 3

**ELSEVIER**

1600 John F. Kennedy Boulevard • Suite 1800 • Philadelphia, Pennsylvania, 19103-2899

http://www.theclinics.com

**THE PEDIATRIC CLINICS OF NORTH AMERICA Volume 60, Number 3**
**June 2013 ISSN 0031-3955, ISBN-13: 978-1-4557-7135-6**

Editor: Kerry Holland
Developmental Editor: Donald Mumford

The Pediatric Clinics of North America (ISSN 0031-3955) is published bimonthly by Elsevier Inc., 360 Park Avenue South, New York, NY 10010-1710. Months of issue are February, April, June, August, October, and December. Periodicals postage paid at New York, NY and additional mailing offices. Subscription prices are $191.00 per year (US individuals), $462.00 per year (US institutions), $259.00 per year (Canadian individuals), $614.00 per year (Canadian institutions), $308.00 per year (international individuals), $614.00 per year (international institutions), $93.00 per year (US students and residents), and $159.00 per year (international and Canadian residents and students). To receive students/resident rare, orders must be accompanied by name of affiliated institution, date of term, and the signature of program/residency coordinator on institution letterhead. Orders will be billed at individual rate until proof of status is received. Foreign air speed delivery is included in all Clinics subscription prices. All prices are subject to change without notice. **POSTMASTER:** Send address changes to The Pediatric Clinics of North America, Elsevier Health Sciences Division, Subscription Customer Service, 3251 Riverport Lane, Maryland Heights, MO 63043. **Customer Service: 1-800-654-2452 (US and Canada). From outside of the US and Canada: 1-314-447-8871. Fax: 1-314-447-8029. For print support, E-mail: JournalsCustomerService-usa@elsevier.com. For online support, E-mail: JournalsOnlineSupport-usa@elsevier.com.**

Reprints. For copies of 100 or more, of articles in this publication, please contact the Commercial Reprints Department, Elsevier Inc., 360 Park Avenue South, New York, NY 10010-1710. Tel.: 212-633-3812; Fax: 212-462-1935; E-mail: reprints@elsevier.com.

The Pediatric Clinics of North America is also published in Spanish by McGraw-Hill Inter-americana Editores S.A., Mexico City, Mexico; in Portuguese by Riechmann and Affonso Editores, Rua Comandante Coelho 1085, CEP 21250, Rio de Janeiro, Brazil; and in Greek by Althayia SA, Athens, Greece.

The Pediatric Clinics of North America is covered in MEDLINE/PubMed (Index Medicus), Excerpta Medica, Current Contents, Current Contents/Clinical Medicine, Science Citation Index, ASCA, ISI/BIOMED, and BIOSIS.

Printed and bound by CPI Group (UK) Ltd, Croydon, CR0 4YY

Transferred to digital print 2013

## PROGRAM OBJECTIVE

The goal of the *Pediatric Clinics of North America* is to keep practicing physicians and residents up to date with current clinical practice in pediatrics by providing timely articles reviewing the state-of-the-art in patient care.

## TARGET AUDIENCE

All practicing pediatricians, physicians and healthcare professionals who provide patient care to pediatric patients.

## LEARNING OBJECTIVES

Upon completion of this activity, participants will be able to:

1. Review advances in critical care of the hematopoietic stem cell transplant patient as well as advances in cardiac intensive care and neurocritical care.
2. Recognize the importance of family-centered care in the pediatric intensive care unit.
3. Describe advances in monitoring and management of shock and pediatric acute lung injury as well as advances in the recognition, resuscitation and stabilization of the critically ill child.

## ACCREDITATION

The Elsevier Office of Continuing Medical Education (EOCME) is accredited by the Accreditation Council for Continuing Medical Education (ACCME) to provide continuing medical education for physicians.

The EOCME designates this journal-based CME activity for a maximum of 15 *AMA PRA Category 1 Credit(s)™*. Physicians should claim only the credit commensurate with the extent of their participation in the activity.

All other health care professionals completing continuing education credit for this activity will be issued a certificate of participation.

## DISCLOSURE OF CONFLICTS OF INTEREST

The EOCME assesses conflict of interest with its instructors, faculty, planners, and other individuals who are in a position to control the content of CME activities. All relevant conflicts of interest that are identified are thoroughly vetted by EOCME for fair balance, scientific objectivity, and patient care recommendations. EOCME is committed to providing its learners with CME activities that promote improvements or quality in healthcare and not a specific proprietary business or a commercial interest.

**The planning committee, staff, authors and editors listed below have identified no financial relationships or relationships to products or devices they or their spouse/life partner have with commercial interest related to the content of this CME activity:**

Kamal Abulebda, MD; Rajesh Aneja, MD; Rajit Basu, MD; Robert A. Berg, MD; Emily Brink, RN, BSN; Joshua Cappell, MD, PhD; Joseph Carcillo, MD; Ranjit Chima, MD; Jeff Clark, MD; Nicole Congleton; Susan Eggly, PhD; James Fortenberry, MD; D. Catherine Fuchs, MD; Kerry Holland; Sonata Jodele, MD; Steven G. Kernie, MD; Indu Kumari; Sandy Lavery; James Marcin, MD; Jill McNair; Kathleen L. Meert, MD; F. Lynne Merk, PhD; Rick Merk; Haifa Mtaweh, MD; Stephen Muething, MD; Vinay Nadkarni, MD; Matthew Niedner, MD; Pratik P. Pandharipande, MD, MSCI; W. Bradley Poss, MD; Carley Riley, MD; Charles Schleien, MD, MBA; Heidi Smith, MD; Erik Su, MD; Kathleen Sutcliffe, PhD; Alexis A. Topjian, MD, MSCE; Erin V. Trakas, MD; Derek S. Wheeler, MD, FAAP, FCCP, FCCM.

**The planning committee, staff, authors and editors listed below have identified financial relationships or relationships to products or devices they or their spouse/life partner have with commercial interest related to the content of this CME activity:**

**Ronald Bronicki, MD** is on speakers bureau for Covidien.

**Paul Checchia, MD** is on speakers bureau for Abbott, and has a research grant from Ikaria Inc.

**Ira Cheifetz, MD** is a consultant/advisor for Philips, Hill-Rom and Teleflex.

**E. Wesley Ely, MD, MPH** is a consultant/advisor for Masimo, and is on speakers bureau for Hospira, Abbott and Orion.

**Stuart L. Goldstein, MD** is on the speaker's bureau for Gambro Renal Products, is a consultant/advisor for Gambro Renal Products, Baxter Healthcare, Ikaria, Inc., Otsuka, Inc., Alexion, and Hemametrics; and has received a research grant from Gambro Renal Products.

**Matthew Paden, MD** has research grants and patents with KIDS CRRT.

## UNAPPROVED/OFF-LABEL USE DISCLOSURE

The EOCME requires CME faculty to disclose to the participants:

1. When products or procedures being discussed are off-label, unlabelled, experimental, and/or investigational (not US Food and Drug Administration [FDA] approved); and

2. Any limitations on the information presented, such as data that are preliminary or that represent ongoing research, interim analyses, and/or unsupported opinions. Faculty may discuss information about pharmaceutical agents that is outside of FDA-approved labelling. This information is intended solely for CME and is not intended to promote off-label use of these medications. If you have any questions, contact the medical affairs department of the manufacturer for the most recent prescribing information.

## TO ENROLL

To enroll in the *Pediatric Clinics of North America* Continuing Medical Education program, call customer service at 1-800-654-2452 or sign up online at http://www.theclinics.com/home/cme. The CME program is available to subscribers for an additional annual fee of USD 261.

## METHOD OF PARTICIPATION

In order to claim credit, participants must complete the following:
1. Complete enrolment as indicated above.
2. Read the activity.
3. Complete the CME Test and Evaluation. Participants must achieve a score of 70% on the test. All CME Tests and Evaluations must be completed online.

## CME INQUIRIES/SPECIAL NEEDS

For all CME inquiries or special needs, please contact elsevierCME@elsevier.com.

# Contributors

## EDITOR

**DEREK S. WHEELER, MD, MMM**
Associate Chief of Staff, Cincinnati Children's Hospital Medical Center; and Associate Professor of Clinical Pediatrics, University of Cincinnati, College of Medicine, Cincinnati, Ohio

## AUTHORS

**KAMAL ABULEBDA, MD**
Clinical Fellow, Division of Critical Care Medicine, Cincinnati Children's Hospital Medical Center, Cincinnati, Ohio

**RAJESH K. ANEJA, MD**
Departments of Critical Care Medicine and Pediatrics, Children's Hospital of Pittsburgh, University of Pittsburgh School of Medicine, Pittsburgh, Pennsylvania

**RAJIT K. BASU, MD, FAAP**
Division of Critical Care, Department of Pediatrics, Cincinnati Children's Hospital and Medical Center, University of Cincinnati, Cincinnati, Ohio

**ROBERT A. BERG, MD**
Department of Anesthesia and Critical Care Medicine, The Children's Hospital of Philadelphia, The University of Pennsylvania, Philadelphia, Pennsylvania

**EMILY BRINK, RN, BSN**
Registered Nurse, Research Coordinator, Research Nurse Specialist III, Department of Anesthesiology, Vanderbilt University, Nashville, Tennessee

**RONALD A. BRONICKI, MD**
Associate Medical Director, Cardiac Intensive Care Unit, Texas Children's Hospital; Associate Professor of Pediatrics, Baylor College of Medicine, Houston, Texas

**JOSHUA CAPPELL, MD, PhD**
Pediatric Critical Care Medicine, Department of Pediatrics, Morgan Stanley Children's Hospital, Columbia University Medical Center, Columbia University College of Physicians and Surgeons; Department of Neurology, Columbia University Medical Center, New York, New York

**JOSEPH A. CARCILLO, MD**
Departments of Critical Care Medicine and Pediatrics, Children's Hospital of Pittsburgh, University of Pittsburgh School of Medicine, Pittsburgh, Pennsylvania

**PAUL A. CHECCHIA, MD, FCCM, FACC**
Medical Director, Cardiac Intensive Care Unit, Texas Children's Hospital; Professor of Pediatrics, Baylor College of Medicine, Houston, Texas

**IRA M. CHEIFETZ, MD, FCCM, FAARC**
Professor of Pediatrics, Division Chief, Pediatric Critical Care Medicine, Duke University Medical Center; Medical Director, Pediatric Intensive Care Unit, Medical Director, Pediatric Respiratory Care and ECMO, Duke Children's Hospital; Director, Pediatric Critical Care Services, Duke University Health System, Durham, North Carolina

**RANJIT S. CHIMA, MD**
Assistant Professor, Division of Critical Care Medicine, Cincinnati Children's Hospital Medical Center; Department of Pediatrics, University of Cincinnati College of Medicine, Cincinnati, Ohio

**JEFF CLARK, MD**
Associate Professor, Department of Pediatrics, Critical Care Medicine, Children's Hospital of Michigan, Detroit, Michigan

**SUSAN EGGLY, PhD**
Associate Professor, Department of Internal Medicine, Karmanos Cancer Institute, Wayne State University, Detroit, Michigan

**EUGENE WESLEY ELY, MD, MPH**
Professor of Medicine, Division of Allergy/Pulmonary/Critical Care Medicine, Center for Health Services Research, Vanderbilt University, VA-GRECC, Nashville, Tennessee

**JAMES D. FORTENBERRY, MD, MCCM, FAAP**
Pediatrician in Chief, Children's Healthcare of Atlanta; Professor of Critical Care, Department of Pediatrics, Emory University School of Medicine, Atlanta, Georgia

**DICKEY CATHERINE FUCHS, MD**
Associate Professor, Division of Child and Adolescent Psychiatry, Department of Psychiatry, Director, Psychological and Counseling Center, Vanderbilt University, Nashville, Tennessee

**STUART L. GOLDSTEIN, MD**
Professor of Pediatrics, University of Cincinnati College of Medicine; Director, Center for Acute Care Nephrology Medical Director, Pheresis Service Nephrology and Hypertension, The Heart Institute, Cincinnati Children's Hospital Medical Center, Cincinnati, Ohio

**SONATA JODELE, MD**
Associate Professor, Division of Bone Marrow Transplantation and Immunodeficiency, Cincinnati Children's Hospital Medical Center; Department of Pediatrics, University of Cincinnati College of Medicine, Cincinnati, Ohio

**STEVEN G. KERNIE, MD**
Director, Pediatric Critical Care Medicine, Department of Pediatrics, Morgan Stanley Children's Hospital, Columbia University Medical Center, Associate Professor of Pediatrics and Pathology & Cell Biology, Columbia University College of Physicians and Surgeons, New York, New York

**JAMES P. MARCIN, MD, MPH**
Professor, Department of Pediatrics, University of California Davis Children's Hospital, Sacramento, California

**KATHLEEN L. MEERT, MD**
Professor, Department of Pediatrics, Critical Care Medicine, Children's Hospital of Michigan, Detroit, Michigan

**LYNNE MERK**
The Pray ~ Hope ~ Believe Foundation, Cincinnati, Ohio

**RICK MERK**
The Pray ~ Hope ~ Believe Foundation, Cincinnati, Ohio

**HAIFA MTAWEH, MD**
Departments of Critical Care Medicine and Pediatrics, Children's Hospital of Pittsburgh, University of Pittsburgh School of Medicine, Pittsburgh, Pennsylvania

**STEPHEN E. MUETHING, MD**
Vice President of Safety, Cincinnati Children's Hospital and Medical Center, Associate Professor of Pediatrics, University of Cincinnati, Cincinnati, Ohio

**VINAY M. NADKARNI, MD, MS**
Endowed Chair, Department of Anesthesia and Critical Care Medicine, The Children's Hospital of Philadelphia, The University of Pennsylvania, Philadelphia, Pennsylvania

**MATTHEW F. NIEDNER, MD**
Director of Quality Improvement and Patient Safety, Pediatric Intensive Care Unit, Division of Critical Care Medicine, Assistant Professor, Department of Pediatrics, Mott Children's Hospital, University of Michigan Medical Center, Ann Arbor, Michigan

**MATTHEW L. PADEN, MD**
Director, Pediatric ECMO, Apheresis, and Advanced Technologies, Children's Healthcare of Atlanta; Assistant Professor of Pediatric Critical Care, Emory University School of Medicine, Atlanta, Georgia

**PRATIK P. PANDHARIPANDE, MD, MSCI**
Associate Professor of Anesthesiology and Surgery, Division of Critical Care, Department of Anesthesiology, Vanderbilt University, Nashville, Tennessee

**W. BRADLEY POSS, MD, MMM**
Medical Director, Pediatric Intensive Care Unit, Division of Pediatric Critical Care Medicine, Primary Children's Medical Center; Professor of Pediatrics, Department of Pediatrics, University of Utah School of Medicine, Salt Lake City, Utah

**CARLEY RILEY, MD, MPP**
Division of Critical Care Medicine, Cincinnati Children's Hospital Medical Center, Cincinnati, Ohio

**CHARLES L. SCHLEIEN, MD, MBA**
Chairman and Professor, Department of Pediatrics, North Shore-LIJ Health System, Hofstra School of Medicine, New York

**HEIDI A.B. SMITH, MD, MSCI, FAAP**
Pediatric Anesthesiology-Fellow and Pediatric Intensivist, Department of Anesthesiology, Vanderbilt University, Nashville, Tennessee

**ERIK SU, MD**
Department of Anesthesia and Critical Care Medicine, Johns Hopkins Hospital, Baltimore, Maryland

**KATHLEEN M. SUTCLIFFE, PhD**
Professor of Business Administration and Professor of Management and Organizations, University of Michigan Ross School of Business, Ann Arbor, Michigan

**ALEXIS A. TOPJIAN, MD**
Department of Anesthesia and Critical Care Medicine, The Children's Hospital of Philadelphia, The University of Pennsylvania, Philadelphia, Pennsylvania

**ERIN V. TRAKAS, MD**
Departments of Critical Care Medicine and Pediatrics, Children's Hospital of Pittsburgh, University of Pittsburgh School of Medicine, Pittsburgh, Pennsylvania

**DEREK S. WHEELER, MD, MMM**
Associate Chief of Staff, Cincinnati Children's Hospital Medical Center; and Associate Professor of Clinical Pediatrics, University of Cincinnati, College of Medicine, Cincinnati, Ohio

# Contents

The past 50 years have witnessed the emergence and evolution of the modern pediatric ICU and the specialty of pediatric critical care medicine. ICUs have become key in the delivery of health care services. The patient population within pediatric ICUs is diverse. An assortment of providers, including intensivists, trainees, physician assistants, nurse practitioners, and hospitalists, perform a variety of roles. The evolution of critical care medicine also has seen the rise of critical care nursing and other critical care staff collaborating in multidisciplinary teams. Delivery of optimal critical care requires standardized, reliable, and evidence-based processes, such as bundles, checklists, and formalized communication processes.

In health care, reliability is the measurable capability of a process, procedure, or health service to perform its intended function in the required time under actual or existing conditions (as opposed to the ideal circumstances under which they are often studied). This article outlines the current state of reliability in a clinical context, discusses general principles of reliability, and explores the characteristics of high-reliability organizations as a desirable future state for pediatric critical care.

Telemedicine technologies involve real-time, live, interactive video and audio communication and allow pediatric critical care physicians to have a virtual presence at the bedside of any critically ill child. Telemedicine use is increasing and will be a common technology in remote emergency departments, inpatient wards, and pediatric intensive care units. There is mounting data that demonstrate that the use of telemedicine technologies can result in higher quality of care, more efficient resource use and improved cost-effectiveness, and higher satisfaction among patients, parents, and remote providers compared to current models of care.

All pediatric intensivists need a primer on ICU finance. The author describes potential alternate revenue sources for the division. Differentiating units by size or academic affiliation, the author describes drivers of expense. Strategies to manage the bottom line including negotiations for

of mortality, but rather on perioperative management strategies intended to improve neurologic outcomes. The care of children with critical cardiac disease will continue to rely on broad and collaborative efforts by specialists and primary care practitioners to build on this foundation of success.

consistently taught to staff and therefore the actual delivery of EOL care is often inconsistent and invariably negatively associated with the long-term mental health of both the patient's family and care providers. This review describes the pertinent aspects of end-of-life care in pediatrics. Finally, a framework to optimize the quality of death is described, which underscores the importance of synchrony between the care team and the family at the end of a child's life.

This review article updates the pediatric medical community on the current literature regarding diagnosis and treatment of delirium in critically ill children. This information will be of value to pediatricians, intensivists, and anesthesiologists in developing delirium monitoring and management protocols in their pediatric critical care units.

Patient-centered and family-centered care (PFCC) has been endorsed by many professional health care organizations. Although variably defined, PFCC is an approach to care that is respectful of and responsive to the preferences, needs, and values of individual patients and their families. Research regarding PFCC in the pediatric intensive care unit has focused on 4 areas including (1) family visitation; (2) family-centered rounding; (3) family presence during invasive procedures and cardiopulmonary resuscitation; and (4) family conferences. Although challenges to successful implementation exist, the growing body of evidence suggests that PFCC is beneficial to patients, families, and staff.

The pediatric intensive care unit (PICU) can be an intimidating and frightening place for parents and family members of critically ill children. Most parents experience a loss of control and feelings of utter helplessness. Many PICUs are working with family members to improve the quality of care provided through patient- and family-centered care, which is in fact 1 of the 6 tenets of the Institute of Medicine's definition of quality health care. However, as highlighted by the tragic and very personal experience described by one family, PICUs can and should be doing more to improve the patient and family experience.

# PEDIATRIC CLINICS OF NORTH AMERICA

**RELATED INTEREST**

*Critical Care Medicine Clinics of North America* January 2013 (Volume 29:1)
**Enhancing the Quality of Care in the ICU**
Available at: http://www.criticalcare.theclinics.com/current
Robert C. Hyzy, MD, *Editor*

**NOW AVAILABLE FOR YOUR iPhone and iPad**

# Preface

# Care of the Critically Ill Pediatric Patient

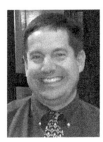

Derek S. Wheeler, MD, MMM
*Editor*

Pediatric critical care medicine is a surprisingly new subspecialty. While pediatric intensive care units (PICUs) were first developed in the late 1950s and early 1960s, pediatric critical care medicine did not emerge as a distinct discipline with its own subspecialty board certification until 1987.[1,2] The field of pediatric critical care medicine has changed considerably over these last 26 years. The modern PICU of today is vastly different, even from as recently as 5 years ago. For example, many pediatric intensivists remember a time when cell phones were prohibited in the PICU, as they interfered with the circuitry of the monitors and life-support devices. Today, pediatric intensivists can often remotely monitor the status of their patients from these same cell phones.[3-6] In fact, it is not hard to imagine that one day soon, pediatric intensivists will be able to remotely monitor and provide treatment recommendations for critically ill children several hundreds of miles away using handheld tablet computers or smart phones. Technological advances in monitoring have similarly changed almost overnight. Near-infrared spectroscopy, continuous venous oximetry, and pulse contour analysis have largely replaced the need for invasive hemodynamic monitoring using the pulmonary artery catheter.[7-9] In the past, pediatric intensivists relied on a diagnostic assessment honed to perfection through years of experience. Now, pediatric intensivists routinely rely on a vast array of condition-specific biomarkers in order to begin treatment even before patients start to manifest classic signs and symptoms.[10] Pediatric critical care medicine has indeed changed for the better and will undoubtedly continue to improve. Yet, even with all of the technological advancements and scientific achievements that will surely come in the future, the human element of what pediatric intensivists do will never change. For all of the science inherent in the specialty of pediatric critical care medicine, there is still art in providing comfort and solace to critically ill children and their families. No technology will ever replace the compassion in the touch of a hand or the soothing words of a calm and gentle voice. Therefore, in the pages that follow, a group of incredibly talented and gifted clinicians discuss both the art

Pediatr Clin N Am 60 (2013) xv–xvi
http://dx.doi.org/10.1016/j.pcl.2013.03.001
0031-3955/13/$ – see front matter © 2013 Published by Elsevier Inc.

**pediatric.theclinics.com**

and the science of pediatric critical care medicine. On behalf of all of them, I give my sincerest and most humble thanks to all of the critically ill children and their families whom we have been blessed to call our patients. It has indeed been our privilege.

Derek S. Wheeler, MD, MMM
Cincinnati Children's Hospital Medical Center
3333 Burnet Avenue
Cincinnati, OH 45229-3039, USA

E-mail address:
Derek.wheeler@cchmc.org

**REFERENCES**

1. Downes JJ. The historical evolution, current status, and prospective development of pediatric critical care. Crit Care Clin 1992;8:1–22.
2. Epstein D, Brill JE. A history of pediatric critical care medicine. Pediatr Res 2005; 58:987–96.
3. Klein AA, Djaiani GN. Mobile phones in the hospital—past, present, and future. Anaesthesia 2003;58:353–7.
4. Lawrentschuk N, Bolton DM. Mobile phone interference with medical equipment and its clinical relevance: A systematic review. Med J Aust 2004;181:145–9.
5. Zhang P, Kogure Y, Matsuoka H, et al. A remote patient monitoring system using a Java-enabled 3G mobile phone. Conf Proc IEEE Eng Med Biol Soc 2007;2007: 3713–6.
6. Zhang P, Kumabe A, Kogure Y, et al. New functions developed for ICU/CCU remote monitoring system using a 3G mobile phone and evaluations of the system. Conf Proc IEEE Eng Med Biol Soc 2008;2008:5342–5.
7. Bronicki RA. Venous oximetry and the assessment of oxygen transport balance. Pediatr Crit Care Med 2011;12:S21–6.
8. Ghanayem NS, Wernovsky G, Hoffman GM. Near-infrared spectroscopy as a hemodynamic monitor in critical illness. Pediatr Crit Care Med 2011;12:S27–32.
9. Gazit AZ, Cooper DS. Emerging technologies. Pediatr Crit Care Med 2011;12: S55–61.
10. Kaplan JM, Wong HR. Biomarker discovery and development in pediatric critical care medicine. Pediatr Crit Care Med 2011;12:165–73.

# The Evolving Model of Pediatric Critical Care Delivery in North America

Carley Riley, MD, MPP[a], W. Bradley Poss, MD, MMM[b],
Derek S. Wheeler, MD, MMM[a,c,d],*

## KEYWORDS

- Pediatric ICU • Critical care medicine • Critical care nursing
- Multidisciplinary teams

## KEY POINTS

- Over the past half century, health care delivery has evolved such that ICUs, including specialized pediatric ICUs (PICUs), have become a vital element in the health care delivery system.
- During this time, both PICUs and the field of pediatric critical care medicine have evolved into their current forms.
- Critical care is now provided to a diverse patient population in a wide array of settings by multidisciplinary teams of physicians, nonphysician providers, nurses, pharmacists, nutritionists, and other ancillary staff members who specialize in pediatric critical care and coordinate with members of other medical and surgical disciplines.
- As the field of pediatric critical care medicine evolves, it seeks to improve so that patients receive reliable, efficient, and evidence-based care with optimal outcomes.
- As the patient population changes, providers adapt, staffing models adjust, technology evolves, therapies advance, and outcomes are transformed.
- The evolution of pediatric critical care over its first 50 years has been tremendous, but the next 50 years will assuredly bring even greater change.

[a] Division of Critical Care Medicine, Cincinnati Children's Hospital Medical Center, 3333 Burnet Avenue, Cincinnati, OH 45229-3039, USA; [b] Division of Pediatric Critical Care Medicine, Department of Pediatrics, University of Utah School of Medicine, 100 North Mario Capecchi Drive, Salt Lake City, UT 84132, USA; [c] Department of Pediatrics, University of Cincinnati College of Medicine, 3333 Burnet Avenue, Cincinnati, OH 45229-3039, USA; [d] The James M. Anderson Center for Health Systems Excellence, Cincinnati Children's Hospital Medical Center, 3333 Burnet Avenue, Cincinnati, OH 45229-3039, USA
* Corresponding author. Division of Critical Care Medicine, Cincinnati Children's Hospital Medical Center, 3333 Burnet Avenue, Cincinnati, OH 45229-3039.
*E-mail address:* derek.wheeler@cchmc.org

Pediatr Clin N Am 60 (2013) 545–562
http://dx.doi.org/10.1016/j.pcl.2013.02.001
0031-3955/13/$ – see front matter © 2013 Elsevier Inc. All rights reserved.

## INTRODUCTION

ICUs are a key element in the overall delivery of health care services. Many patients receive care in an ICU (or in some cases, by an ICU team outside an ICU) at some point during their hospital stay. ICU care also accounts for a significant proportion of total health care costs.[1] For example, recent studies suggest that ICU care represents between 17.4% and 39.0% of all hospital costs[1–4] and between 0.56% and 1% of the United States' gross domestic product.[5] These statistics highlight the importance of providing safe, effective, patient-centered and family-centered, efficient, timely, and equitable care in an ICU.[6,7] One of the challenges faced by every ICU today is to minimize costs of care while maintaining quality (ie, increasing the value). This article provides a brief overview of the current state of pediatric critical care delivery and discusses some of the recent changes in the overall evolution of pediatric critical care delivery in North America, starting with a brief historical description of the field of pediatric critical care medicine as an important backdrop to where the field is likely to move in the future.

## A BRIEF HISTORY OF PEDIATRIC CRITICAL CARE MEDICINE

Evolution of the modern PICU and evolution of the specialty of pediatric critical care medicine have occurred approximately in tandem over the last 50 years. The roots of pediatric critical care medicine, as a specialty, include adult respiratory care, neonatology, pediatric general surgery, pediatric cardiac surgery, and pediatric anesthesiology. ICUs first developed in response to the global epidemic of polio, which was a universally fatal disease until the development of the iron lung in the late 1920s. The knowledge gained in artificial ventilation was then generalized to other conditions, and pediatric critical care medicine began to develop as a specialty to provide care for other types of patients, including neonatal ICU graduates.

The first known PICU was established in Sweden in 1955, whereas the first US PICU opened in 1967 at the Children's Hospital of Philadelphia, a 6-bed unit with a separate nursing staff and 24-hour in-house physician coverage provided by pediatric anesthesia fellows.[8] PICUs began to spread throughout the United States and by the mid-1970s were located in most hospitals that had a pediatric residency program. The Pediatrics Section of the Society of Critical Care Medicine and Section on Critical Care of the American Academy of Pediatrics were established in 1981 and 1984, respectively. In 1987, the first American Board of Pediatrics certification examination for pediatric critical care medicine was offered (182 of the 242 first-time takers passed).[9] The first pediatric critical care medicine textbook was also published that same year.[10] *Pediatric Critical Care Medicine*, a journal devoted exclusively to the specialty of pediatric critical care, began publication in 2000.[11]

## CURRENT STATE OF PEDIATRIC CRITICAL CARE MEDICINE
### Number of Pediatric ICUs

The exact number of pediatric critical care beds in the United States is unknown, but several studies have attempted to clarify the issue. A 2004 report estimated that there were 350 PICU units, although more than half of them had fewer than 8 beds.[12] A 2003 survey of PICUs in the United States demonstrated 337 PICUs with a total of 4044 beds, a median bed number of 12 beds, and 58 admissions per bed.[13] Although the number of PICU beds in the United States varies based on which survey data are used, the number is lower than the estimated 67,357 adult critical care beds and 20,000 neonatal intensive care beds.[1–3]

Dedicated pediatric cardiac ICUs (CICUs) have been a more recent development in larger children's hospitals, along with creation of educational conferences and a professional society devoted to this field (Pediatric Cardiac Intensive Care Society). It is estimated that approximately half of pediatric cardiac surgery centers operate dedicated CICUs,[14] although the overall impact on patient care outcomes[15] and pediatric critical care education[16] is uncertain. Specialized PICUs, such as CICUs, are discussed later.

### Pediatric Critical Care Medicine Specialists

In a 2008 survey, slightly more than 10,000 physicians reported their practice as adult critical care medicine or pediatric critical care medicine.[17] This study emphasized, however, that the actual number of physicians practicing full-time critical care was likely significantly less than what was reported. The American Board of Pediatrics reported 1881 board-certified pediatric intensivists in the United States in 2011, with an average age of 49 years. Of the board-certified pediatric intensivists, 25% were 56 years of age or older. Significant geographic variation exists for board-certified pediatric critical care physicians, resulting in wide variation in available specialist-to-child ratios across the United States (**Fig. 1**).[18] The exact number of physicians practicing pediatric critical care medicine is unknown due to both board-certified physicians no longer practicing pediatric critical care and non–board-certified practitioners, such as pediatric anesthesiologists and pediatric cardiologists, among others, who do.

### Pediatric Critical Care Medicine Trainees

Completion of a 3-year pediatric critical care fellowship (after completion of a pediatric residency or an internal medicine–pediatric residency) at 1 of the 70 Canadian or United States accredited training programs is currently the only pathway to become board certified by the American Board of Pediatrics. The Royal College of Physicians and Surgeons of Canada has less-restrictive requirements for both fellowship admission and board certification. The mid-1990s showed a decreasing number of critical care trainees (adult and pediatric), but more recent trends have been encouraging, with an overall increase in critical care trainees of 11% during the period from 2001 to 2006 and an increase of 18% in pediatric critical care trainees.[19] This upward trend has continued (**Fig. 2**). Pediatric critical care training programs, like all training programs, have had to adjust to changing requirements and duty hour regulations, and the ideal curriculum[20] and method of delivering this content[21] remain uncertain.

## MODELS OF CRITICAL CARE DELIVERY

Avedis Donabedian,[22] considered the founder of the study of health care quality and outcomes research, proposed that the evaluation of health care delivery be conceptualized in 3 dimensions—structure, processes, and outcomes (**Fig. 3**). *Structure* refers to the setting in which care is delivered, whose elements can be easily recalled by *P's* and *T's*. The 2 *P's* refer to the people in ICUs (patients and providers). The types of patients cared for in a particular ICU (trauma, solid organ transplant, bone marrow transplant, neurointensive care, cardiac intensive care, and so forth) as well as the providers working in an ICU (background, level of education, training, and certification of individuals who provide care in ICUs) have an impact on ICU outcomes. The 2 *T's* refer to the technology (ventilators, physiologic monitors, and so forth) and therapy. *Processes* refer to how care is provided in ICUs, which encompasses how different

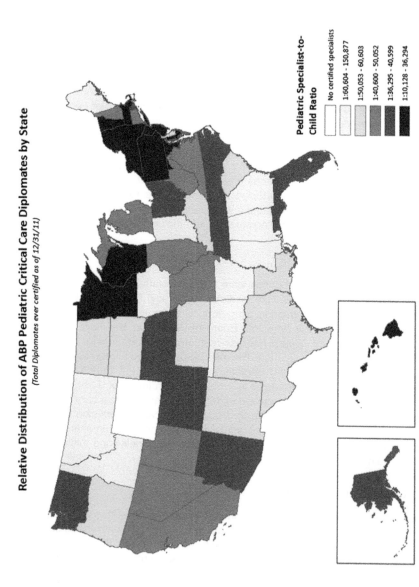

**Relative Distribution of ABP Pediatric Critical Care Diplomates by State**

*(Total Diplomates ever certified as of 12/31/11)*

**Pediatric Specialist-to-Child Ratio**

No certified specialists
1:60,604 - 150,877
1:50,053 - 60,603
1:40,600 - 50,052
1:36,295 - 40,599
1:10,128 - 36,294

**Fig. 1.** Relative distribution of American Board of Pediatrics Pediatric Critical Care Diplomates by state. (*Courtesy of* the American Board of Pediatrics.)

**Critical Care Medicine**
**Training Level Tracking Data**

| Year Starting July 1 | Training Level 1 | Training Level 2 | Training Level 3 | Total |
|---|---|---|---|---|
| 1998 | 90 | 62 | 85 | 237 |
| 1999 | 96 | 82 | 50 | 228 |
| 2000 | 99 | 88 | 75 | 262 |
| 2001 | 99 | 88 | 84 | 271 |
| 2002 | 112 | 82 | 83 | 277 |
| 2003 | 116 | 99 | 85 | 300 |
| 2004 | 135 | 107 | 74 | 316 |
| 2005 | 127 | 122 | 96 | 345 |
| 2006 | 164 | 113 | 105 | 382 |
| 2007 | 147 | 140 | 109 | 396 |
| 2008 | 142 | 135 | 118 | 395 |
| 2009 | 168 | 131 | 118 | 417 |
| 2010 | 163 | 147 | 123 | 433 |
| 2011 | 172 | 145 | 131 | 448 |

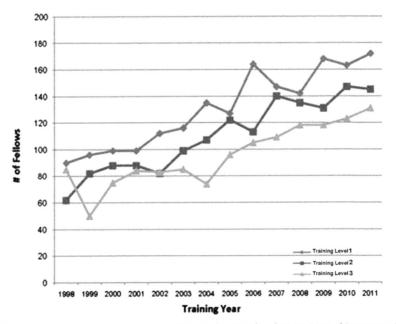

**Fig. 2.** Number of pediatric critical care trainees by year level 1998–2011. (*Courtesy of* the American Board of Pediatrics.)

providers interact and work together to take care of critically ill patients. *Outcomes* refer to the endpoints of care, encompassing survival and quality of life as well as other important outcomes, such as complications (adverse drug events, unplanned extubation, hospital-acquired infections, and so forth), length of stay (LOS), patient/family experience, staff satisfaction, and costs. Donabedian suggested that processes are effective only when the appropriate structures are in place to support them and when outcomes are measured, so that processes can be evaluated for effectiveness and modified to produce better outcomes.[22]

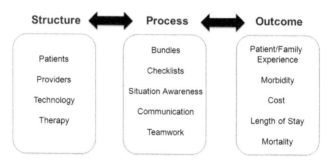

**Fig. 3.** Donabedian's model for quality.

## Structure

### Patients

As discussed previously, an important structural consideration driving outcomes is the type of patients who receive care in a particular ICU. Critical illness stems from a diverse range of conditions that can affect just one or even multiple organ systems. This diversity in the type and severity of critical illness (ie, case mix) is one of the most commonly cited reasons why it is so difficult to compare outcomes among multiple different ICUs.[23–27] The particular case mix is an important consideration even in specialized organ-specific or disease-specific ICUs (eg, neuro-ICUs and CICUs). These ICUs take advantage of economies of scope and scale to care for critically ill patients with a specific disease type or organ dysfunction. Although previously limited to adult centers, there are now several specialized ICUs or critical care teams in cardiac intensive care[14,15,28] and neurointensive care[29–33] at several large children's hospitals in North America. Whether or not these specialized ICUs or critical care teams improve outcomes is a matter of debate.[15,34–37]

Over the past few decades, a new population of patients has emerged in the PICU. Children with diseases once considered uniformly fatal are surviving into late adolescence and early adulthood.[38,39] These children are surviving but develop complex, chronic medical conditions that frequently require admission to the hospital. The number of children with complex, chronic medical conditions requiring PICU care is increasing.[40,41] Advances in intensive care are also enabling children to survive acute critical illness in greater numbers, many of whom develop long-term dependence on technology to support chronic organ dysfunction (eg, long-term mechanical ventilator support and renal replacement therapy). Many of these patients may remain dependent on intensive care for sustained organ dysfunction that persists for weeks to months, even before discharge to home. These patients have been described as chronically critically ill and will continue to pose challenges for critical care medicine and for the overall system of health care delivery.[42–44]

### Providers

**Staffing shortages in ICUs** The critical care team is one of the key structural elements driving quality of care in an ICU. Unfortunately, there is a growing shortage of adequately trained critical care physicians, nurses, respiratory therapists, and pharmacists in the United States.[17,45–48] These shortages are especially relevant with regard to physician staffing in ICUs, as demonstrated by studies showing that no more than 1 of every 3 adult ICU patients is managed by an intensivist.[45,48] The situation becomes even more worrisome because of the trend of early retirement of current intensivists, because less than 1% of medical school graduates are choosing to enter the field of critical care medicine, and because an increasing number of patients will require ICU care.[17,45,47–49] Early retirement is a real concern, with results of studies revealing burnout as a common occurrence in critical care medicine.[50–52] As Krell[17] states in his essay on the critical care workforce, "finding new drugs or devices to treat the critically ill will have little effect compared with solving our manpower problems."

Telemedicine has been proposed as one potential solution to the growing shortage of trained critical care providers. With merely 5500 intensivists practicing in the United States and only one-third of ICU patients cared for by an intensivist, telemedicine makes it possible for more patients to be managed or triaged by intensivists, especially in underserved areas.[53] The use of telemedicine in ICUs is reviewed extensively in the accompanying article by Dr. Marcin in this volume. Regionalization of services is another solution. In examining staffing of PICUs, in particular, Randolph and colleagues[12] demonstrated that resources for PICUs in the United States continue to be "spread out across diverse PICUs, with highly variable staffing and subspecialist availability patterns." This reality, coupled with the high cost associated with critical care medicine, has prompted many policy experts to advocate for regionalization of PICU care. This position is supported by evidence that centralization of PICU resources in tertiary centers corresponds with improved health outcomes.[12]

**High-intensity versus low-intensity physician staffing** Another important structural consideration driving outcomes in ICUs is the critical care providers themselves. The American College of Critical Care Medicine Task Force on Models of Critical Care Delivery published a summary of the relevant literature on this topic in 2001[54] and suggested that critically ill patients should be cared for by a multidisciplinary team of critical care providers led by a physician specifically trained and certified in the field of critical care medicine (ie, an intensivist). The Task Force further suggested that a "closed" model of ICU organization (now more commonly referred to as *high-intensity staffing*), in which this dedicated team is directly responsible for all aspects of care in ICUs, is superior to the more traditional and ubiquitous "open" model of ICU organization (now more commonly referred to as *low-intensity staffing*), in which patients are admitted to an ICU and are cared for by their primary care or subspecialty physician, often with little or no input from the critical care team. Multiple studies have demonstrated better outcomes—including improved mortality—in ICUs with high-intensity physician staffing.[49,55] Based on these studies, the Leapfrog Group[48,49] published a report in 2007 that upheld ICU staffing as the most important safety standard by which to measure a hospital's quality of care. The group outlined a standard for adult ICU and PICU staffing that included an intensivist dedicated to an ICU to manage the care of patients through direct, on-site care during daytime hours every day of the week and as needed via page at other times.[56,57] Unfortunately, more recent studies suggest that a large percentage of ICUs across the United States are unable to comply with the Leapfrog Group recommendations.[48]

**24/7 Intensivist staffing** Several hospitals and organizations are taking the Leapfrog Group's recommendations a step further by suggesting that ICUs should be staffed by an in-house intensivist 24 hours per day, 7 days per week (24/7 intensivist staffing).[56] Historically, the vast majority of hospitals have not staffed their ICUs in this manner. For example, a survey of 2900 ICUs at more than 1700 US hospitals in 1991 found that only 6% of hospitals provided attending coverage with 24/7 intensivist staffing. On average, ICUs were only staffed for 6 hours per day by an intensivist.[58]

A pediatric study published in 2001 showed that less than 1 in 5 (17%) of all PICUs had 24/7 intensivist staffing.[12] In this particular study, larger PICUs (>20 beds) were more likely to have 24/7 intensivist staffing compared with smaller PICUs.[12] In a more recent study, limited to ICUs at academic medical centers, only 33% of those responding stated that they provided 24/7 intensivist staffing; 24/7 intensivist staffing was more common in PICUs and surgical ICUs.[59]

Unfortunately, the results from studies comparing outcomes in ICUs with 24/7 intensivist staffing versus those without are mixed. For example, Arias and colleagues[60] retrospectively reviewed their single-center experience and found a higher risk-adjusted mortality rate for patients admitted to the PICU during evening hours compared with those admitted during daytime hours. Although staffing was not directly assessed in this study, one of the concerns is that differential staffing from day to night may have correlated with and contributed to this significant difference in outcomes. Peeters and colleagues,[61] however, did not find any significant differences in risk-adjusted mortality during off-hours admission to their PICU. Coverage at night in this PICU was provided by a resident physician, although all of the intensivists lived within 15 minutes of the hospital. Numa and colleagues[62] reported similar findings in their retrospective, single-center review of a 10-year period. Subsequently, in their retrospective review of approximately 6000 admissions to a single PICU with 24/7 in-house staffing of pediatric intensivists, Hixson and colleagues[63] found no significant differences in outcomes between weekend and/or evening admission versus weekday admissions. Finally, Nishisaki and colleagues[64] reported that duration of mechanical ventilation and ICU LOS significantly decreased, although risk-adjusted mortality did not change, after introduction of 24/7 intensivist staffing in their single-center PICU. Unfortunately, single-center studies and retrospective, multicenter cohort studies are not adequate to address this issue, due largely to the heterogeneity in physician coverage models across the country, as suggested by a recent systematic review and meta-analysis based on 10 adult cohort studies that failed to show a significant differences in outcome between daytime versus nighttime admission to an ICU.[65]

Wallace and colleagues[66] recently conducted a multicenter, retrospective cohort analysis that attempted to address the issue of heterogeneity of coverage models in the United States. These investigators used the Acute Physiology and Chronic Health Evaluation clinical information system (2009–2010 data) combined with a survey of ICU staffing practices, which combined data from more than 65,000 critically ill adults admitted to 49 ICUs at 25 different hospitals. In ICUs with high-intensity daytime staffing, nighttime (ie, 24/7 intensivist staffing) was not associated with improved outcomes. Conversely, among ICUs with low-intensity daytime staffing, nighttime intensivist coverage significantly improved outcomes. These findings are similar to the available pediatric data, but as of yet, there are no multicenter pediatric studies exploring this issue.

**Physician assistants, nurse practitioners, and hospitalists** The shortage of critical care physicians and coverage demands (discussed previously) have led to the growing use of so-called physician extenders (ie, physician assistants [PAs] and advanced practice nurses) in critical care medicine.[21,57,67–69] The proper term for such providers (physician extenders, midlevel providers, affiliated providers, or licensed independent providers), however, is under debate, with the term, *physician extenders*, currently the most commonly used term by health care organizations. A national survey of PICUs in 2005 found that nurse practitioners (NPs) worked an average of 50 hours per week, with responsibilities including direct patient management, coordination of care, education, research, and consultation. NPs also performed procedures, including venipuncture, intravenous placement, endotracheal intubation, central venous and arterial catheterization, and peripherally inserted central catheter insertion.[70] In that same year, Mathur and colleagues[71] described their experience with PAs in their PICU in New York. After completing a 6-month to 1-year orientation, PAs primarily serve as providers of bedside care. Like NPs, they also manage a variety of other responsibilities, including assistance with procedures, education, research, and quality assurance.

NPs and PAs bring strengths different from those of resident physicians. Although residents typically possess a greater fund of knowledge and understanding of pathophysiology, PAs (and likely also NPs), with increasing experience in ICUs, possess knowledge of unit-specific policies, practices, and common diagnoses.[71] If managed well, these 2 roles may complement each other to the benefit of the individuals, the patients, and the unit as a whole. Current literature, although limited, suggests that retention of NPs and PAs has proved a challenge to units that seek to use them and requires thoughtful attention given the labor-intensive nature of orientation and the disruption to the function of the unit by turnover.[71] The trend toward using NPs and PAs in pediatric critical care continues, with anticipation of greater numbers in the future. As a result, the body of literature that examines the preparation, use, and retention of NPs and PAs is mounting.[57,70–74]

In recent years, the specialty of pediatric hospital medicine has evolved rapidly, and the hospitalist has become an increasingly prominent figure. Increasing numbers of patients admitted to hospitals receive care from hospitalists—or house physicians—rather than from primary care physicians, who provide care in both outpatient and inpatient settings. In many hospitals, in particular those in less well-served areas, a hospitalist cares for patients not only in general wards but also in low-level ICUs.[57] For example, Tenner and colleagues[75] demonstrated improved outcomes with hospitalists providing after-hours coverage instead of residents in a PICU. A single-center, prospective, cohort study suggested that adjusted mortality and LOS were not significantly different between a hospitalist-led ICU versus intensivist-led ICU. LOS was shorter and mortality was better, however, when mechanically ventilated patients with intermediate severity of illness were cared for by an intensivist-led team.[76] Pediatric critical care is just beginning to wrestle with how best to train, use, and incorporate hospitalists into the evolving discipline of pediatric critical care.[74]

**Critical care pharmacist** The critical care pharmacist is a key member of an ICU team. Several studies show that the addition of a critical care pharmacist to an ICU team reduces the incidence of adverse drug events, improves antibiotic stewardship, and improves compliance with evidence-based medication practices, all of which are associated with improved outcomes.[54,77–80] Ideally, a critical care pharmacist should join bedside rounds with the rest of the ICU team.

**Nursing and ancillary staff** The critical care nurse represents the front line in an ICU and is a key member of the critical care team. ICU nursing staff should work closely with the intensivists, pharmacists, and other members of the ICU team (pharmacist, respiratory therapist, dietician, social worker, chaplain, physical/occupational therapists, psychologist, and so forth) to meet all of the needs of critically ill children and their families. All members of an ICU team (including the intensivists) should meet on a regular basis to discuss difficult cases and ethical issues, review current performance on key outcome and process measures, share and discuss best practices, and provide continuous education and training. These regular meetings also serve to build a culture of mutual respect, trust, and camaraderie in ICUs. Multiple studies conducted over the past 20 years suggest that an organizational culture of mutual respect, trust, and teamwork significantly improves outcomes in ICUs.[81–88] Some investigators have suggested that the proper organizational culture may be more important than the ongoing controversies and issues related to staffing (discussed previously).[55,66,84,87]

**Optimal staffing ratios** The optimal physician staffing ratio in ICUs is not known. Dara and Afessa[89] conducted a retrospective cohort study at a single center to determine whether there was an association between the intensivist-to-bed ratio and outcome. Four different staffing ratios were used over time (1:7.5, 1:9.5, 1:12, and 1:15). Differences in intensivist-to–ICU bed ratios were not associated with differences in either ICU or hospital mortality. A 1:15 intensivist-to–ICU bed ratio was associated with increased ICU LOS. This is an important area that has not been adequately studied. Most critically ill children warrant a nurse-to-patient ratio of 1:1 or 1:2, depending on their underlying severity of illness.[90,91] Several studies have linked nursing workload to nurse retention, burnout, patient safety, and outcomes in ICUs.[52,92,93] The qualification and training of the nurses also must be considered when determining staffing ratios.

### Technology and therapy
Aside from the physical design and layout of ICUs (not discussed in this article[90,94–96]), the other key structural elements driving quality of care in ICUs are technology and therapy. Technologic advances in monitoring, information systems and clinical decision support, and end-organ support have advanced the care of critically ill patients over the past decade. In addition, translational research continues to bring the latest and most advanced treatments from bench to bedside. Many of these advances are discussed elsewhere in this issue and, therefore, are not discussed further in this article.

### Processes

Structural elements (discussed previously) interact with key processes in ICUs to drive improved outcomes. Structural elements, however, cannot make up for lack of an appropriate organizational climate that supports implementation of standardized, reliable, evidence-based processes.[97] For example, the mere presence of an intensivist in an ICU is not likely to improve patient outcomes if the intensivist is not effectively communicating with other physicians, with the nursing staff, and with the patients and their families. Similarly, optimal nurse-to-patient staffing ratios are not likely to reduce medical errors or hospital-acquired infections unless standardized, reliable processes are in place. A retrospective analysis of a large, prospective database (Project IMPACT), involving more than 101,000 critically ill patients receiving care at 123 ICUs in 100 US hospitals, showed that after adjusting for severity of illness and propensity score, hospital mortality rates were higher for those patients cared for exclusively by intensivists compared with patients cared for entirely by nonintensivists.[98] Rather than calling for a moratorium on intensivists, most critical care policy experts suggest that the results of this study put into sharp focus the need for reliable processes in ICUs.[87,99,100]

### Bundles and checklists
There are several studies that have shown significant reductions in adverse drug events, unplanned extubations, central line–associated bloodstream infections, ventilator-associated pneumonia, catheter-associated urinary tract infections, pressure ulcers,

surgical site infections, and other errors in PICUs through the implementation of standardized, reliable processes, or bundles (**Box 1**). A bundle is a small set of standardized, evidence-based interventions (or, if there is insufficient evidence, best practice interventions) for a specific patient population or disease condition, that, when implemented reliably and consistently, leads to improvements in outcomes. Certain cultural elements (eg, communication, teamwork, leadership, and accountability) are also necessary to assure that these improvements are sustainable for the long term. Many of these cultural elements are found in so-called high-reliability organizations. High-reliability organizations are discussed in greater detail in an accompanying article by Niedner and colleagues.

Checklists are another important process for improving the overall care of critically ill children admitted to PICUs. Gawande[101] and Pronovost,[102] the leading pioneers in patient safety, popularized the use of checklists in the operating room and ICU, respectively.[103,104] Daily goal sheets are another way of improving communication and collaboration between different members of a critical care team.[105,106] Finally, structured communication during multidisciplinary rounds[107] and handoffs[108–111] are additional key process driving quality and improved outcomes in the PICU.

### Critical care as an emergent system
The ICU is just one component of the overall hospital system. The old adage, "the sum is greater than the parts," is true here. Borrowing a term from the industrial engineering

---

**Box 1**
**Key processes in the PICU**

Daily multidisciplinary rounds (including medical and surgical subspecialists)

Daily goals sheet

Daily shift huddles

Primary nursing assignments

PICU leadership walk rounds

Central line insertion bundle

Central line maintenance bundle

Ventilator-associated respiratory infection bundle

Urinary catheter care bundle

Pressure ulcer bundle

Peripheral intravenous care bundle

Medication reconciliation

Operating room to ICU handoffs

Handoffs

Transitions of care

Discharge planning

Standard care protocols (eg, extubation readiness testing and sedation/analgesia protocols)

Condition-specific protocols (status asthmaticus, sepsis, diabetic ketoacidosis, traumatic brain injury, and so forth)

Clinical pathways

and operations research literature, hospital care, in particular, critical care, is an *emergent system*.[112,113] The overall quality of care provided in an emergent system is manifest only when viewed in its entirety. The whole system (critical care) is greater than the sum of the individual components or parts (eg, emergency department, operating room suite, medical/surgical inpatient unit, interhospital transport, ICU, and rehabilitation unit). Therefore, improvements at the system level should be made only when viewing the whole system in its entirety rather than merely as a collection of multiple, individual parts. As McQuillan and colleagues stated several years ago, "the greatest impact on the outcome for intensive care units may come from improvements in input to intensive care, particularly in the quality of acute care."[114] These concepts, as applied to improving processes in ICUs, are most visible with the improved outcomes observed in association with the implementation of rapid response systems in pediatrics.[115–118]

## *Outcomes*

As discussed previously, comparing outcomes between different PICUs is limited by the heterogeneity in case mix and severity of illness between PICUs as well as other organizational factors that can have an impact on different outcomes. Currently, there are no widely accepted, standard PICU outcome measures, although multiple candidate measures have been proposed.[119,120] It is likely that no single measure can adequately summarize the overall quality of care that a critically ill child receives in any individual PICU. Rather, a panel of measures, including process measures (eg, compliance with evidence-based practices and bundle compliance), measures of organizational culture (eg, safety culture surveys and communication), and outcome measures (hospital-acquired infections, rate of unplanned extubation, adverse drug events, pressure ulcers, PICU LOS, duration of mechanical ventilation, PICU and hospital survival, and so forth), is likely to be the most effective way of benchmarking PICU performance internally. Trends in each individual measure should be tracked over time using statistical process control methodology.[121,122] The standardized mortality ratio, defined as observed deaths divided by expected deaths (based on a validated severity of illness score), may allow for internal benchmarking of outcomes over time, although problems with statistical imprecision preclude its utility as an external benchmark.[123]

## SUMMARY

Over the past half century, health care delivery has evolved such that ICUs, including specialized PICUs, have become a vital element in the health care delivery system. During this time, both PICUs and the field of pediatric critical care medicine have evolved into their current forms. Critical care is now provided to a diverse patient population in a wide array of settings by multidisciplinary teams of physicians, nonphysician providers, nurses, pharmacists, nutritionists, and other ancillary staff members who specialize in pediatric critical care and coordinate with members of other medical and surgical disciplines. As the field of pediatric critical care medicine evolves, it seeks to improve so that patients receive reliable, efficient, and evidence-based care with optimal outcomes. As the patient population changes, providers adapt, staffing models adjust, technology evolves, and therapies advance, outcomes are transformed. The evolution of pediatric critical care over its first 50 years has been tremendous, but the next 50 years will assuredly bring even greater change.

**REFERENCES**

1. Halpern NA, Pastores SM. Critical care medicine in the United States 2000-2005: an analysis of bed numbers, occupancy rates, payer mix, and costs. Crit Care Med 2010;38:65–71.
2. Halpern NA, Pastores SM, Greenstein RJ. Critical care medicine in the United States 1985-2000: an analysis of bed numbers, use, and costs. Crit Care Med 2004;32:1254–9.
3. Halpern NA, Pastores SM, Thaler HT, et al. Critical care medicine use and cost among Medicare beneficiaries 1995-2000: major discrepancies between two United States federal Medicare databases. Crit Care Med 2007;35:692–9.
4. Coopersmith CM, Wunsch H, Fink MP, et al. A comparison of critical care research funding and the financial burden of critical illness in the United States. Crit Care Med 2012;40:1072–9.
5. Ward NS, Levy MM. Rationing and critical care medicine. Crit Care Med 2007; 35:S102–5.
6. Institute of Medicine, editor. Crossing the quality chasm: a new health system for the twenty-first century. Washington, DC: National Academy Press; 2001.
7. Slonim AD, Pollack MM. Integrating the Institute of Medicine's six quality aims into pediatric critical care: relevance and applications. Pediatr Crit Care Med 2005;6:264–9.
8. Downes J. Development of pediatric critical care. In: Wheeler DS, Wong HR, Shanley T, editors. Pediatric critical care medicine. New York: Springer; 2007. p. 3–30.
9. The AAP Section on Critical Care 25th Anniversary 1984-2009: American Academy of Pediatrics Section on Critical Care 2009.
10. Rodgers M, editor. Textbook of pediatric intensive care. Baltimore (MD): Williams & Wilkins; 1987.
11. Parrillo JE. Pediatric critical care medicine: another member of the critical care family. Pediatr Crit Care Med 2000;1:1.
12. Randolph AG, Gonzales CA, Cortellini L, et al. Growth of pediatric intensive care units in the United States from 1995 to 2001. J Pediatr 2004;144:792–8.
13. Odetola FO, Clark SJ, Freed GL, et al. A national survey of pediatric critical care resources in the United States. Pediatrics 2005;115:e382–6.
14. Burstein DS, Rossi AF, Jacobs JP, et al. Variation in models of care delivery for children undergoing congenital heart surgery in the United States. World J Pediatr Congenit Heart Surg 2010;1:8–14.
15. Burstein DS, Jacobs JP, Li JS, et al. Care models and associated outcomes in congenital heart surgery. Pediatrics 2011;127:e1482–9.
16. Su L, Munoz R. Isn't it the right time to address the impact of pediatric cardiac intensive care units on medical education? Pediatrics 2007;120:e1117–9.
17. Krell K. Critical care workforce. Crit Care Med 2008;36:1350–3.
18. Workforce and research: American Board of Pediatrics.
19. Chandler E, LP. Are there more critical care physician trainees today? SCCM Critical Connections. June 2006.
20. Morrison WE, Helfaer MA, Nadkarni VM. National survey of pediatric critical care medicine fellowship clinical and research time allocation. Pediatr Crit Care Med 2009;10:397–9.
21. Chudgar SM, Cox CE, Que LG, et al. Current teaching and evaluation methods in critical care medicine: has the Accreditation Council for Graduate Medical Education affected how we practice and teach in the intensive care unit? Crit Care Med 2009;37:49–60.

22. Donabedian A. Evaluating the quality of medical care. Milbank Mem Fund Q 1966;44:166–206.
23. Glance LG, Osler TM, Dick A. Rating the quality of intensive care units: is it a function of the intensive care unit scoring system? Crit Care Med 2002;30:1976–82.
24. Garland A. Improving the ICU: part 1. Chest 2005;127:2151–64.
25. Garland A. Improving the ICU: part 2. Chest 2005;127:2165–79.
26. Terblanche M, Adhikari NK. The evolution of intensive care unit performance assessment. J Crit Care 2006;21:19–22.
27. Bakhshi-Raiez F, Peek N, Bosman RJ, et al. The impact of different prognostic models and their customization on institutional comparison of intensive care units. Crit Care Med 2007;35:2553–60.
28. Chang AC. How to start and sustain a successful pediatric cardiac intensive care program: a combined clinical and administrative strategy. Pediatr Crit Care Med 2002;3:107–11.
29. Bell MJ, Carpenter J, Au AK, et al. Development of a pediatric neurocritical care service. Neurocrit Care 2009;10:4–10.
30. Lee JC, Riviello JJ. Education of the child neurologist: pediatric neurocritical care. Semin Pediatr Neurol 2011;18:128–30.
31. Murphy S. Pediatric neurocritical care. Neurotherapeutics 2012;9:3–16.
32. Scher M. Proposed cross-disciplinary training in pediatric neurointensive care. Pediatr Neurol 2008;39:1–5.
33. Tasker RC. Pediatric neurocritical care: is it time to come of age? Curr Opin Pediatr 2009;21:724–30.
34. Balachandran R, Nair SG, Gopalraj SS, et al. Dedicated pediatric cardiac intensive care unit in a developing country: does it improve the outcome? Ann Pediatr Cardiol 2011;4:122–6.
35. Eldadah M, Leo S, Kovach K, et al. Influence of a dedicated paediatric cardiac intensive care unit on patient outcomes. Nurs Crit Care 2011;16:281–6.
36. Pineda JA, Leonard JR, Mazotas IG, et al. Effect of implementation of a paediatric neurocritical care programme on outcomes after severe traumatic brain injury: a retrospective cohort study. Lancet Neurol 2013;12:45–52.
37. Lott JP, Iwashyna TJ, Christie JD, et al. Critical illness outcomes in specialty versus general intensive care units. Am J Respir Crit Care Med 2009;179:676–83.
38. Simon TD, Berry J, Feudtner C, et al. Children with complex chronic conditions in inpatient hospital settings in the United States. Pediatrics 2010;126:647–55.
39. Burns KH, Casey PH, Lyle RE, et al. Increasing prevalence of medically complex children in US hospitals. Pediatrics 2010;126:638–46.
40. Odetola FO, Gebremariam A, Davis MM. Comorbid illnesses among critically ill hospitalized children: impact on hospital resource use and mortality, 1997-2006. Pediatr Crit Care Med 2010;11:457–63.
41. Edwards JD, Houtrow AJ, Vasilevskis EE, et al. Chronic conditions among children admitted to U.S. pediatric intensive care units: their prevalence and impact on risk for mortality and prolonged length of stay. Crit Care Med 2012;40:2196–203.
42. Nelson JE, Cox CE, Hope AA, et al. Chronic critical illness. Am J Respir Crit Care Med 2010;182:446–54.
43. MacIntyre NR. Chronic critical illness: the growing challenge to health care. Respir Care 2012;57:1021–7.
44. Peterson-Carmichael SL, Cheifetz IM. The chronically critically ill patient: pediatric considerations. Respir Care 2012;57:993–1003.

45. Angus DC, Kelley MA, Schmitz RJ, et al, (COMPACCS) CoMfPaCCS. Caring for the critically ill patient. Current and projected workforce requirements for care of the critically ill and patients with pulmonary disease: can we meet the requirements of an aging population? JAMA 2000;284:2762–70.
46. Ewart GW, Marcus L, Gaba MM, et al. The critical care medicine crisis: a call for federal action: a white paper from the critical care professional societies. Chest 2004;125:1518–21.
47. Grover A. Critical care workforce: a policy perspective. Crit Care Med 2006;34: S7–11.
48. Angus DC, Shorr AF, White A, et al. Critical care delivery in the United States: distribution of services and compliance with Leapfrog recommendations. Crit Care Med 2006;34:1016–24.
49. Pronovost PJ, Angus DC, Dorman T, et al. Physician staffing patterns and clinical outcomes in critically ill patients: a systematic review. JAMA 2002;288: 2151–62.
50. Donchin Y, Seagull FJ. The hostile environment of the intensive care unit. Curr Opin Crit Care 2002;8:316–20.
51. Levy MM. Caring for the caregiver. Crit Care Clin 2004;20:541–7.
52. Embriaco N, Papazian L, Kentish-Barnes N, et al. Burnout syndrome among critical care healthcare workers. Curr Opin Crit Care 2007;13:482–8.
53. Lustbader D, Fein A. Emerging trends in ICU management and staffing. Crit Care Clin 2000;16:735–48.
54. Brilli RJ, Spevetz A, Branson RD, et al. Critical care delivery in the intensive care unit: defining clinical roles and the best practice model. Crit Care Med 2001;29: 2007–19.
55. Kim MM, Barnato AE, Angus DC, et al. The effect of multidisciplinary care teams on intensive care unit mortality. Arch Intern Med 2010;170:369–76.
56. Banerjee R, Naessens JM, Seferian EG, et al. Economic implications of nighttime attending intensivist coverage in a medical intensive care unit. Crit Care Med 2011;39:1257–62.
57. Cramer CL, Orlowski JP, DeNicola LK. Pediatric intensivist extenders in the pediatric ICU. Pediatr Clin North Am 2008;55:687–708, xi–xii.
58. Groeger JS, Strosberg MA, Halpern NA, et al. Descriptive analysis of critical care units in the United States. Crit Care Med 1992;20:846–63.
59. Diaz-Guzman E, Colbert CY, Mannino DM, et al. 24/7 In-house intensivist coverage and fellowship education: a cross-sectional survey of academic medical centers in the United States. Chest 2012;141:959–66.
60. Arias Y, Taylor DS, Marcin JP. Association between evening admissions and higher mortality rates in the pediatric intensive care unit. Pediatrics 2004;113: e530–4.
61. Peeters B, Jansen NJ, van Vught AJ, et al. Off-hours admission and mortality in two pediatric intensive care units without 24-h in-house senior staff attendance. Intensive Care Med 2010;36:1923–7.
62. Numa A, Williams G, Awad J, et al. After-hours admissions are not associated with increased risk-adjusted mortality in pediatric intensive care. Intensive Care Med 2008;34:148–51.
63. Hixson ED, Davis S, Morris S, et al. Do weekends or evenings matter in a pediatric intensive care unit? Pediatr Crit Care Med 2005;6:523–30.
64. Nishisaki A, Pines JM, Lin R, et al. The impact of 24-hr, in-hospital pediatric critical care attending physician presence on process of care and patient outcomes. Crit Care Med 2012;40:2190–5.

65. Cavallazzi R, Marik PE, Hirani A, et al. Association between time of admission to the ICU and mortality: a systematic review and metaanalysis. Chest 2010;138: 68–75.

66. Wallace DJ, Angus DC, Barnato AE, et al. Nighttime intensivist staffing and mortality among critically ill patients. N Engl J Med 2012;366:2093–101.

67. Ward NS, Read R, Afessa B, et al. Perceived effects of attending physician workload in academic medical intensive care units: a national survey of training program directors. Crit Care Med 2012;40:400–5.

68. Kleinpell RM, Ely EW, Grabenkort R. Nurse practitioners and physician assistants in the intensive care unit: an evidence-based review. Crit Care Med 2008;36:2888–97.

69. Gershengorn HB, Johnson MP, Factor P. The use of nonphysician providers in adult intensive care units. Am J Respir Crit Care Med 2012;185:600–5.

70. Verger JT, Marcoux KK, Madden MA, et al. Nurse practitioners in pediatric critical care: results of a national survey. AACN Clin Issues 2005;16:396–408.

71. Mathur M, Rampersad A, Howard K, et al. Physician assistants as physician extenders in the pediatric intensive care unit setting-A 5-year experience. Pediatr Crit Care Med 2005;6:14–9.

72. Caffin CL, Linton S, Pellegrini J. Introduction of a liaison nurse role in a tertiary paediatric ICU. Intensive Crit Care Nurs 2007;23:226–33.

73. Sorce L, Simone S, Madden M. Educational preparation and postgraduate training curriculum for pediatric critical care nurse practitioners. Pediatr Crit Care Med 2010;11:205–12.

74. Siegal EM, Dressler DD, Dichter JR, et al. Training a hospitalist workforce to address the intensivist shortage in American hospitals: a position paper from the Society of Hospital Medicine and the Society of Critical Care Medicine. Crit Care Med 2012;40:1952–6.

75. Tenner PA, Dibrell H, Taylor RP. Improved survival with hospitalists in a pediatric intensive care unit. Crit Care Med 2003;31:847–52.

76. Wise KR, Akopov VA, Williams BR, et al. Hospitalists and intensivists in the medical ICU: a prospective observational study comparing mortality and length of stay between two staffing models. J Hosp Med 2012;7:183–9.

77. Kane SL, Weber RJ, Dasta JF. The impact of critical care pharmacists on enhancing patient outcomes. Intensive Care Med 2003;29:691–8.

78. Durbin CG. Team model: advocating for the optimal method of care delivery in the intensive care unit. Crit Care Med 2006;34:S12–7.

79. Horn E, Jacobi J. The critical care clinical pharmacist: evolution of an essential team member. Crit Care Med 2006;34:S46–51.

80. Erstad BL. A primer on critical care pharmacy services. Ann Pharmacother 2008;42:1871–81.

81. Shortell SM, LoGerfo JP. Hospital medical staff organization and quality of care: results for myocardial infarction and appendectomy. Med Care 1981;19: 1041–55.

82. Shortell SM, Rousseau DM, Gillies RR, et al. Organizational assessment in intensive care units (ICUs): construct development, reliability, and validity of the ICU nurse-physicain questionnaire. Med Care 1991;29:709–25.

83. Zimmerman JE, Shortell SM, Rousseau DM, et al. Improving intensive care: observations based on organizational case studies in nine intensive care units: a prospective, multicenter study. Crit Care Med 1993;21:1443–51.

84. Knaus WA, Draper EA, Wagner DP, et al. An evaluation of outcome from intensive care in major medical centers. Ann Intern Med 1986;104:410–8.

85. Curry LA, Spatz E, Cherlin E, et al. What distinguishes top-performing hospitals in acute myocardial infarction mortality rates? A qualitative study. Ann Intern Med 2011;154:384–90.

86. Huang DT, Clermont G, Kong L, et al. Intensive care unit safety culture and outcomes: a U.S. multicenter study. Int J Qual Health Care 2010;22:151–61.

87. Nguyen YL, Wunsch H, Angus DC. Critical care: the impact of organization and management on outcomes. Curr Opin Crit Care 2010;16:487–92.

88. Manthous CA, Hollingshead AB. Team science and critical care. Am J Respir Crit Care Med 2011;184:17–25.

89. Dara SI, Afessa B. Intensivist-to-bed ratio: association with outcomes in the medical ICU. Chest 2005;128:567–72.

90. Valentin A, Ferdinande P. Imrpovement EWGoQ. Recommendations on basic requirements for intensive care units: structural and organizational aspects. Intensive Care Med 2011;37:1575–87.

91. Bray K, Wren I, Baldwin A, et al. Standards for nurse staffing in critical care units determined by: the British Association of Critical Care Nurses, The Critical Care Networks National Nurse Leads, Royal College of Nursing Critical Care and In-flight Forum. Nurs Crit Care 2010;15:109–11.

92. Numata Y, Schulzer M, van der Wal R, et al. Nurse staffing levels and hospital mortality in critical care settings: literature review and meta-analysis. J Adv Nurs 2006;55:435–48.

93. Carayon P, Gurses AP. A human factors engineering conceptual framework of nursing workload and patient safety in intensive care units. Intensive Crit Care Nurs 2005;21:284–301.

94. Bartley J, Streifel AJ. Design of the environment of care for safety of patients and personnel: does form follow function or vice versa in the intensive care unit? Crit Care Med 2010;38:S388–98.

95. Rashid M. A decade of adult intensive care unit design: a study of the physical design features of the best-practice examples. Crit Care Nurs Q 2006;29:282–311.

96. Thompson DR, Hamilton DK, Cadenhead CD, et al. Guidelines for intensive care unit design. Crit Care Med 2012;40:1586–600.

97. Gajic O, Afessa B. Physician staffing models and patient safety in the ICU. Chest 2009;135:1038–44.

98. Levy MM, Rapoport J, Lemeshow S, et al. Association between critical care physician management and patient mortality in the intensive care unit. Ann Intern Med 2008;148:801–9.

99. Rubenfeld GD, Angus DC. Are intensivists safe? Ann Intern Med 2008;148:877–9.

100. Khan M, Dubose JJ. Improving trauma care in the ICU: best practices, quality improvement initiatives, and organization. Surg Clin North Am 2012;92:893–901.

101. Gawande A. The checklist manifesto. New York: Metropolitan Books; 2009.

102. Pronovost P, Vohr E. Safe patients, smart hospitals: How one doctor's checklist can help us change health care from the inside out. New York: Hudson Street Press; 2010.

103. Gawande A. The checklist: if something so simple can transform intensive care, what else can it do? New Yorker 2007;10:86–101.

104. Hales BM, Pronovost PJ. The checklist - a tool for error management and performance improvement. J Crit Care 2006;21:231–5.

105. Phipps LM, Thomas NJ. The use of a daily goals sheet to improve communication in the paediatric intensive care unit. Intensive Crit Care Nurs 2007;23:264–71.

106. Agarwal S, Frankel L, Tourner S, et al. Improving communication in a pediatric intensive care unit using daily patient goal sheets. J Crit Care 2008;23:227–35.

107. Vats A, Goin KH, Villareal MC, et al. The impact of a lean rounding process in a pediatric intensive care unit. Crit Care Med 2012;40:608–17.

108. Catchpole KR, de Leval MR, McEwan A, et al. Patient handover from surgery to intensive care: using Formula 1 pit-stop and aviation models to improve safety and quality. Paediatr Anaesth 2007;17:470–8.

109. Joy BF, Elliot E, Hardy C, et al. Standardized multidisciplinary protocol improves handover of cardiac surgery patients to the intensive care unit. Pediatr Crit Care Med 2011;12:304–8.

110. Zavalkoff SR, Razack SI, Lavoie J, et al. Handover after pediatric heart surgery: a simple tool improves information exchange. Pediatr Crit Care Med 2011;12: 309–13.

111. Chen JG, Wright MC, Smith PB, et al. Adaptation of a postoperative handoff communication process for children with heart disease: a quantitative study. Am J Med Qual 2011;26:380–6.

112. Sobo EJ, Bowman C, Gifford AL. Behind the scenes in health care improvement: the complex structures and emergent strategies of Implementation Science. Soc Sci Med 2008;67:1530–40.

113. Paina L, Peters DH. Understanding pathways for scaling up health services through the lens of complex adaptive systems. Health Policy Plan 2012;27: 365–73.

114. McQuillan P, Pilkington S, Allan A, et al. Confidential inquiry into quality of care before admission to intensive care. BMJ 1998;316:1853–8.

115. Brilli RJ, Gibson R, Luria JW, et al. Implementation of a medical emergency team in a large pediatric teaching hospital prevents respiratory and cardiopulmonary arrests outside the intensive care unit. Pediatr Crit Care Med 2007;8:236–46.

116. Sharek PJ, Parast LM, Leong K, et al. Effect of a rapid response team on hospital-wide mortality and code rates outside the ICU in a Children's Hospital. JAMA 2007;298:2267–74.

117. Tibballs J, Kinney S. Reduction of hospital mortality and of preventable cardiac arrest and death on introduction of a pediatric medical emergency team. Pediatr Crit Care Med 2009;10:306–12.

118. Brady PW, Muething S, Kotagal U, et al. Improving situation awareness to reduce unrecognized clinical deterioration and serious safety events. Pediatrics 2012;131(1):e298–308.

119. Scanlon MC, Mistry KP, Jeffries HE. Determining pediatric intensive care unit quality indicators for measuring pediatric intensive care unit safety. Pediatr Crit Care Med 2007;8:S3–10.

120. LaRovere JM, Jeffries HE, Sachdeva RC, et al. Databases for assessing the outcomes of the treatment of patients with congenital and paediatric cardiac disease—the perspective of critical care. Cardiol Young 2008;18:130–6.

121. Pronovost PJ, Berenholtz SM, Ngo K, et al. Developing and pilot testing quality indicators in the intensive care unit. J Crit Care 2003;18:145–55.

122. Krimsky WS, Mroz IB, McIlwaine JK, et al. A model for increasing patient safety in the intensive care unit: increasing the implementation rates of proven safety measures. Qual Saf Health Care 2009;18:74–80.

123. Feudtner C, Berry JG, Parry G, et al. Statistical uncertainty of mortality rates and rankings for children's hospitals. Pediatrics 2011;128:e966–72.

# The High-Reliability Pediatric Intensive Care Unit

Matthew F. Niedner, MD[a],*, Stephen E. Muething, MD[b],
Kathleen M. Sutcliffe, PhD[c]

## KEYWORDS

- Reliability • High-reliability organization • Quality improvement • Patient safety
- Safety culture • Psychological safety

## KEY POINTS

- Define high reliability.
- Describe contexts wherein high reliability is crucial, including critical care.
- Describe characteristics of high-reliability organizations.
- Define the characteristics of a high-reliability pediatric intensive care unit.

## INTRODUCTION TO RELIABILITY

Principles of organizational and process reliability are used extensively in numerous high-risk and high-tech industries to help compensate for the natural limits of human performance and attention, thereby improving operational performance and safety. Reliability can be defined in several ways. Hollnagel and other engineers have described reliability as the absence of unwanted variance in performance, whereas others have considered it a measure of failure-free operation over time.[1,2] The importance of reducing variation and failures varies greatly, depending on the outcome at stake. In health care, reliability is the measurable capability of a process, procedure, or health service to perform its intended function in the required time under actual or existing conditions (as opposed to the ideal circumstances under which they are often studied).[1] Reliability is commonly expressed as the inverse of the system's failure rate, which may be referred to as unreliability. Thus, a process that has a failure or defect rate of 1 in 10 (10%) performs at a reliability level of $10^{-1}$. Many studies confirm that the

[a] Pediatric Intensive Care Unit, Division of Critical Care Medicine, Department of Pediatrics, Mott Children's Hospital, University of Michigan Medical Center, F-6894 Mott #0243, 1500 East Medical Center Drive, Ann Arbor, MI 48109-0243, USA; [b] Department of Pediatrics, Cincinnati Children's Hospital and Medical Center, University of Cincinnati, 3333 Burnet Avenue, Cincinnati, OH 45229, USA; [c] University of Michigan Ross School of Business, 701 Tappan Street, Ann Arbor, MI 48109, USA
* Corresponding author.
*E-mail address:* mniedner@med.umich.edu

Pediatr Clin N Am 60 (2013) 563–580
http://dx.doi.org/10.1016/j.pcl.2013.02.005
0031-3955/13/$ – see front matter Published by Elsevier Inc.

pediatric.theclinics.com

majority of health care in the United States operates roughly at this level, although some specific domains in health care have improved to higher orders of reliability.[3–7] A reliability scale with corresponding real-world and health care examples is outlined in **Table 1**. This article outlines the current state of reliability in a clinical context, discusses general principles of reliability, and finally explores the characteristics of high-reliability organizations (HROs) as a desirable future state for pediatric critical care.

## CURRENT STATE OF RELIABILITY IN CLINICAL CARE AND THE PEDIATRIC INTENSIVE CARE UNIT

The health care industry has a fairly woeful track record of reliably delivering contemporary best practice while simultaneously avoiding harm, struggling in the domains of both quality and safety. It is estimated that adults typically receive recommended, evidence-based care about 55% of the time, with little variation among acute, chronic, and preventive care.[3] General pediatric data from a similar analysis suggest performance that is comparable with adult care on average, but more variability exists based on the type of care environment.[11] Children receive an estimated 68% of indicated care for acute medical problems, 53% for chronic medical conditions, and 41% for preventive care. Furthermore, data derived from such performance reviews do not include many errors unrelated to widely accepted best practices, nor those invisible to the measurement methodology. In a survey of pediatric physicians and nurses, half filed incident reports on less than 50% of their own errors, and a third did so less than 20% of the time.[12] It is reasonable to conclude that most medical practitioners are only aware of the tip of the iceberg when it comes to unsafe conditions, near misses, preventable harm, and opportunities for improving the quality and safety of health care.

Although pediatric intensive care unit (PICU)-specific data are scarce, several studies provide support that the intensive care unit (ICU) is no exception. Two

**Table 1**
**Levels of reliability**

| Level | Reliability | Success | Opportunities Per Failure | Real-World Example | Health Care Example |
|---|---|---|---|---|---|
| Chaotic | $<10^{-1}$ | <90% | <10 | Annual mortality if >90 y old | Achievement of best-practice processes in outpatient care |
| 1 | $10^{-1}$ | 90% | 10 | Mortality of climbing Mt Everest | Achievement of best-practice processes in inpatient care |
| 2 | $10^{-2}$ | 99% | 100 | Mortality of Grand Prix racing | Deaths in risky surgery (American Society of Anesthesiologists grades 3–5) |
| 3 | $10^{-3}$ | 99.9% | 1000 | Helicopter crashes | Deaths in general surgery |
| 4 | $10^{-4}$ | 99.99% | 10,000 | Mortality of canoeing | Deaths in routine anesthesia |
| 5 | $10^{-5}$ | 99.999% | 100,000 | Chartered-flight crashes | Deaths from blood transfusions |
| 6 | $10^{-6}$ | 99.9999% | 1,000,000 | Commercial airline crashes | — |

*Data from Refs.[3,8–10]*

prospective studies in the 1990s estimated that iatrogenic adverse complications occurred in 5% to 8% of PICU admissions.[13,14] In 2000, the Institute of Medicine (IOM) cited the ICU as one of the health care environments most prone to errors and preventable harm.[15] More recently, the use of hospital-wide trigger tools to systematically identify harm in the health care setting demonstrated greater sensitivity than self-reporting and retrospective chart review.[16] This finding was again demonstrated in the PICU setting by Larsen and colleagues,[17] whose study team found approximately 1 preventable adverse event for every 5 patient-days, 3% of which were considered to be serious. In a 20-bed PICU at full occupancy for a year, this would translate to 1416 minor to moderate adverse events and 44 serious ones. So the PICU, like other health care settings, has a great deal of opportunity to improve reliability.

Current efforts by many ICUs to enhance reliability represent a good beginning, but an unacceptable end point. Evidence-based consensus guidelines from professional organizations, when transformed into local protocols and pathways, help to guide care toward best or preferred practices of which there are many now for the PICU practitioner, from traumatic brain injury, to septic shock, to the prevention of central-line infections.[18–20] Beyond basic standardization, Gawande[21,22] and Pronovost and colleagues[23] have championed the use of checklists to help manage some of the complexity of modern medicine. Identifying a minimum set of high-value practices immediately before an action or in real time during a process has helped prevent errors of ineptitude (ie, the failure to apply knowledge) and mitigate errors of ignorance (ie, the absence of knowledge). Protocolized care and checklists reduce unnecessary variation, which can promote predictability and thereby reduce errors of communication, teamwork, and supervision (ie, the lack thereof). Improved performance reliability through the use of checklists has been demonstrated in many ICUs, including PICUs, with examples of reducing central-line infections, reducing ventilator-associated pneumonias, and increasing daily harm-prevention practices, to name but a few.[24–26]

However, in achieving highly reliable health care, there are some problems with standardized care, use of checklists, implementation of protocols, and automation of decision-support tools. Experienced by many providers as "cookbook medicine," such tools do not always accommodate the wide range of practitioner or team experience nor facilitate innovation and creative problem solving in the face of unusual or unexpected circumstances. As the old NASA saying goes about astronauts, "There are two ways to die in space: (1) not following the procedure exactly as written and (2) following the procedure *exactly* as written." For PICUs to achieve high reliability, we will have to transcend the implementation of isolated tools or techniques and instead arrive at a state of continuous, mindful organizing whereby the quality of organizational attention enables a coordinated capacity to perceive, understand, and act on opportunities to prevent, intercept, mitigate, and learn from all undesired phenomena.[1,27,28]

## PRINCIPLES OF RELIABILITY

The Institute for Healthcare Improvement (IHI) has put forward a stepwise model for applying principles of reliability to health care systems: prevention, identification/mitigation, and redesign.[1] Prevention strategies, such as Failure Modes and Effects Analysis, are the furthest upstream, but eliminating latent vulnerabilities in complex and interdependent systems can become more theoretical than empirical, and cannot anticipate all possibilities. Process simplification and process control reduce opportunities for failures to occur or propagate downstream, and are common methods used in the current quality and safety movement in American health care, as evidenced by lean engineering as well as bundles and checklists. However, situations do not always unfold the same way each time, so each opportunity for a failure is slightly different. This aspect requires that performance adapts in real time to achieve reliability. So in a loosely coupled system such as health care, prevention strategies have significant shortcomings, and increasing attention is being placed on effective identification and mitigation, as evidenced by contemporary work around failure to rescue.[29] Identification of failures and emerging risk is crucial, but insufficient for situational awareness to be created.[30] Yet even when problems are perceived there are issues with misperception, misconception, and misunderstanding, confounding the ability to adapt to or invent countermeasures for harm propagating through the system. **Fig. 1** outlines a range of strategies that are targeted at different levels where risk and harm emerge in complex systems.

The IHI also describes levels of reliability to help distinguish design characteristics of systems, and a proposed grouping of such traits is outlined in **Table 2**.[1,31] It should be noted that occurrence rates of failed processes (eg, compliance with best practice) and catastrophic outcomes (eg, death) can differ by orders of magnitude. Reliability of $10^{-1}$ or less typically represents systems whereby there is no articulated common process and reliability strategies are no more sophisticated than training and reminders. Performance relies on individuals' intent, vigilance, and hard work. Reliability of $10^{-2}$ on key process measures is more consistent with systems using intentionally designed quality and safety tools as well as evidence-based procedures that are implemented using principles of human factors engineering. Reliability of $10^{-3}$ or better on key process measures typically reflects well-designed systems with attention to structure, processes, context, human psychology, and their collective relationship to performance and outcomes.[28,31,32]

## HIGH-RELIABILITY ORGANIZATIONS

During the growing movement of quality improvement and patient safety in health care over the last 2 decades, there has been increasing interest in adapting successful

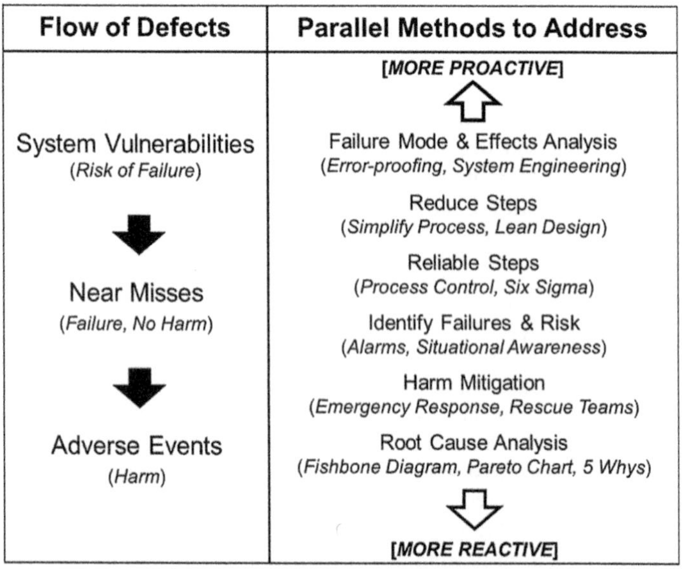

| Flow of Defects | Parallel Methods to Address |
|---|---|
|  | *[MORE PROACTIVE]* ⬆ |
| System Vulnerabilities *(Risk of Failure)* | Failure Mode & Effects Analysis *(Error-proofing, System Engineering)* |
|  | Reduce Steps *(Simplify Process, Lean Design)* |
| ⬇ | Reliable Steps *(Process Control, Six Sigma)* |
| Near Misses *(Failure, No Harm)* | Identify Failures & Risk *(Alarms, Situational Awareness)* |
| ⬇ | Harm Mitigation *(Emergency Response, Rescue Teams)* |
| Adverse Events *(Harm)* | Root Cause Analysis *(Fishbone Diagram, Pareto Chart, 5 Whys)* |
|  | ⬇ *[MORE REACTIVE]* |

**Fig. 1.** Flow of defects in systems and parallel methods to address them.

**Table 2**
**System characteristics as they relate to differing levels of reliability**

| Low Reliability (Generally More Basic and Inconsistent) | ← Reliability → | High Reliability (Generally More Robust and Effective) |
|---|---|---|
| Individual preference prevails | Personnel informed by reliability science | Sophisticated organizational design |
| Intent to perform well | | Integrated hierarchies, processes, teams |
| Individual excellence rewarded | Implementation of human factors | Error-proofing: forced function, shutdown |
| Human vigilance for risk, error, harm | Standardization of processes is the norm | Failure modes and effects analysis |
| Hard work, trying harder after failures | Ambiguities in standard work eliminated | Routine simulation for training/reinforcing |
| Codified policies, procedures, guidelines | "Work-around" solutions eliminated | Strong teamwork climate |
| Personal checklists | Reminders and decision support built-in | Strong safety culture |
| Retrospective performance feedback | Standard checklists (real-time compliance) | Staff perception of psychological safety |
| Didactic training/retraining | Good habits/behaviors leveraged | Preoccupation with failure |
| Awareness-raising | Error-proofing: warnings, sensory alerts | Reluctance to simplify interpretations |
| Basic standardization (equipment, brands, forms) | Deliberate redundancy in critical steps | Sensitivity to operations |
| | Key tasks are scheduled/assigned | Deference to expertise |
| | Some simulation training for emergencies | Commitment to resilience |
| | Real-time performance feedback | |

*Data from* Refs.[1,28,31]

safety and quality models from other industries, such as lean engineering, Six Sigma process control, and failure mode analysis. Similarly, clinical enterprises have become increasingly interested in applying principles of HROs; namely, those organizations operating in complex and high-risk industries where errors and accidents are expected, yet where harm and catastrophe are effectively anticipated and mitigated in nearly all cases.[33] It is fair to state that no health care enterprise has fully implemented all aspects of an HRO nor realized their spectacularly low incidence of harm from human errors and system failures. Whether the vexing complexity of health care can be conquered through HRO principles is yet to be determined, but the sound principles surely move us closer to the goal of medical care free from preventable harm. Indeed, high reliability has come to be a phrase not only of high-reliability achieving organizations, but high-reliability seeking organizations, to which all ICUs ought to aspire.[33,34]

The early characterization of HROs in the 1980s was motivated by observations of a few American industries that seemed to defy normal accident theory and human reliability, such as flight decks of aircraft carriers, commercial aviation, and nuclear power plants. Before the advent of HRO models, normal accident theory (NAT) represented the dominant thinking about how disasters occur in complex sociotechnical systems despite high vigilance and explicit countermeasures, such as with nuclear power plant meltdowns.[35,36] In NAT, processes that are tightly coupled, time dependent, and have little slack or flexibility can allow impending aberrant events to propagate invisibly and with sufficient complexity so as to make real-time comprehension impossible. NAT pessimistically argues that in such systems, accidents are inevitable or "normal" regardless of management and operational effectiveness. This attitude is akin to the prevalent mindset in health care whereby hospital-acquired conditions and deaths from errors are fatalistically viewed as just "a cost of doing business." By contrast, HROs take a more optimistic perspective about continuously seeking effective management of inherently complex and risky systems through organizational control of both hazard and probability, primarily through collective mindfulness.[33]

Numerous industries are faced with the need to regularly perform complex and inherently hazardous tasks dependent on highly technical skill sets in time-critical and unforgiving contexts. However, unlike most other industries (including health care), HROs' devotion to a zero rate of failure has been nearly matched by performance.[28,37,38] Some HRO industries, such as the Federal Aviation Administration's Air Traffic Control system, have used strategies very familiar to medical professionals: extensive and continuous training, selection of individuals with fitting aptitude, performance auditing, and cumulative team experience. But some HRO industries, such as US naval aircraft operations, seem to fly in the face of conventional wisdom, such as the launching and landing of multi-million dollar warbirds on a pitching deck of a carrier at sea in the dark that is faithfully executed by a young, inexperienced, and transient crew.[39]

But whereas HROs tend to be high risk and high reliability, health care tends to be high risk and low reliability. Cook and Rasmussen[40] have described a dynamic safety model that helps contrast high- and low-reliability organizations (**Fig. 2**). In this model, complex sociotechnical systems operate within a zone bounded by certain forces such as economic failure, unacceptable workload, and unacceptable performance. As unreliability increases, the probability of operations unintentionally crossing one of these boundaries also increases, leading to financial losses, workforce overload, and/or adverse events. Compared with high-risk low-reliability organizations, HROs can safely exist in the high-risk zone near the boundary of harm. In part this is because performance is so reliable that there is little likelihood of operations violating intended thresholds, but also in part because when operations slip or drift in the direction toward harm, HROs are aware and adaptive enough to intercept or mitigate threatening events and circumstances. It must be noted that high reliability in performance and outcomes does not mean invariance in processes or procedures. On the contrary, lack of flexibility can create brittle systems. What requires the upmost consistency in an HRO is the collective cognitive process that makes sense of events and changing circumstances.[27,41] Managing unexpected events requires revised inputs and tactics that are predicated on a shared understanding and prioritization of safety. What must be reliable is the detection of threats and errors; what must remain flexible is the adaptive response to the unexpected.

So what is it that unifies such HRO industries and enterprises as disparate as air traffic control, nuclear power plants, and aircraft carriers? Just as necessity is the mother of invention, HROs emerge in the kind of contexts that demand them, in settings where "failure" is neither affordable nor tolerable, stakes are high, and learning is difficult.[41,42] While numerous industries share these contextual features, key adaptive features set HROs apart.[43] HROs create collective mindfulness through several processes: preoccupation with failure, reluctance to simplify interpretations, sensitivity to operations, deference to expertise, and commitment to resilience.[27] These contexts and characteristics are outlined in **Table 3** and are further described here.

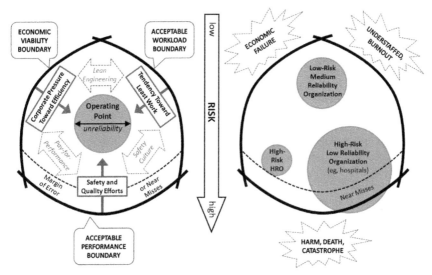

**Fig. 2.** Dynamic safety model, opposing versus realigning forces, and organizational reliability. A system's operating point is constrained by boundaries (*heavy black lines*) of economic viability, acceptable workload, and acceptable performance. Corporate financial pressures and human tendency toward least work push the operating point in a riskier direction, whereas safety and quality efforts push the operating point away from unacceptable outcomes and harm. Several mechanisms of health care quality and safety (*dashed arrows*) realign these opposing forces: lean engineering reduces workload while saving money; pay-for-performance creates economic incentives to engage safe practices; and a strong safety culture alters staff effort toward safety work. The operating point can shift within a zone of reliability (as reflected by *gray circle* where the diameter corresponds to the degree of unreliability). High-reliability organizations (HROs) have an operating point that shifts very little and can therefore exist close to the boundary of acceptable performance without harming. Low-reliability organizations, such as hospitals, cannot exist close to high-risk outcomes without failures and harm, because the operating point can exhibit large, rapid shifts across the boundary of acceptable performance. (*Modified from* Cook R, Rasmussen J. "Going solid": a model of system dynamics and consequences for patient safety. Qual Saf Health Care 2005;14:131; with permission.)

### Shared Contexts of HROs and PICUs: Socially and/or Politically Unforgiving Environments

HROs reside in environments that are socially or politically unforgiving, and it is fair to say that health care is becoming increasingly so.[15] Historically the social intolerance

| Table 3 | |
|---|---|
| **High-reliability organizations: contexts and adaptive characteristics** | |
| **Contexts** | **Characteristics** |
| There is marked complexity in systems, processes, technology, and work | Preoccupation with failure |
| | Reluctance to simplify interpretations |
| The environment is socially and/or politically unforgiving | Sensitivity to operations |
| | Deference to expertise |
| The consequences for failure are potentially catastrophic | Commitment to resilience |
| The cost of failure precludes learning through trial and error or traditional experimentation | |

toward medical error and harm is reflected in the scale of litigation, in terms of the high volume of lawsuits as well as the large awards. Further evidence of intolerability is the high degree of regulation. Like commercial aviation and nuclear power plants, health care is highly regulated. With *To Err is Human*, the IOM powerfully summarized of the scope of errors, failures, and preventable harm in modern health care, raising awareness as much for the medical industry as for the American population at large.[15] Over recent decades, medical errors and preventable harm have been increasingly unacceptable to consumers, regulators, and providers. From patients' bills of rights to mandatory public reporting to never events, the American social and political milieu has brought the practice of medicine under the heaviest scrutiny and accountability since the words *primum non nocere* were first uttered. The PICU, in particular, is a target for this intense scrutiny. Of all the pediatric hospital-based measures endorsed by the National Quality Forum, approximately half are PICU specific, and of all of Medicare's never events are highly relevant in pediatric critical care (**Fig. 3**).

### Shared Contexts of HROs and PICUs: Consequences of Failure are Potentially Catastrophic

Although life-or-death human catastrophes can occur in almost any context (eg, driving down the freeway), there are some settings in which failures can become particularly catastrophic (eg, jumbo jet crash, nuclear power plant meltdown). HROs have evolved in such high-stakes situations, although clearly not all such contexts have produced HROs. Health care, by its very nature, often concerns life-or-death circumstances, with a particular focus on averting death that might otherwise be imminent. This milieu is distinct from that of most high-risk industries; the starting conditions are those of health instability. Even when life does not seem to be on the line in health care (eg, preventive medicine), many minor health care activities have the potential to become lethal (eg, an acetaminophen prescription becoming an accidental overdose). And for all the challenges that adult medicine has in defining, measuring, and improving the quality of health care, this is amplified in pediatrics, where evidence for best practice is more limited, the data infrastructure less robust, and the potential loss of quality-adjusted life-years greater.[44] More children die in PICUs than in any other inpatient setting, not only because of their severity of illness but also their intolerance to further insults that healthier patients might weather better.

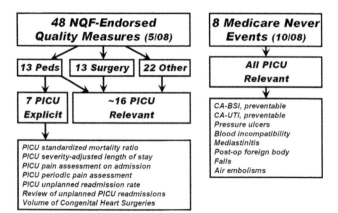

**Fig. 3.** Quality and safety measures endorsed by national bodies. CA-BSI, catheter-associated bloodstream infection; CA-UTI, catheter-associated urinary tract infection; NQF, National Quality Framework; Peds, pediatrics; PICU, pediatric intensive care unit.

### Shared Contexts of HROs and PICUs: Costs of Failure Preclude Learning Through Traditional Experimentation

For an HRO, the high-stakes consequences preclude learning through trial and error or traditional experimentation. Society does not tolerate randomized controlled trials of airliners or nuclear power plant designs to see which ones crash or melt down more frequently. Yet with untold lives on the line, academic experimentation and trial-and-error management has been the status quo. More recently, health systems (and ICUs in particular) have started moving more in the direction of HRO learning mechanisms, such as the increased use of high-fidelity simulation, more deliberate prebriefings and debriefings, and industry-wide learning through patient safety organizations.

### Shared Contexts of HROs and PICUs: Marked Complexity in Systems, Processes, Technology, and Work

Gawande[21] has described in a single word the greatest threat to safe and high-quality health care: complexity. All known HROs function in highly complex systems whereby there are many opportunities for errors and failures to begin propagating toward calamity. The interaction of numerous complexities makes emerging harm opaque, as the interactions can have hidden, unanticipated, or unintended consequences.[35] The IOM cites areas of greatest complexity and time sensitivity (ICUs, emergency departments, and operating rooms) as the locations where defects in care delivery are most prolific.[15] Sequential and dependent steps in complex operations are often a basis for the gap between intended practice and actual execution, especially in low-reliability industries such as health care. If one were to start with valid, evidence-based health care guidelines, many steps must be executed correctly for the best care to reach a patient. Staff must be aware of the evidence, accept it sufficiently, know how to apply it, work in a care environment that makes it feasible, remember to do it in real time, have agreement from the care team and consumer, and ensure that the care is actually performed in the right time, place, and manner. If each of these steps were to occur with 95% fidelity, best care would be delivered only about 70% of the time.

In the PICU, work flow is unpredictable, diverse, complex, technical, stressful, fast-paced, and invasive. Care must be multidisciplinary, with no one role—physician, nurse, respiratory therapist, pharmacist, social worker, or parent—able to have mastery of all the information and skills necessary to treat the patient optimally. Because the work requires many individuals and teams coordinating efforts effectively in short and fast-paced time frames, the ICU becomes critically dependent on teamwork and communication, which are 2 of the most common sources of errors and sentinel events.[45,46]

## THE CONTRAST BETWEEN HROS AND THE CURRENT STATE OF HEALTH CARE: WHAT WOULD A HIGH-RELIABILITY PICU LOOK LIKE?

As noted earlier, the best HROs are characterized by patterns of mindful organizing, resulting in a quality of organizational attention that increases the likelihood that people will notice unique details of situations and be able to act on them appropriately.[27,28] Five interrelated processes constitute mindful organizing: preoccupation with failure, reluctance to simplify interpretations, sensitivity to operations, commitment to resilience, and flexible decision structures. Collectively these processes and associated practices help people focus attention on perceptual details that are typically lost when they coordinate their actions and share their interpretations.[28] This strategy expands capabilities to both anticipate and defend against foreseeable risks or surprises, and to bounce back from dangers after they have become manifest.[47] More simply, processes of mindfulness increase the likelihood that organizational members will be able to detect and correct or cope with errors and unexpected events more swiftly. This section describes these processes in more detail, and contrasts them with common practice in the modern American health care system. Just as a living organism is more than an assemblage of organs, so too is an HRO more than the characteristics outlined herein. This dissected model is easier to articulate and understand, but the characteristics are interdependent. Although any of the many reliability principles might represent incremental organizational improvement over a current state, true organizational transformation occurs when all aspects of the HRO are in full force simultaneously and harmoniously.

### Preoccupation with Failure

Within HROs, small, seemingly inconsequential errors, mishaps, or surprises are regarded as symptomatic of something that may be seriously wrong in the system. There is a commitment to finding and analyzing the "half-events," and to treat all failures as learning opportunities in a nonpunitive and transparent manner.[27,43] A constant sense of vulnerability to failure is maintained across the organization, from the front line through leadership, and there is commitment to continuous improvement in operations. Performance data are available as near to real time as possible, as are failure analyses. HROs have largely overcome the culture of individual blame, and maintain humility about the universal imperfections in human performance.[48] In addition, HROs are preoccupied with imagining and understanding, prospectively, what might go wrong and how it could happen.

Contrast this with modern health care. Despite the known risks to patients from deficits in quality and safety countermeasures, most clinicians do not deliberately use or leverage quality and safety principles in their work, often believing that the responsibility for "systems issues" resides with the hospital administration.[12,49] Most clinicians focus on an understanding of pathophysiology and evidence, then apply this knowledge to the best of their ability to one patient at a time. In low-reliability health care, near misses are commonly regarded as evidence of their successful ability to avert disaster, reinforcing the belief that current operations are adequate and that no systems changes are needed. The ongoing perception of success (ie, luck) breeds overconfidence in current operations and intolerance to opposing views. When failures occur, it is common to see medical personnel fall back on the ABCs of a punitive safety culture: Accuse, Blame, Criticize.

The PICU in particular has a very high volume of "sharp-end" activities, namely the point of care at which all propagated defects emerging from the system actually reach the patient: a medicine injected, a catheter inserted, a chest shocked. Yet despite the pervasive risks in this setting, adverse outcomes from errors are camouflaged. More deaths occur in PICUs than in any other care units within a pediatric hospital, and adverse outcomes, although unwanted, are not unexpected. A death in a general care unit stands out in bold relief and is scrutinized deeply for what went wrong, but how is it clearly discerned when morbidity or mortality in the PICU is the consequence of progressive refractory critical illness or unrecognized (or unreported) medical errors slipping under the radar of awareness? Deaths and adverse events would still occur in a high-reliability PICU that was operating perfectly—but which ones?

Imagine a high-reliability PICU preoccupied with failure. Every error or unexpected discrepancy would be identified and made visible to the multiprofessional team and unit leadership, be it a medication-dose error, a delay in antibiotics for a septic child, or a dissatisfied parent. Subtle deviations from the norm and unexpected surprises would be revealed, to combat misconceptions and misunderstandings; for example, through closed-loop communication and open-minded inquiry into each other's mental models. Nonpunitive response to error would be maintained by leadership and frontline alike, treating each error, glitch, or adverse outcome as a learning opportunity. Seemingly minor near misses, such as noncompliance with hand hygiene or evidence-based bundles, would be viewed as symptomatic of deeper causes, and root-cause analyses would be meaningfully engaged by the most relevant staff. Despite harm-free operations over long periods of time, staff would not become less vigilant for medical errors, threats, or unsafe conditions. Frontline staff, project teams, and unit leadership would have real-time data measuring operational variables, process performance, and outcomes, rates of hospital-acquired infections, compliance with best practices, and workload and staffing projections. Compliance with routine processes would exceed 95% reliability in audits, and safety critical processes would operate at 99.9% reliability. This information would be highly visible via dashboards, and emerging trends would be broadcast with expert interpretation to promote situational awareness. Change of shift handoffs would be thorough and standardized. Prebriefings before procedures would always occur, and inquiry would be invited. Debriefings would occur after every procedure to identify deviations from expectations. There would be no preventable deaths or harm.

### Sensitivity to Operations

HROs are able to maintain a heightened quality of attention across the enterprise, enabled by a sensitivity to operations at all levels, particularly the front line. Sensitivity to operations means creating and maintaining an integrated "big picture" of current situations through ongoing attention to real-time information. Organizations that have real-time information and situational understanding can forestall the compounding of small problems or failures by making several small adjustments. Small adjustments are opportunities to stop mistakes and errors from lining up in such a way that they grow into a bigger crisis. These data on processes and system performance reflect daily work, and emerge visibly to both leaders and the front line. This situation promotes a shared mental model for how operations should be performing and situational awareness when they are not. Clear alignment of purpose is maintained throughout the organization; everyone understands what is happening and why.

"Attention is the currency of leadership," as the axiom goes. Leaders within HROs maintain awareness of and actively shape the social and interactive infrastructure of the organization to promote strong teamwork and create a context of respect and trust, so that people feel safe in voicing concerns. Both enable a robust safety culture and also seek to refine and balance nonpunitive responses to error, while maintaining a strong sense of responsibility and accountability at every level: individual, team, unit, and organization. HROs work to flatten decision hierarchies so that they are neither bureaucratic nor authoritarian. Discovery of defects in complex systems with transparent, nonpunitive dissemination of findings is crucial for organizational learning.[50,51]

Contrasting this to many health care settings, we find errors and defects are underreported for many reasons: fear of reprisal, the concern of lawsuits, time constraints, uncertainty of which incidents to report, concerns of implicating others, and lack of feedback and evidence that information was valued and used for system change.[12,49] Historically, the focus has rested on the frontline clinician's error, with blame being followed by punishment. However, punitive responses reinforce the behavior of hiding errors, preventing the recognition, analysis, and correction of the root causes and systemic problems.[15,51] Such punitive response is but one dimension of safety culture, which is broken in many health care settings. Huang and colleagues[52] stated that poor frontline perceptions of management were associated with hospital mortality rates, and that low measures of safety culture correlated with increased length of stay. Similarly, Hutchinson and colleagues[53] demonstrated a positive association between incident reporting rates and measures of safety culture when comparing institutions. Because of this, many health care settings lack situational awareness and lose opportunities to keep small problems from becoming large ones.

Imagine a high-reliability PICU exquisitely sensitive to operations. Leaders and staff know what is going on in the PICU and why. Everyone is able to keep their attention focused on the key tasks within their role, but do not lose sight of the whole PICU or colleagues' priorities. Frontline staff has immediate access to expert supervision and informational resources to support its daily work. Unsafe conditions, such as strained staffing or contradictory information, are recognized, acknowledged, and swiftly addressed. Leaders show inquiry into frontline work and proactively look for ways to support it organizationally. The safety culture is palpable, with easily visible psychological safety. People are asking questions about the diagnosis, sharing insights into the latest evidence, using closed-loop communication, double-checking syringe pumps, and not interrupting attention-critical activities. Strong teamwork practices are self-evident: everyone knows everyone's name, or introduces themselves; there is role clarity with seamless and fluid leadership and followership; mutual accountability is respectful, constructive, and just. The PICU is transparent with, and supported by, the broader organization, without disciplinary or professional silos. Everyone is situationally aware, and everyone is constantly focused on what is correct and best for the patient.

### Reluctance to Simplify

Occam and Einstein were in agreement that everything should be made as simple as possible, but not simpler. In the face of complexity, simplification is often adaptive by enhancing understanding. However, oversimplification can yield tragically incorrect conclusions and a false sense of security or comprehension. Oversimplification reduces sensitivity to threats and unintended consequences, undermining situational awareness. It sweeps under the rug weak signals as mere noise. It is difficult to recognize a unique problem no one has ever seen before. Therefore, HROs proactively seek out differing viewpoints to reveal the unknown, challenge assumptions, and cultivate loyal dissent as a norm.[27,54] Excusing or explaining away discrepancies and surprises is avoided. Diversity in experience, perspective, and opinion are encouraged. And there is a kind of trust in the wisdom of crowds: that all of us together are smarter than any one of us, whatever one's rank. HROs are organizationally self-aware of their intrinsic sociotechnical complexity, and therefore seek to understand all aberrant phenomena in the context of that complexity.

Reason's[36] "Swiss cheese model" emphasizes that many latent defects, technical failures, and/or human errors must align for risk to propagate toward actual harm. Yet it is characteristic among low-reliability organizations for causes to be ascribed to system defects proximate to the harm. In much of health care, the underpinnings of failure are commonly oversimplified and assigned to people or processes late in the chain of events. Near misses are considered by many as "no harm, no foul," and therefore do not get reported. Incident reports are frequently cited as "writing someone up" rather than articulating what would have been best for the patient.

Morbidity and mortality case reviews are commonly confounded by hindsight bias, absence of first-hand historians, and a lack of systematic analysis by personnel expertise in human factors and complex systems. The PICU is a particularly vexing environment with a high volume of hands-on and invasive activities (eg, blood transfusion, bedside procedures, intravenous medications) but is also an environment of low-frequency, high-complexity care (eg, extracorporeal membrane oxygenation, cardiac arrest, therapeutic hypothermia). The profound variation in day-to-day clinical and technical work in a PICU would tempt even the most detail-oriented staff into heuristics that underappreciate the full complexity at hand.

Imagine a high-reliability PICU reluctant to simplify interpretations. Leaders and staff would not only have clinical content expertise but also be familiar with human factors engineering. Participants would be able to use language to accurately describe the PICU environment with sufficient nuance to reflect its actual complexity socially, psychologically, and technically. Ambiguities and work-arounds would be anathema. Personal "to do" lists would be replaced by standardized checklists, continuously refined by consensus. Staff and leaders would welcome having their assumptions questioned or verified. The youngest nurse could ask the most seasoned intensivist to explain the rationale for a procedure. Diverse opinions would be sought actively when seeking to understand performance variation. Doctors, nurses, parents, and infection preventionists would weigh in together on every hospital-acquired infection. Staff would always consider worse-case scenarios and assume Murphy's Law is true: that if something could go wrong, it probably will. Excuses like "I won't let it happen again" are replaced with "how can we ensure this will never happen in the future?" Failures would not be attributed to sharp end processes without exploring the underpinnings further upstream in the Swiss cheese model: no nurse administering a medication overdose would be alone in owning the process failures that include the prescriber, dispensing pharmacy, electronic order entry, countermeasures, and double-checker. Staff would not be overconfident in their understanding of PICU operations, but seek always to understand others before being understood. Every morbidity and mortality would be reviewed deeply not only for iatrogenic complications, but to discern missed opportunities whereby care might have adhered to a higher standard of care or whereby potential opportunities were missed. For expected pediatric death from terminal progressive illness, the standards to achieve a comfortable and dignified death would be analyzed with vigor equal to that exercised for unexpected deaths.

## Deference to Expertise

HROs resist inflexible command-and-control hierarchies whereby leaders "may be wrong but are never in doubt." In an HRO, decision making and problem solving deeply engage people with the most related knowledge and expertise, typically the frontline workers. Vertical chains of command are flattened when and where possible, especially in high-tempo times, creating dynamic and flexible decision-making teams that shift authority to those most expert in the aspect or process of the system.[27] In the setting of time-critical crises, it is the reflex of many organizations to become more vertical, but HROs act collectively as a cohesive organism, with awareness, engagement, and input from all levels, regardless of rank. This process is particularly adaptive in the face of novel problems or unexpected crises for which solutions must be invented.

In health care, organization is typically more hierarchical, be it from the C-suite to unit managers, from the attending to the medical student, or from the charge nurse to the nursing orientee. Not only are there steep hierarchies within professional domains, there are marked inequalities between professionals, most notably between physicians and nurses (as well as other allied health care providers). The belief that the decisions of the medical team leader should not be questioned is common among physicians, in stark contrast to captains in commercial aviation.[55] The mental model of the highly trained doctor or health care leader is that important actions are decided by important decision makers, and not necessarily by the most knowledgable decision makers for that problem. The growing trend toward patient-centered and family-centered care is partly a recognition of the foibles of paternalistic medicine. Erudite education and functional expertise are not always distinguished in health care. No one has greater insight into the nuances of a child more than the parent, and when this insight is working synergistically with medically trained professionals' efforts, superior outcomes are achieved.[56]

Imagine a high-reliability PICU with exquisite decision-making flexibility. The PICU leaders and staff know who are particularly knowledgable or adept in particular domains. Personnel put forth their unique skill sets to the benefit of patients: the nurse who is skillful in the deployment of peripheral intravenous lines in babies, the surgeon who is experienced with operating on patients on extracorporeal membrane oxygenation, the intensivist with training in palliative care. Parents' voices are central to interpreting their children's needs and cues. During crises, teams pool talents and skills to solve problems or adapt to the unexpected. Egos and rank are checked at the door, and orders are not barked by physicians to nurses. Authority flows from trust, respect, experience, and a shared mental model of what is happening, what needs to happen, and who best can make the difficult call.

### Commitment to Resilience

HROs understand that errors and unforeseen situations will arise, and that it is impossible to write procedures to cover every situation. One cannot have specific standard work for events that have never been encountered or anticipated. However, HROs have evolved adaptive strategies for approaching unexpected events, system failures, and harm. HROs have a self-expectation of swift adaptation, speedy communication, and creative problem solving.[27,47] These traits are often exercised through simulation whereby the focus is not only on the operational outcome of the simulation but also the dynamic processes of the team: respectful interactions, assertive information sharing, flat hierarchies, cooperation, attentiveness, contingency planning, and so forth. Though seemingly a paradox, HROs achieve dynamic stability not through rigid invariance in operations and processes, but from highly effective management of performance variation and unexpected perturbations of the system.[27,43] In addition to being poised to bounce back from mishaps, resilience also refers to the capacity to maintain operations under constant stress. Because stress largely derives from what one cannot control and cannot predict, HROs help build resilience to stress through many other HRO traits alluded to, such as data streams and situational awareness that help people predict emerging threats, as well as effective teamwork, communication, and training that help people feel more in control of inherently risky work. Finally, resilience is generated by constructively learning from anomalies and failures to better understand the system and to develop response repertoires more capable of response to unexpected contingencies in the future. HROs and low-reliability organizations will both experience failures, but HROs are not disabled by errors and failures.

Whereas HROs would interpret a fail-safe system as one whereby one can assume that eventually someone or something will fail and, thus, have a plan to ensure everyone remains safe regardless, health care has historically interpreted fail-safe as failure free, meaning "nobody fail!" Health care systems have sought to reduce errors though more education, selection of smarter trainees, and trying harder to make humans be more perfect, all of which are strategies of $10^{-1}$ reliability organizations that are considered ineffective on their own.[1,15]

Imagine a high-reliability PICU truly committed to resilience. The staff talks regularly about mishaps, sharing historical failures as a reminder of what could go wrong today to serve as a learning opportunity and prevent repetitions in the future. Leaders, in particular, demonstrate their fallibility, role-modeling humility for more junior staff. All members of staff can tell you about the last dozen mishaps with patient harm in the PICU. Simulations in situ are routine, with mock-codes going on daily alongside regular patient care. Members of staff cross-train in simulations to learn each other's roles. Dismissals such as "it's a risk we have to take" are replaced by "what is the contingency plan for this unavoidable risk?" Plans are reviewed and drills undertaken around unlikely scenarios, such as mass casualties, evacuations, and pandemics. Team-building exercises outside the scope of medicine are pursued. Staff nurture and mentor one another professionally.

## SUMMARY

Safety is neither an accomplishment nor a destination, but rather an emergent state derived from characteristics of the system, agents within it, and management of it. This tenet is one reason why health care has struggled so much with safety, because there are no silver bullets, be they aimed at leaders, the front line, the processes, or the technologies, that ensure safe and reliable care. To pursue high reliability requires a continuous and dynamic process of organizing because, just as HROs demand perfection, they know they cannot ultimately achieve it. While HROs constantly seek to reduce errors, failures, and harm, they also remain perpetually poised to cope with and quickly recover when things go awry. High reliability requires an insightful balance of many dyads: accountability and nonpunitive response, teamwork and autonomy, prevention and resilience, consistency and flexibility, to name but a few. Although examples exist of specific HROs in non–health care industries that are inspirational for the health care community, there are no hospitals or clinical units that can be held up as a high-reliability health care organization. It may be said that some health care systems have begun their high-reliability–seeking journey. But even if high reliability of performance were achieved, the crucial point remains: you never get it behind you. Organizing for high reliability is continually repeated to maintain it, every minute of every day.

At no other time have quality and recognition of patient safety in health care been of greater import than they are now. The modern patient-safety movement continues to grow at an unprecedented pace, at both pragmatic and academic levels. The PICU is an environment rich with the potential for risk, error, and harm. It is also full of dedicated, bright, vigilant people who have a wealth of clinical and operational information at their fingertips. This situation creates a very fertile environment to be able to engage in and pioneer quality and safety science. PICUs across the United States have reduced historical rates of central-line infections, ventilator-associated pneumonias, harmful medication errors, and unplanned extubations, and have even standardized mortality.[57–60] Sustainability of such improvements is patchy, and enhancements of positive dimensions of care more elusive.[61,62] If the PICU is to be the canary in the coal mine for pediatrics, then it can also be an incubator of innovation. The same contextual realities that helped forge the first HROs also exist for the PICU, making a PICU out there somewhere a good candidate to become the first health care HRO.

## REFERENCES

1. Nolan T, Rear R, Haraden C, et al. Improving the reliability of health care. IHI Innovation Series white paper. Boston: Institute for Healthcare Improvement; 2004.
2. Hollnagel E. Cognitive reliability and error analysis method: CREAM. Oxford (United Kingdom), New York: Elsevier; 1998. p. 287, xiv.
3. McGlynn EA, Asch SM, Adams J, et al. The quality of health care delivered to adults in the United States. N Engl J Med 2003;348:2635–45.
4. Kerr EA, McGlynn EA, Adams J, et al. Profiling the quality of care in twelve communities: results from the CQI study. Health Aff (Millwood) 2004;23:247–56.
5. Baker GR, Norton PG, Flintoft V, et al. The Canadian Adverse Events Study: the incidence of adverse events among hospital patients in Canada. CMAJ 2004; 170:1678–86.
6. Davis P, Lay-Yee R, Briant R, et al. Adverse events in New Zealand public hospitals I: occurrence and impact. N Z Med J 2002;115:U271.
7. Vincent C, Neale G, Woloshynowych M. Adverse events in British hospitals: preliminary retrospective record review. BMJ 2001;322:517–9.
8. Dismukes K. Human error in aviation. Critical essays on human factors in aviation. Farnham (Surrey), Burlington (VT): Ashgate; 2009. p. 579, xxiv.
9. Amalberti R, Auroy Y, Berwick D, et al. Five system barriers to achieving ultrasafe health care. Ann Intern Med 2005;142:756–64.
10. Your chances of dying. 2011. Available at: http://www.besthealthdegrees.com/health-risks. Accessed November 1, 2012.
11. Mangione-Smith R, DeCristofaro AH, Setodji CM, et al. The quality of ambulatory care delivered to children in the United States. N Engl J Med 2007;357:1515–23.
12. Taylor JA, Brownstein D, Christakis DA, et al. Use of incident reports by physicians and nurses to document medical errors in pediatric patients. Pediatrics 2004;114:729–35.
13. Stambouly JJ, McLaughlin LL, Mandel FS, et al. Complications of care in a pediatric intensive care unit: a prospective study. Intensive Care Med 1996;22:1098–104.
14. Stambouly JJ, Pollack MM. Iatrogenic illness in pediatric critical care. Crit Care Med 1990;18:1248–51.
15. Kohn LT, Corrigan J, Donaldson MS. To err is human: building a safer health system. Washington, DC: National Academy Press; 2000. p. 287, xxi.
16. Rozich JD, Haraden CR, Resar RK. Adverse drug event trigger tool: a practical methodology for measuring medication related harm. Qual Saf Health Care 2003;12:194–200.
17. Larsen GY, Donaldson AE, Parker HB, et al. Preventable harm occurring to critically ill children. Pediatr Crit Care Med 2007;8:331–6.
18. Kochanek PM, Carney N, Adelson PD, et al. Guidelines for the acute medical management of severe traumatic brain injury in infants, children, and adolescents—second edition. Pediatr Crit Care Med 2012;1(Suppl 13):S1–82.
19. Dellinger RP, Levy MM, Carlet JM, et al. Surviving Sepsis Campaign: international guidelines for management of severe sepsis and septic shock: 2008. Crit Care Med 2008;36:296–327.
20. Warady BA, Bakkaloglu S, Newland J, et al. Consensus guidelines for the prevention and treatment of catheter-related infections and peritonitis in pediatric patients receiving peritoneal dialysis: 2012 update. Perit Dial Int 2012;2(Suppl 32):S32–86.
21. Gawande A. The checklist manifesto: how to get things right. New York: Metropolitan Books; 2009.

22. Gawande A. The checklist: if something so simple can transform intensive care, what else can it do? New Yorker 2007;86–101.
23. Pronovost P, Needham D, Berenholtz S, et al. An intervention to decrease catheter-related bloodstream infections in the ICU. N Engl J Med 2006;355: 2725–32.
24. Miller MR, Niedner MF, Huskins WC, et al. Reducing PICU central line-associated bloodstream infections: 3-year results. Pediatrics 2011;128:e1077–83.
25. Bigham MT, Amato R, Bondurrant P, et al. Ventilator-associated pneumonia in the pediatric intensive care unit: characterizing the problem and implementing a sustainable solution. J Pediatr 2009;154:582–587.e2.
26. Halm MA. Daily goals worksheets and other checklists: are our critical care units safer? Am J Crit Care 2008;17:577–80.
27. Weick KE, Sutcliffe KM, Obstfeld D. Organizing for high reliability: processes of collective mindfulness. In: Sutton R, Staw B, editors. Research in organizational behavior. Greenwich (CT): JAI Press; 1999. p. 81–124.
28. Weick KE, Sutcliffe KM. Managing the unexpected: resilient performance in an age of uncertainty. San Francisco (CA): Jossey-Bass; 2007. p. 194, xii.
29. Watkinson PJ, Tarassenko L. Current and emerging approaches to address failure-to-rescue. Anesthesiology 2012;116:1158–9 [author reply: 1159].
30. McCarthy G. Situational awareness in medicine. Qual Saf Health Care 2006;15: 384 [author reply: 384].
31. AHRQ. Becoming a high reliability organization: operational advice for hospital leaders. AHRQ Publication No. 08–0022. Rockville (MD): Agency for Healthcare Research and Quality; 2008. Available at: http://www.ahrq.gov/qual/hroadvice/. Accessed July 1, 2012.
32. Donabedian A. Evaluating the quality of medical care. Milbank Mem Fund Q 1966;44(Suppl):166–206.
33. Rochlin GI. Defining high reliability organizations in practice: a taxonomic prologue. In: Roberts KH, editor. New challenges to understanding organizations. New York: Macmillan; 1993. p. 11–32.
34. Sutcliffe KM. High reliability organizations (HROs). Best Pract Res Clin Anaesthesiol 2011;25:133–44.
35. Perrow C. Normal accidents: living with high risk. Princeton (NJ): Princeton University Press; 1999.
36. Reason JT. Managing the risks of organizational accidents. Aldershot (England), Brookfield (VT): Ashgate; 1997. p. 252, xvii.
37. Nance JJ. Why hospitals should fly: the ultimate flight plan to patient safety and quality care. Bozeman (MT): Second River Healthcare Press; 2008. p. 225, ix.
38. United States, Agency for Healthcare Research and Quality, Lewin Group. Becoming a high reliability organization: operational advice for hospital leaders. Rockville (MD): Agency for Healthcare Research and Quality; 2008. p. 33.
39. Rochlin GI, Porte TR, Roberts KH. The self-designing high-reliability organization: aircraft carrier flight operations at sea. Nav War Coll Rev 1987;40:76–90.
40. Cook R, Rasmussen J. "Going solid": a model of system dynamics and consequences for patient safety. Qual Saf Health Care 2005;14:130–4.
41. Schulman P. The negotiated order of organizational reliability. Adm Soc 1993;25: 353–72.
42. Weick KE, Roberts KH. Collective mind in organizations: heedful interrelating on flight decks. Adm Sci Q 1993;38:357–81.
43. Schulman PR. General attributes of safe organisations. Qual Saf Health Care 2004;13(Suppl 2):ii39–44.

44. Shaller D. Implementing and using quality measures for children's health care: perspectives on the state of the practice. Pediatrics 2004;113:217–27.
45. Donchin Y, Gopher D, Olin M, et al. A look into the nature and causes of human errors in the intensive care unit. Crit Care Med 1995;23:294–300.
46. Sutcliffe KM, Lewton E, Rosenthal MM. Communication failures: an insidious contributor to medical mishaps. Acad Med 2004;79:186–94.
47. Wildavsky A. Searching for safety. New Brunswick (NJ): Transaction; 1991. p. 77.
48. Landau M, Chisholm D. The arrogance of optimism: notes on failure avoidance management. J Contingencies Crisis Manag 1995;3:67–80.
49. Lehmann DF, Page N, Kirschman K, et al. Every error a treasure: improving medication use with a nonpunitive reporting system. Jt Comm J Qual Patient Saf 2007; 33:401–7.
50. Conway J. Getting boards on board: engaging governing boards in quality and safety. Jt Comm J Qual Patient Saf 2008;34:214–20.
51. Ginsburg LR, Chuang YT, Berta WB, et al. The relationship between organizational leadership for safety and learning from patient safety events. Health Serv Res 2010;45:607–32.
52. Huang DT, Clermont G, Kong L, et al. Intensive care unit safety culture and outcomes: a US multicenter study. Int J Qual Health Care 2010;22:151–61.
53. Hutchinson A, Young TA, Cooper KL, et al. Trends in healthcare incident reporting and relationship to safety and quality data in acute hospitals: results from the National Reporting and Learning System. Qual Saf Health Care 2009;18:5–10.
54. Fiol CM, O'Connor EJ. Waking up! mindfulness in the face of bandwagons. Acad Manage Rev 2003;28(1):54–70.
55. Sexton JB, Thomas EJ, Helmreich RL. Error, stress, and teamwork in medicine and aviation: cross sectional surveys. BMJ 2000;320:745–9.
56. Kuhlthau KA, Bloom S, Van Cleave J, et al. Evidence for family-centered care for children with special health care needs: a systematic review. Acad Pediatr 2011; 11:136–43.
57. Miller MR, Griswold M, Harris JM 2nd, et al. Decreasing PICU catheter-associated bloodstream infections: NACHRI's quality transformation efforts. Pediatrics 2010;125:206–13.
58. Brilli RJ, Sparling KW, Lake MR, et al. The business case for preventing ventilator-associated pneumonia in pediatric intensive care unit patients. Jt Comm J Qual Patient Saf 2008;34:629–38.
59. Abstoss K, Shaw B, Owens T, et al. Increasing medication error reporting rates while reducing harm through simultaneous cultural and system-level interventions in an intensive care unit. BMJ Qual Saf 2011;20:914–22.
60. Sadowski R, Dechert RE, Bandy KP, et al. Continuous quality improvement: reducing unplanned extubations in a pediatric intensive care unit. Pediatrics 2004;114:628–32.
61. How-to guide: sustainability and spread. Cambridge (MA): Institute for Healthcare Improvement; 2011.
62. Improvement leader's guide to sustainability and spread. Cambridge (MA): Institute for Healthcare Improvement; 2011.

# Telemedicine in the Pediatric Intensive Care Unit

James P. Marcin, MD, MPH

## KEYWORDS

- Telemedicine • Telehealth • Tele-ICU • Remote monitoring

## KEY POINTS

- Telehealth technologies can address disparities in care, allowing critical care providers an immediate presence at the bedside of critically ill children in remote locations.
- Telehealth technologies can improve remote diagnostic, therapeutic, and transport decisions among children receiving care in nonpediatric referral centers.
- The use of telehealth technologies has been shown to positively impact intensive care units' quality of care and the cost-effectiveness of care.
- The use of telehealth technologies has the potential to improve the efficiency of pediatric critical care workflows and help address shortages in the workforce.

## INTRODUCTION

In the past 2 decades, it has become increasingly evident that the quality of care provided in the pediatric intensive care unit (ICU) is improved when patients are actively cared for by pediatric critical care physicians. Research has demonstrated in both adult and pediatric ICUs that critically ill patients have a lower risk of death, shorter ICU and hospital length of stay, and receive higher care quality when critical care physicians are involved in their management.[1–5] Specifically, researchers estimate that ICU mortality can be reduced by some 10% to 25% when critical care physicians direct patient care compared with ICUs whereby critical care physicians have little to no involvement in patient care.[1,2,6]

Unfortunately, not all critically ill children are cared for in regionalized pediatric ICUs and they are not uniformly treated by pediatric critical care physicians. This circumstance is in part explained by the fact that regionalization of pediatric ICUs, although increasing quality and efficiencies of care, by its design, also creates disparities in access. Critically ill children from nonurban areas are frequently treated and cared for, by necessity, in hospitals that may lack the full spectrum of pediatric ICU services and/or pediatric critical care expertise.[7,8] Magnifying this problem is the continued

Department of Pediatrics, University of California Davis Children's Hospital, 2516 Stockton Boulevard, Sacramento, CA 95817, USA
E-mail address: jpmarcin@ucdavis.edu

Pediatr Clin N Am 60 (2013) 581–592
http://dx.doi.org/10.1016/j.pcl.2013.02.002
0031-3955/13/$ – see front matter
pediatric.theclinics.com

shortages of critical care physicians, for both adult and pediatric ICUs, which is expected to worsen in future years.[9-11] Combined, regionalization and physician shortages make it difficult to guarantee that all critically ill patients are treated in a timely manner by qualified physicians in an appropriate full-service ICU.

Telemedicine, defined as the provision of health care over a distance using telecommunications technologies, can enable specially trained critical care physicians' participation in the care all of critically ill patients in remote locations while simultaneously maintaining the regionalization of ICU services. This model of care, referred to as Tele-ICU, can be used to more efficiently increase access to specialty care services, including critical care physicians, to patients living in underserved and remote communities and in community hospitals where the full spectrum of ICU and critical care services is not available.[12,13] By importing specialty expertise using telemedicine, emergency departments (EDs), inpatient wards, and nonspecialty ICUs are given the means to increase their capacity to provide higher quality of care to critically ill patients. Critical care physicians can also increase their efficiency with these technologies so that their expertise can be disseminated to more patients at more than one ICU or hospital at a time. The use of telemedicine technologies can also reduce the need to transfer less ill children to referral centers, reserving the limited pediatric ICU beds to those most in need of a regionalized center.[14,15] For these reasons, the use of telemedicine by hospitals and physicians providing critical care services will continue to increase and be individualized to best fit the needs of the patients that they serve.

Although the use of Tele-ICU can help providers of critical care services address disparities in access to care, improve quality of care, and reduce overall health care costs, it will never replace the bedside pediatric critical care physician or eliminate the need to transfer critically ill children to regional pediatric ICUs. Instead, pediatric critical care physicians can use telemedicine and telehealth technologies as a tool to assist in the remote monitoring and treatment of patients where their services may not otherwise be immediately available. Herein, the author reviews how telemedicine can be used by pediatric critical care physicians and pediatric ICUs, focusing particularly on the delivery of care in remote hospital EDs, in critical care transport, in remote hospital inpatient wards, and in remote ICUs where pediatric critical care specialists are not immediately available.

## TELEMEDICINE FOR CRITICALLY ILL CHILDREN IN REMOTE EDS

It is well documented that without pediatric expertise, critically ill children presenting to EDs receive poorer quality of care compared with the care provided in EDs with pediatric expertise.[16-20] These EDs are also, at times, inadequately equipped to care for pediatric emergencies.[16,17,21-24] In addition, the staff working in smaller, general EDs, including physicians, nurses, pharmacists, and support staff, are often less experienced in caring for critically ill children. Combined, the relative lack of equipment, infrastructure and experienced personnel can result in delayed or incorrect diagnoses, suboptimal therapies, and imperfect medical management.[3,18,25,26] As a consequence, acutely ill or injured children receive lower quality of care than children presenting to EDs in regionalized children's hospitals.[18,27-30]

The use of telemedicine technologies for disaster victims[31] or in remote or underserved EDs can be a means of obtaining subspecialty expertise by consultation.[32-38] The benefit of using this technology as opposed to using the telephone (the current standard of care) is that the consultant (ie, the pediatric critical care physician) has the ability to have a virtual presence at the patients' bedside. The consultant has access to high-definition patient views, the treating providers, the family, as well as monitors and equipment. Previous studies have demonstrated that the use of telemedicine in the ED to deliver consultations is similar to in-person consultations when comparing diagnostic accuracy, treatment plans, and plans for disposition.[33,39–42] The use of telemedicine to urgently obtain a consultation from a neurologist in the ED to treat patients with an acute stroke is now common practice.[41–44] Similarly, telemedicine is used to provide emergency medicine consultations to critical access hospitals, which are staffed by physician assistants.[45] Both of these examples have been shown to result in high-quality, cost-effective care.[45–47]

With regard to providing pediatric critical care consultations to remote EDs for critically ill children, there is increasing acceptance and evidence that this model of care can improve the quality of care and increase provider, patient, and parent-guardian satisfaction.[40,48] Two studies have describe how pediatric critical care physicians use telemedicine to provide consultations to critically ill children presenting to rural EDs.[40,48] Heath and colleagues,[40] at the University of Vermont, concluded that the use of telemedicine was associated with improved patient care and was superior to telephone consultations.[49] In another study by Dharmar and colleagues,[48,50] it was shown that patients receiving telemedicine consultations in remote EDs received higher overall care quality when compared with similar patients receiving telephone consultations. Both of these programs also reported that referring ED physicians more frequently changed their diagnosis and/or therapeutic interventions compared with when consultations were provided by telephone. Finally, the use of telemedicine to provide critical care consultations has also been shown to result in significantly higher parent-guardian satisfaction and perceived quality when compared with telephone consultations.[48]

Overall, although more research is needed, there is mounting evidence that pediatric critical care consultations to rural and underserved EDs using telemedicine can be used to help address disparities in access to specialists and, in doing so, improve the overall quality of care. It is also likely that because of better care and the reduction in unnecessary transports, telemedicine consultations to rural and underserved EDs can be provided in a cost-efficient manner that reduces the health care costs that would otherwise be encumbered if telemedicine were not used.

## TELEMEDICINE DURING TRANSPORT OF CRITICALLY ILL PEDIATRIC PATIENTS

The use of telemedicine by physicians to assist in the care of critically ill patients during transport could have the potential to improve processes of care at several levels. For example, telemedicine could allow physicians to be an immediate part of the monitoring, identification, and management of changes in the patients' status that occur during transport. With more immediate physician supervision using telemedicine, medical decisions, including new medication orders, have the potential to occur more rapidly and efficiently than without direct physician supervision.

Currently, mobile telephone technologies are used to transmit 2-way audio as well as data, including electrocardiogram data. However, to create a model of care that uses telemedicine during transport, much more robust, mobile broadband telecommunications are needed. Only a handful of transport programs in the United States use these technologies because high-quality broadband mobile telecommunications is expensive and not always or easily available.[51] This circumstance is particularly true if continuous video transmission or large data streaming is desired. Two common methods of transmitting video include the use of high-fidelity cell-phone service (sometimes combining several cell-phone lines) and the use of the Internet that can be available with citywide Wi-Fi or satellite services.[52,53] Although satellite technologies can be used to provide mobile telemedicine connections, this technology is most often prohibitively expensive.

There have been anecdotal reports documenting the feasibility of cell-phone and Wi-Fi transmitted telemedicine consultations during transport. In one study, the outcomes of simulated adult trauma patients were compared among scenarios that used telemedicine and scenarios that used telephone communications during transport.[54] The researchers found that use of telemedicine resulted in a reduction in adverse clinical events, including fewer episodes of desaturation, hypotension, and less tachycardia compared with identical simulated patients without telemedicine use. In addition, the researchers found that recognition rates for key physiologic signs and the need for critical interventions were higher in the transport simulations that used telemedicine.[54] These data are encouraging and support the possibility that telemedicine can be used during patient transport. However, until more reliable and affordable mobile telecommunications are available to implement telemedicine during transport and more research is conducted on the impact that telemedicine has during transport, the effectiveness and benefit of this technology remain undetermined.

## CRITICAL CARE TELEMEDICINE CONSULTATIONS FOR HOSPITALIZED CHILDREN

Pediatric critical care services are more regionalized and fewer than adult critical care services. As a result, children living in nonurban communities that may need critical care services have to be transferred a sometimes lengthy and risky transport to a pediatric ICU. Often, pediatric patients that are not critically ill are overtriaged and transferred to the regional center because there may be the potential for needing the specialty services provided by the pediatric ICU.[55] This practice is particularly inefficient given the fact that regionalized quaternary pediatric ICUs are frequently running at full capacity. In fact, the transfer of some pediatric patients to a quaternary pediatric referral center is often not necessary if there is a closer hospital with adequate pediatric capabilities, such as a level II or community pediatric ICU, an intermediate or step-down pediatric care unit, or general ICU with pediatric expertise.[56]

Admitting some of the less-ill children to hospitals other than regional, quaternary referral centers can result in high quality of care provided with similar length of stays, less resource use, and lower costs.[57–59] It is, therefore, logical that some mildly or moderately ill children (eg, a child with asthma who requires continuous albuterol or a child with known diabetes and mild diabetic ketoacidosis) can be cared for in a level II or community pediatric ICU or other non–children's hospital's ICU under the care of pediatric nurses and physicians with supervision from a regional children's hospital pediatric critical care team using telemedicine and remote monitoring.

Telemedicine can be used by pediatric critical care clinicians using a broad range of applications to assist in the care of hospitalized children in a variety of clinical scenarios.[60] Physician consultations, nurse and physician monitoring, and medical oversight can range from a simple model of intermittent, need-based consultations (consultative model) to a model that integrates continuous monitoring and proactive medical decision making (continuous care model). In a consultative model, a pediatric critical care physician can provide bedside telemedicine consultations to patients in a remote inpatient ward, high-acuity unit, or ICU. Such consultations could prompt a variety of clinical interventions, including recommendations on diagnostic studies, medications, or other therapies. The consultation may also conclude that the patient should be transported to the regional pediatric ICU. This type of model could result in a range of interventions from a one-time consultation to multiple videoconferencing interactions during the course of the day or hospital stay.[61,62]

In the continuous care model, telemedicine can be used in combination with comprehensive electronic remote monitoring as well as oversight by critical care physicians and nurses. In such a model, a remote team of physicians and nurses are able to monitor many patient beds, sometimes several ICUs. This continuous care model of telemedicine is more proactive with medical interventions and can involve nontelemedicine guidelines, such as the implementation of evidence-based standards. This Tele-ICU model is created by centralizing electronic health records, ICU monitoring technologies and nurse/physician video oversight. Continuous care Tele-ICUs can be created internally by a large health system, or can be contracted out to a third party technology and physician organizations that specialize in remote ICU monitoring services.

## Consultative Model

A pediatric critical care telemedicine program based on the consultative model has been successfully used in caring for mildly to moderately ill children in remote ICUs by several programs.[61] One such model could involve pediatric critical care physicians from a regional pediatric ICU connecting to the bedside for consultations to a referring neonatologist, general pediatrician, adult critical care physician, and/or surgeon caring for an infant, child, or adolescent in a community or combined pediatric-adult ICU. The bedside nurse or physician could initiate a request for consultation either from the regional pediatric critical care nurse or physician. Such a model would also require compliance with critical care best practices and maintenance of pediatric critical care training, advanced life support certifications, and participation in quality-assurance programs.[61,62]

In this model of care, telemedicine consultations from pediatric critical care physicians should be available 24 hours per day, 7 days per week. Consultations should consist of a full history (with referring physician, nurse, and/or parent-guardian) and physical examination, which may require the use of telemedicine peripheral devices (such as a stethoscope, otoscope, ophthalmoscope, and/or general examination camera) or reported physical findings from the bedside clinical staff. The consultation should include the review of pertinent radiographs, medical records, and laboratories. Follow-up consultations can be conducted at the discretion of the consulting critical care physician or as requested by the referring physician or bedside nurse. At any time after the initial or follow-up consultation, patients can be transported to the regional pediatric ICU based on the specialty needs of the patients, the discretion of the referring or consulting physicians with considerations to nurse and physician comfort, and/or parental preference.

Published data from a consultative telemedicine program demonstrates excellent clinical outcomes, including mortality and length of stay, similar to severity-adjusted benchmark data from a set of national pediatric ICUs.[61,62] This program has reported a high degree of satisfaction among remote providers and parents-guardians and has allowed patients to remain in their local community, which lessens the burden of family members. In addition, implementation of this consultative telemedicine model resulted in an overall reduction in health care costs because of more appropriate transport use and the decreased use of the more costly, regional pediatric ICU.[63] This consultative telemedicine model has also been reported by other specialists to provide inpatient consultations, including cardiology consultations and ethics consultations.[64,65]

## Continuous Care Model

When telemedicine is integrated with continuous remote electronic monitoring and electronic health records, the result is a tele-presence ICU system. This model is a more comprehensive and proactive care model that involves around-the-clock monitoring by critical care nurses and physicians. In this model of care, the role of the critical care specialist can range from involvement only during patient emergencies to more active involvement, including ongoing communication with remote providers directing changes in care and therapies. Using this continuous care model, initial research studies comparing preintervention to postintervention outcomes suggested a nonstatistically significant reduction in severity-adjusted ICU mortality, severity-adjusted hospital mortality, incidence of some ICU complications, and decreased ICU length of stay.[66,67] However, the studies found no significant reduction in overall hospital length of stay and were conducted by teams of investigators affiliated with the proprietary remote ICU telemedicine company used in the investigations.

There have been several subsequent studies evaluating the impact of the continuous care Tele-ICU model in a variety of adult ICU settings. In a large study conducted at 6 ICUs in a large US health care system, a similar preintervention versus postintervention study found that the implementation of an integrated telemedicine and remote monitoring program did not have a large impact on evaluated care.[68] This study reported no difference in ICU mortality, hospital mortality, ICU length of stay, or hospital length of stay. However, the researchers found that among the subset of patients with higher involvement of remote telemedicine providers, outcomes, including survival, were improved.[68] Using the data from this study, another group of investigators researched the costs and cost-effectiveness of the tele-ICU program.[69] They found that the daily average ICU and hospital costs after the implementation of the program increased by 28% and 34%, respectively. The investigators concluded that the cost-effectiveness of the continuous care program was limited to the most severely ill patients.[69]

Several more recent studies in smaller hospital settings found conflicting results.[70–72] In one report whereby the Tele-ICU was used to monitor 4 ICUs in 2 community hospitals, investigators found no reduction in ICU mortality, hospital mortality, ICU length of stay, or hospital length of stay.[72] In the same year, in a similarly designed study of a single academic community hospital, the continuous remote oversight ICU telemedicine model resulted in a statistically significant reduction in mortality from 21.4% at baseline to 14.7%. These investigators also found a significant reduction in ICU length of stay from 4.06 days at baseline to 3.77 days, which remained significant even after adjustment for case mix and severity of illness.[71]

In one of the largest studies to date, researchers evaluated 7 adult ICUs on 2 campuses of a single academic medical center where a similar continuous care telemedicine program was implemented. These researchers found that the Tele-ICU program was associated with significant improvements in several clinical outcomes.[73] The adherence to critical care best practices, including guidelines for the prevention of deep vein thrombosis, stress ulcers, ventilator-associated pneumonia, catheter-related bloodstream infections, and guidelines for cardiovascular protection, all significantly improved. In addition, there was a relative reduction in unadjusted and risk-adjusted ICU mortality by 13% and 20%, respectively. Further, both risk-adjusted hospital mortality ICU and hospital length of stay were significantly decreased.[73,74]

There have been at least 2 meta-analyses that have combined published data evaluating ICU telemedicine impact on patient outcomes. In one meta-analysis, researchers found that among 13 eligible studies involving 35 ICUs, there was a significant reduction in ICU mortality (pooled odds ratio, 0.80) but found no impact on in-hospital mortality for patients admitted to the ICU.[75] They also found that remote ICU telemedicine coverage was associated with a reduction in ICU length of stay by

1.3 days but found no statistically significant reduction in hospital length of stay.[75] In another, researchers reviewed 11 eligible studies and found that the continuous care telemedicine model resulted in statistically significant reductions in ICU and hospital mortality (pooled risk ratio, 0.79 and 0.89, respectively) as well as ICU and hospital length of stay.[76] All studies included in both of these meta-analyses were combined assessments that compared pretelemedicine outcomes to post-telemedicine outcomes, which are subject to significant bias. As demonstrated by the fact that inconsistent conclusions were made by 2 different meta-analyses that analyzed virtually identical data, there is the real need to conduct more rigorous studies whereby timelines are concurrent and/or patients and ICUs are randomized as part of a larger trial.[77,78]

The reasons why some continuous care telemedicine programs have resulted in significantly improved outcomes and others have not is likely multifactorial and related to how the programs were implemented and supported. In general, when ICUs experienced improvements in clinical outcomes, the centralized monitoring critical care teams seemed to work more proactively and were involved in the care of a greater proportion of patients. On the other hand, when ICUs did not experience improvements in clinical outcomes, the ICUs often limited the participation of the centralized monitoring critical care teams. In addition, some studies that did not find improvements in clinical outcomes often did not simultaneously implement clinical improvement programs. In other words, the degree of benefit seems to be related to the extent to which the telemedicine, remote monitoring, and collaboration between the monitoring and monitored teams are mutually embraced and whether the program is supported as a means of creating sustainable improvements in ICU care.[73,79,80]

Collectively, the studies suggest that the utility of a care model that uses telemedicine to assist in the treatment of infants and children hospitalized in remote hospitals or ICUs is promising but remains controversial because of a lack of evidence. It is known that telemedicine technologies, in and of itself, will not result in improved care. Rather, telemedicine is a technological tool that can enable providers to provide better care. Telemedicine needs to be thoughtfully integrated into partnering institutions in a well-defined and collaborative effort; in these cases, it can result in improvements in access and quality for mildly or moderately ill children.[81,82] Similar to other quality improvement efforts, for the success of a telemedicine partnership, there must be firm support from administrators, physicians, nurses, and other clinical providers on both sides of telemedicine.

## THE FUTURE OF TELEMEDICINE IN THE PEDIATRIC ICU

It is very likely that the use of telemedicine in pediatric critical care and in the pediatric ICU will increase. Telehealth technologies can allow specialists, including pediatric critical care physicians, to extend their expertise more quickly and easily to locations in need of their service more than ever before. The potential advantages are numerous and include improved access, improved efficiencies, improved quality, and more cost-effective care. All of these work to the advantage of our patients, our patients' families, remote clinicians, and regional health care systems.

In addition, telemedicine connections between remote hospitals and regionalized pediatric ICUs can be enhanced because pediatric critical care physicians can better educate remote providers in the care of critically ill children. Telemedicine technologies will become more integrated into our practice of medicine, similar to computerized physician order entry and the electronic health record. Different models of care will require different technologies depending on the needs of the patients, the remote hospitals, and the regional pediatric ICUs. More data will help us determine where, when, and for whom the telemedicine technologies are most clinically and economically effective.

## REFERENCES

1. Pronovost PJ, Angus DC, Dorman T, et al. Physician staffing patterns and clinical outcomes in critically ill patients: a systematic review. JAMA 2002;288(17):2151–62.
2. Blunt MC, Burchett KR. Out-of-hours consultant cover and case-mix-adjusted mortality in intensive care. Lancet 2000;356(9231):735–6.
3. Pollack MM, Alexander SR, Clarke N, et al. Improved outcomes from tertiary center pediatric intensive care: a statewide comparison of tertiary and nontertiary care facilities. Crit Care Med 1991;19(2):150–9.
4. Pollack MM, Cuerdon TT, Patel KM, et al. Impact of quality-of-care factors on pediatric intensive care unit mortality. JAMA 1994;272(12):941–6.
5. Goh AY, Lum LC, Abdel-Latif ME. Impact of 24 hour critical care physician staffing on case-mix adjusted mortality in paediatric intensive care. Lancet 2001;357(9254):445–6.
6. Wallace DJ, Angus DC, Barnato AE, et al. Nighttime intensivist staffing and mortality among critically ill patients. N Engl J Med 2012;366(22):2093–101.
7. Odetola FO, Miller WC, Davis MM, et al. The relationship between the location of pediatric intensive care unit facilities and child death from trauma: a county-level ecologic study. J Pediatr 2005;147(1):74–7.
8. Kanter RK. Regional variation in child mortality at hospitals lacking a pediatric intensive care unit. Crit Care Med 2002;30(1):94–9.
9. Angus DC, Kelley MA, Schmitz RJ, et al. Caring for the critically ill patient. Current and projected workforce requirements for care of the critically ill and patients with pulmonary disease: can we meet the requirements of an aging population? JAMA 2000;284(21):2762–70.
10. American Academy of Pediatrics Committee on Pediatric Workforce. Pediatrician workforce statement. Pediatrics 2005;116(1):263–9.
11. Kelley MA, Angus D, Chalfin DB, et al. The critical care crisis in the United States: a report from the profession. Chest 2004;125(4):1514–7.
12. Marcin J, Ellis J, Mawis R, et al. Telemedicine and the medical home: providing pediatric subspecialty care to children with special health care needs in an underserved rural community. Pediatrics 2004;113(1):1–6.
13. Marcin JP, Ellis J, Mawis R, et al. Using telemedicine to provide pediatric subspecialty care to children with special health care needs in an underserved rural community. Pediatrics 2004;113(1 Pt 1):1–6.
14. Haskins PA, Ellis DG, Mayrose J. Predicted utilization of emergency medical services telemedicine in decreasing ambulance transports. Prehosp Emerg Care 2002;6(4):445–8.
15. Tsai SH, Kraus J, Wu HR, et al. The effectiveness of video-telemedicine for screening of patients requesting emergency air medical transport (EAMT). J Trauma 2007;62(2):504–11.
16. Athey J, Dean JM, Ball J, et al. Ability of hospitals to care for pediatric emergency patients. Pediatr Emerg Care 2001;17(3):170–4.
17. McGillivray D, Nijssen-Jordan C, Kramer MS, et al. Critical pediatric equipment availability in Canadian hospital emergency departments. Ann Emerg Med 2001;37(4):371–6.

18. Dharmar M, Marcin JP, Romano PS, et al. Quality of care of children in the emergency department: association with hospital setting and physician training. J Pediatr 2008;153:783–9.
19. Bowman SM, Zimmerman FJ, Christakis DA, et al. Hospital characteristics associated with the management of pediatric splenic injuries. JAMA 2005;294(20):2611–7.
20. Li J, Monuteaux MC, Bachur RG. Interfacility transfers of noncritically ill children to academic pediatric emergency departments. Pediatrics 2012;130(1):83–92.
21. Middleton KR, Burt CW. Availability of pediatric services and equipment in emergency departments: United States, 2002-03. Adv Data 2006;(367):1–16.
22. Gausche-Hill M, Schmitz C, Lewis RJ. Pediatric preparedness of US emergency departments: a 2003 survey. Pediatrics 2007;120(6):1229–37.
23. Bourgeois FT, Shannon MW. Emergency care for children in pediatric and general emergency departments. Pediatr Emerg Care 2007;23(2):94–102.
24. Burt CW, Middleton KR. Factors associated with ability to treat pediatric emergencies in US hospitals. Pediatr Emerg Care 2007;23(10):681–9.
25. Tilford JM, Roberson PK, Lensing S, et al. Improvement in pediatric critical care outcomes. Crit Care Med 2000;28(2):601–3.
26. Keeler EB, Rubenstein LV, Kahn KL, et al. Hospital characteristics and quality of care. JAMA 1992;268(13):1709–14.
27. Seidel JS, Henderson DP, Ward P, et al. Pediatric prehospital care in urban and rural areas. Pediatrics 1991;88(4):681–90.
28. Seidel JS, Hornbein M, Yoshiyama K, et al. Emergency medical services and the pediatric patient: are the needs being met? Pediatrics 1984;73(6):769–72.
29. Durch J, Lohr KN, Institute of Medicine (U.S.), Committee on Pediatric Emergency Medical Services. Emergency medical services for children. Washington, DC: National Academy Press; 1993.
30. Durch JS, Lohr KN. From the Institute of Medicine. JAMA 1993;270(8):929.
31. Burke RV, Berg BM, Vee P, et al. Using robotic telecommunications to triage pediatric disaster victims. J Pediatr Surg 2012;47(1):221–4.
32. Lambrecht CJ. Emergency physicians' roles in a clinical telemedicine network. Ann Emerg Med 1997;30(5):670–4.
33. Brennan JA, Kealy JA, Gerardi LH, et al. Telemedicine in the emergency department: a randomized controlled trial. J Telemed Telecare 1999;5(1):18–22.
34. Brennan JA, Kealy JA, Gerardi LH, et al. A randomized controlled trial of telemedicine in an emergency department. J Telemed Telecare 1998;4(Suppl 1):18–20.
35. Stamford P, Bickford T, Hsiao H, et al. The significance of telemedicine in a rural emergency department. IEEE Eng Med Biol Mag 1999;18(4):45–52.
36. Rogers FB, Ricci M, Caputo M, et al. The use of telemedicine for real-time video consultation between trauma center and community hospital in a rural setting improves early trauma care: preliminary results. J Trauma 2001;51(6):1037–41.
37. Latifi R, Hadeed GJ, Rhee P, et al. Initial experiences and outcomes of telepresence in the management of trauma and emergency surgical patients. Am J Surg 2009;198(6):905–10.
38. Hicks LL, Boles KE, Hudson ST, et al. Using telemedicine to avoid transfer of rural emergency department patients. J Rural Health 2001;17(3):220–8.
39. Kofos D, Pitetti R, Orr R, et al. Telemedicine in pediatric transport: a feasibility study. Pediatrics 1998;102(5):E58.
40. Heath B, Salerno R, Hopkins A, et al. Pediatric critical care telemedicine in rural underserved emergency departments. Pediatr Crit Care Med 2009;10:588–91.

41. Meyer BC, Raman R, Hemmen T, et al. Efficacy of site-independent telemedicine in the STRokE DOC trial: a randomised, blinded, prospective study. Lancet Neurol 2008;7(9):787–95.
42. Demaerschalk BM, Raman R, Ernstrom K, et al. Efficacy of telemedicine for stroke: pooled analysis of the Stroke Team Remote Evaluation Using a Digital Observation Camera (STRokE DOC) and STRokE DOC Arizona telestroke trials. Telemed J E Health 2012;18(3):230–7.
43. Emsley H, Blacker K, Davies P, et al. Telestroke. When location, location, location doesn't matter. Health Serv J 2010;120(6227):24–5.
44. Pervez MA, Silva G, Masrur S, et al. Remote supervision of IV-tPA for acute ischemic stroke by telemedicine or telephone before transfer to a regional stroke center is feasible and safe. Stroke 2010;41(1):e18–24.
45. Galli R, Keith JC, McKenzie K, et al. TelEmergency: a novel system for delivering emergency care to rural hospitals. Ann Emerg Med 2008;51(3):275–84.
46. Henderson K. TelEmergency: distance emergency care in rural emergency departments using nurse practitioners. J Emerg Nurs 2006;32(5):388–93.
47. Nelson RE, Saltzman GM, Skalabrin EJ, et al. The cost-effectiveness of telestroke in the treatment of acute ischemic stroke. Neurology 2011;77(17):1590–8.
48. Dharmar M, Romano PS, Kuppermann N, et al. Impact of pediatric telemedicine consultations on critically ill children in rural emergency departments. Crit Care Med, in press.
49. Dharmar M, Marcin JP. A picture is worth a thousand words: critical care consultations to emergency departments using telemedicine. Pediatr Crit Care Med 2009;10(5):606–7.
50. Dharmar M, Marcin JP, Kuppermann N, et al. A new implicit review instrument for measuring quality of care delivered to pediatric patients in the emergency department. BMC Emerg Med 2007;7:13.
51. Liman TG, Winter B, Waldschmidt C, et al. Telestroke ambulances in prehospital stroke management: concept and pilot feasibility study. Stroke 2012;43(8):2086–90.
52. Qureshi A, Shih E, Fan I, et al. Improving patient care by unshackling telemedicine: adaptively aggregating wireless networks to facilitate continuous collaboration. AMIA Annu Symp Proc 2010;2010:662–6.
53. Hsieh JC, Lin BX, Wu FR, et al. Ambulance 12-lead electrocardiography transmission via cell phone technology to cardiologists. Telemed J E Health 2010;16(8):910–5.
54. Charash WE, Caputo MP, Clark H, et al. Telemedicine to a moving ambulance improves outcome after trauma in simulated patients. J Trauma 2011;71(1):49–55.
55. Wakefield DS, Ward M, Miller T, et al. Intensive care unit utilization and interhospital transfers as potential indicators of rural hospital quality. J Rural Health 2004;20(4):394–400.
56. Rosenberg DI, Moss MM. Guidelines and levels of care for pediatric intensive care units. Crit Care Med 2004;32(10):2117–27.
57. Merenstein D, Egleston B, Diener-West M. Lengths of stay and costs associated with children's hospitals. Pediatrics 2005;115(4):839–44.
58. Odetola FO, Gebremariam A, Freed GL. Patient and hospital correlates of clinical outcomes and resource utilization in severe pediatric sepsis. Pediatrics 2007;119(3):487–94.
59. Gupta RS, Bewtra M, Prosser LA, et al. Predictors of hospital charges for children admitted with asthma. Ambul Pediatr 2006;6(1):15–20.

60. Dharmar M, Smith AC, Armfield NR, et al. Telemedicine for children in need of intensive care. Pediatr Ann 2009;38(10):562–6.
61. Marcin JP, Nesbitt TS, Kallas HJ, et al. Use of telemedicine to provide pediatric critical care inpatient consultations to underserved rural Northern California. J Pediatr 2004;144(3):375–80.
62. Marcin JP, Schepps DE, Page KA, et al. The use of telemedicine to provide pediatric critical care consultations to pediatric trauma patients admitted to a remote trauma intensive care unit: a preliminary report. Pediatr Crit Care Med 2004;5(3):251–6.
63. Marcin JP, Nesbitt TS, Struve S, et al. Financial benefits of a pediatric intensive care unit-based telemedicine program to a rural adult intensive care unit: impact of keeping acutely ill and injured children in their local community. Telemed J E Health 2004;10:1–5.
64. Huang T, Moon-Grady AJ, Traugott C, et al. The availability of telecardiology consultations and transfer patterns from a remote neonatal intensive care unit. J Telemed Telecare 2008;14(5):244–8.
65. Kon AA, Rich B, Sadorra C, et al. Complex bioethics consultation in rural hospitals: using telemedicine to bring academic bioethicists into outlying communities. J Telemed Telecare 2009;15(5):264–7.
66. Rosenfeld BA, Dorman T, Breslow MJ, et al. Intensive care unit telemedicine: alternate paradigm for providing continuous intensivist care. Crit Care Med 2000;28(12):3925–31.
67. Breslow MJ, Rosenfeld BA, Doerfler M, et al. Effect of a multiple-site intensive care unit telemedicine program on clinical and economic outcomes: an alternative paradigm for intensivist staffing. Crit Care Med 2004;32(1):31–8.
68. Thomas EJ, Lucke JF, Wueste L, et al. Association of telemedicine for remote monitoring of intensive care patients with mortality, complications, and length of stay. JAMA 2009;302(24):2671–8.
69. Franzini L, Sail KR, Thomas EJ, et al. Costs and cost-effectiveness of a telemedicine intensive care unit program in 6 intensive care units in a large health care system. J Crit Care 2011;26(3):329.e1–6.
70. Kohl BA, Fortino-Mullen M, Praestgaard A, et al. The effect of ICU telemedicine on mortality and length of stay. J Telemed Telecare 2012;18(5):282–6.
71. McCambridge M, Jones K, Paxton H, et al. Association of health information technology and teleintensivist coverage with decreased mortality and ventilator use in critically ill patients. Arch Intern Med 2010;170(7):648–53.
72. Morrison JL, Cai Q, Davis N, et al. Clinical and economic outcomes of the electronic intensive care unit: results from two community hospitals. Crit Care Med 2010;38(1):2–8.
73. Lilly CM, Cody S, Zhao H, et al. Hospital mortality, length of stay, and preventable complications among critically ill patients before and after tele-ICU reengineering of critical care processes. JAMA 2011;305(21):2175–83.
74. Kahn JM. The use and misuse of ICU telemedicine. JAMA 2011;305(21):2227–8.
75. Young LB, Chan PS, Lu X, et al. Impact of telemedicine intensive care unit coverage on patient outcomes: a systematic review and meta-analysis. Arch Intern Med 2011;171(6):498–506.
76. Wilcox ME, Adhikari NK. The effect of telemedicine in critically ill patients: systematic review and meta-analysis. Crit Care 2012;16(4):R127.
77. Smith AC, Armfield NR. A systematic review and meta-analysis of ICU telemedicine reinforces the need for further controlled investigations to assess the impact of telemedicine on patient outcomes. Evid Based Nurs 2011;14:102–3.

78. Kahn JM. Intensive care unit telemedicine: promises and pitfalls. Arch Intern Med 2011;171(6):495–6.

79. Rogove HJ, McArthur D, Demaerschalk BM, et al. Barriers to telemedicine: survey of current users in acute care units. Telemed J E Health 2012;18(1):48–53.

80. Boots RJ, Singh S, Terblanche M, et al. Remote care by telemedicine in the ICU: many models of care can be effective. Curr Opin Crit Care 2011;17(6):634–40.

81. Reynolds HN, Bander J, McCarthy M. Different systems and formats for tele-ICU coverage: designing a tele-ICU system to optimize functionality and investment. Crit Care Nurs Q 2012;35(4):364–77.

82. Rogove H. How to develop a tele-ICU model? Crit Care Nurs Q 2012;35(4): 357–63.

# The Pediatric Intensive Care Unit Business Model

Charles L. Schleien, MD, MBA

## KEYWORDS

- Pediatric intensive care unit • Business model • Relative value unit • Revenue
- Full time eqivalent (FTE) • Medical services agreement (MSA) • Clinical productivity

## KEY POINTS

- Most pediatric intensive care units (PICUs) have a limited number of revenue sources that should be maximize.
- There are various financial models or types of PICUs in existence ranging from smaller to larger and non-academic to academic.
- Other revenue sources include medical service agreements for clinical or administrative services in other ICUs.
- The use of relative value units to assess physician productivity has become a widespread practice, and understanding it conceptually is a necessity for all practicing ICU physicians.
- The use of more granular productivity data has been shown to improve critical care clinical revenue.

## INTRODUCTION

Like the sub-division of any large business entity, typically each intensive care unit (ICU) must stand alone and exhibit solvency from quarter to quarter and year to year. Rare is an organization like Apple Inc, whereby divisions are not stand-alone business entities and the whole organization's or corporate entity's bottom line is the only important metric. Like the hospital industry, Steve Jobs recognized that at times, when certain product lines or divisions were strengthened, other divisions or products might be weakened by cannibalization. As long as the aggregate bottom line was improved, he thought that this is what gave heft to the company as a whole and made the development and rollout of a new product a worthwhile endeavor.[1] Unfortunately for most of us in the pediatric ICU (PICU), we need to show a healthy bottom line independent of the performance of other divisions within the department or hospital. The concept that decisions that may further the cause of the hospital as a whole (financial or otherwise) but may hurt the division specifically are okay is not necessarily acceptable within the specific hospital system. Thus, understanding the components of the bottom line for the professional side of the PICU and taking the

Department of Pediatrics, North Shore-LIJ Health System, Hofstra School of Medicine, New Hyde Park, NY 11040, USA
E-mail address: cschleien@nshs.edu

Pediatr Clin N Am 60 (2013) 593–604
http://dx.doi.org/10.1016/j.pcl.2013.02.003
0031-3955/13/$ – see front matter © 2013 Elsevier Inc. All rights reserved.

mystery out of these finances is critical to maintaining economic health. In this article, the author discusses ways to enhance revenue, decrease costs, and improve the bottom line. The relationship between the hospital's support of the PICU and the overall profit and loss statement is discussed because it is an important feature. The hospital financial executives need to be or remain convinced that the division needs support when necessary to enhance its bottom line and keep it solvent to support good personnel at competitive salaries. Although not serving as a complete treatise on every possible source of revenue enhancement or cost savings, the author concentrates on topical issues that do enhance the bottom line and are what hospital executives are concentrating on in this era of financial duress. The author also discusses some of the current trends in the hospital business related to changes at the federal level as well as the push for capitation, bundling, enhanced productivity, and other issues.

## BASIC SOURCES AND USES

Most PICUs have a limited number of revenue sources. These sources include mostly clinically produced revenue and revenue derived from contracts or medical service agreements for critical care physicians to perform either clinical or administrative services outside the home institution. The services include the coverage of other ICUs and other services both inside and outside the main hospital or hospital system (see later discussion). Other sources of revenue include grants and direct hospital support. It is clear that in most cases clinical revenue does not cover all of the costs associated with running an academic, large pediatric critical care division with high overhead expenses. These expenses are caused by generous fringe benefit packages, high billing costs, rent, depreciation of expensive new buildings, other capital expenditures for advanced technology, as well as general taxes to deans, chairs, practice organizations, and others that typically outstrip all revenue sources. This level of overhead does not exist at the same level in the private sector or with smaller nonacademic critical care divisions (**Box 1**). Additionally, there remains misalignment between the PICU division and the hospital entity in areas of revenue generation. For example, hospitals in an attempt to decrease costs with a diagnosis-related group (DRG)–based payment system are incentivized to not only discharge patients from the hospital in as short a time frame possible but also to move patients out of the higher-priced ICU environment into a lower-cost floor setting. With an ongoing

---

**Box 1**
**PICU overhead**

Physician salary

Fringe benefit

Malpractice insurance

Space rent

Administrative salaries

Ancillary medical personnel (eg, nurse practitioner, hospitalists)

Billing

Capital expense: equipment

Taxes: dean, chair, practice organization

fee-for-service model still in place in most localities in the United States, the intensivist group remains intent on keeping the unit full while being paid a per diem rate for professional care. The irony, of course, is that as intensivists we are fully invested in supporting hospital priorities, such as shorter lengths of stay and efficient throughput. As discussed later, this fee-for-service model will most likely fade away over the coming years but remains the present reality.

## Types of Units

As mentioned earlier, there are various financial models or types of PICUs in existence. Understanding that any scheme to represent these types of models is an oversimplification, it does help to understand the various incentives and factors that affect the bottom line both positively and negatively. For example, larger, academically based ICUs are driven by the number of beds with a high acuity basis of payment for hospital entities. Professional fees as charged by physician groups are largely driven by the number of beds and the right mix between those beds and the number of ICU attendings. However, in these large ICU settings, there is generally a high volume of patients with government-based (low revenue producing) insurance (ie, a large Medicaid population). Although Medicaid revenue may increase modestly in an Affordable Care Act system matching Medicare rates, these fees remain modest.[2] These units also have other high-cost features, including the large number of trainees, such as critical care fellows being paid at a high resident level who do not have the ability to generate an invoice and collect revenue. A busy PICU with 9 attendings, for example, will typically cost the division over $3 million in salary, fringe benefits, travel, books and dues, administrative graduate medical education support, and other fixed costs (assistants, rent, and so forth). Because of the busy and acute nature of these units, many divisions also have a collection of nurse practitioners and/or hospitalists to supplement resident-level duties. In most cases, these individuals do not bill but work under the attending intensivist, which adds to the expense line without additional accrued revenue. Typically, in larger institutions, nurse practitioners do not work independently, as they more typically do in smaller nonacademic ICU settings. In these larger academic ICUs, as in every other academic department, nonclinical time is often mandated for faculty and often not supplemented by dollars to offset the time taken away from clinical duties. Sources of these dollars could include both federal- and industry-derived clinical research support or financial resources given to faculty for serving other duties within the hospital or medical school. These duties might include time for teaching, covering other services (eg, step-down, emergency department), sedation, or other clinical services. Unfortunately, as we know too well, many of these services, when delivered within a large academically oriented hospital, go unfunded or only partially funded, leaving a bottom-line loss for the division. It is a rare occurrence when research or teaching medical students, residents, or fellows does not generate a loss, even if partially funded by outside sources. As discussed earlier, there are several other overhead items adding to a negative bottom line, including billing costs, rent, and other administrative issues.

Alternatively, the smaller, less academic ICU has several items that add positively (or at least not as negatively) to the financial bottom line. These issues include a lower administrative overhead with fewer administrative assistants, lower billing costs, and smaller offices associated with lower rent. Generally, the clinical work is done with more bed coverage per attending (lower aggregate salary and fringe overhead), with many fewer other clinical personnel (eg, fellows). There is also less research and teaching time, thus fewer unfunded mandates. Of course, the number of beds could be a limitation in these settings, especially when the number of beds is so few that the financial infrastructure cannot support multiple attendings. Thus, the model of small versus large and academic versus nonacademic, although frequently not a pure model, does allow for conceptualizing the issues in managing an ICU from a financial perspective (**Box 2**).

As a consequence, revenue generation depends on several factors. Clinical revenue is generated by billing professional fees. Using the *International Classification of Diseases, Ninth Revision* coding for diagnoses in the ICU is the basic building block of the hospital bill, which is now basically linked to the all patient refined (APR)-DRG system.[3,4] Hospital systems that want to enhance ICU revenue (and any other service for that matter) sometimes use coders that assist physicians, so that the most complex and highest acuity coding could be used, resulting in maximizing revenue.[5] The physician generates a current procedural terminology (CPT) code, which is linked to a relative value unit (RVU). For a full description of CPT coding, see the work by Ackerman and Harrison.[6] The use of RVUs to incentivize physicians in the ICU and to benchmark productivity is discussed later.

### Other Revenue Sources

Other revenue sources include medical service agreements for clinical or administrative services in other ICUs. These contracts are generally negotiated by the physician group itself or by their practice organization. In negotiating the price of the service, it is prudent to include not only the proper clinical coverage and fringe benefits prorated for the portion of the coverage for the individual practitioner but also other overhead, including the cost of billing (if it is being performed), a prorated share of malpractice costs and administrative costs at the home institution, travel and parking, and other expenses. Additionally, it is also typical to build in profit to the contract in the same way that any service builds profit into the price of the service. This profit can range from 5% to 50%.

---

**Box 2**
**Large versus small PICU**

*Large units/academic*

Large number of beds: increase revenue

Higher acuity: increase revenue

Poor payer mix: decrease revenue

More trainees: increase expense

Research time: increase expense

Ancillary health care workers: increase expense

Overhead higher: increase expense

Taxes: increase expense

Office space plentiful: increase expense

*Smaller units/nonacademic*

Smaller number of beds: decrease revenue

Low overhead: decrease expense

No academic taxes: decrease expense

Smaller space: decrease expense

Other sources of revenue for clinical services, as mentioned earlier, include in-hospital services, such as coverage of step-down units, hospitalist services for floor coverage, and sedation services (eg, magnetic resonance imaging, peripherally inserted central catheter lines, and biopsies). Other types of services that some hospitals are willing to build into the pay structure of physician leadership includes administrative oversight of the unit or pediatric service and quality officers overseeing both quality improvement and patient safety. Sometimes it is easier to be paid for teaching responsibilities in outside institutions than for any teaching efforts within one's own institution. Grants and royalties are particularly desirable in terms of defraying the costs of research. Each institution has its own set of rules for indirect costs of the grant. The National Institutes of Health and other federal agencies carry a large indirect cost rate of 50% to 80%.[6] Whether the investigator or the division may receive a portion of these indirect costs is specific to the particular organization. So, for example, some organizations return a large proportion of indirect costs to the investigator, division, or department; however, in those cases, the individual or division is then responsible for paying the high overhead costs for performing that research (eg, rent). In these situations, it is prudent for the investigator/division to be frugal with its use of space, hiring of administrators, and other expense issues. Those investigators who learn how to scavenge equipment and supplies often do well in maintaining a healthy budget. There are several granting agencies that should be considered for pediatric critical care clinical trials research, such as the American Heart Association, American Lung Association, March of Dimes, and many others. Also, it is hoped that the number of private companies in the pharmaceutical and device space that may be willing to fund clinical trials at a time when federal funding is lagging will increase.[7]

Two other major sources of revenue include gifts and hospital support. Hiring a gifts officer to help deal with philanthropy can be money wisely spent, if the development officer and the attending staff are on the same page and aligned in dealing with large gifts from grateful patients. ICUs are notorious for not being able to attract large gifts because of the overlapping nature of subspecialty care in the unit. Often, a grateful patient will be philanthropic toward the primary subspecialist (eg, oncologist, cardiologist), without giving directly to the ICU group. Clearly, a development officer that is aligned to the needs and strengths of the ICU group in terms of capital (eg, high-technology equipment) and scholarly needs can overcome this barrier.

Hospital support is another potential and major source of funding for the critical care division. Even though professional fees can be modest, especially when government insurance is used, downstream revenue to the hospital often represents the profit center for the organization. When the ICU helps support well-reimbursed surgical cases, most of that revenue goes to the hospital. This support of patients, who generate large amounts of downstream revenue, makes a solid discussion point with hospital executives, helping to defray losses on the part of the critical care division. Other groups have worked out the marginal cost for each attending and applied a fixed subsidy from hospital to division for each new attending hired. For a large group of intensivists, this support could amount to more than a million dollars of financial support. The home institution may also be willing to support other services not already mentioned, including transport oversight, quality, and clinical coverage of other areas in the hospital. Other duties that can be performed for the hospital that are typically nonreimbursable but that could be subsidized include residency and fellowship directorship and teaching duties, such as directing a simulation center, which is a growing area in many hospitals.

## PHYSICIAN PRODUCTIVITY

The use of RVUs to assess physician productivity has become a widespread practice, and understanding it conceptually is a necessity for all practicing ICU physicians. Using the Faculty Practice Solutions Center (FPSC) of UHC or any system that easily evaluates and benchmarks RVUs can deliver to hospitals, divisions, and even individual practitioners data that reflect their clinical effort relative to others practicing in that specialty. Work RVUs are calculated for a given time period. An imputed clinical full-time equivalent (CFTE) is then calculated by dividing the work RVUs by a benchmark (all annualized).

Imputed CFTE = work RVU/benchmark

So, for example (See **Table 1**, doctor [Dr] 1), an intensivist with 9233 RVUs and using a benchmark of 8207 would have an imputed CFTE of 9233/8207 equaling 1.12.

The next step in calculating productivity, and often the most difficult, is determining a reported CFTE. This calculation takes into account all other (nonclinical) activities for the specific individual practitioner. Fractions of time are subtracted from 1.0 for time spent in other major activities. So, for example, if you have 20% of your time funded by research, you would subtract 0.2 from 1.0. Other time that could be considered includes major administrative duties, such as division director or business director; fellowship director; or chairs of major committees, such as the Institutional Review Board or quality and safety officer. The last step in the calculation is to divide the imputed CFTE (previously calculated) by the reported CFTE to determine the RVUs imputed/reported ratio.

RVUs imputed/reported ratio = imputed CFTE/reported CFTE

Thus, for an individual with an imputed CFTE of 1.12 (see previous example) and 25% of their time serving as the quality officer, we would divide 1.12 by 0.75, resulting in an imputed/reported ratio of 149%. Ratios greater than 100% typically represent high-productivity physicians; lower numbers (those less than 100%) represent lower productivity. In looking, then, at **Table 1**, the first example (Dr 1) represents a physician with high productivity. In the second example (Dr 2), the individual physician has a modest number of RVUs generated and, with almost the same reported CFTE, a much lower imputed/reported ratio of 43%. In the third example (Dr 3), although the number of RVUs generated is also quite low, because the individual has a much lower reported CFTE (because of their many major administrative positions

**Table 1**
Assessing clinical productivity using work RVUs

|       | Work RVUs | Benchmark | Imputed CFTE | Reported CFTE | Imputed/Reported (%) |
|-------|-----------|-----------|--------------|---------------|----------------------|
| Dr 1  | 9233      | 8207      | 1.12         | 0.88          | 127                  |
| Dr 2  | 2929      | 8207      | 0.36         | 0.84          | 43                   |
| Dr 3  | 3164      | 8207      | 0.39         | 0.50          | 78                   |
| Dr 4  | 1200      | 8207      | 0.15         | 0.10          | 146                  |

The 4 examples of Dr 1, 2, 3, and 4 used in the text are shown along the right border.
*Abbreviation:* Dr, doctor.
*Data from* Faculty Practice Solutions Center, UHC; As presented to the CHCA CMO forum on Oct 28, 2011 and SCCM annual meeting 2012 by Dr Schleien.

and grant funding), the imputed/reported ratio is higher than in example 2, equaling 78%. In the fourth example (Dr 4), the physician has few RVUs but also a very low reported CFTE because of robust grant funding and a major administrative position running the neuroscience research center, so that the imputed/reported ratio equals 146%.

It is important to perform both internal and national comparisons because of the idiosyncratic nature of the specific division and specific hospital. For example, if nurse practitioners are working alongside physicians and billing on their own, then physician productivity by the RVU calculation might be falsely depressed, even though oversight for those patients might still fall under the auspices of the intensivist. However, in the situation whereby the nurse practitioner is working with the intensivist billing under the physician's name, then productivity might be falsely elevated. Other specific situations might account for differences among a specific group. The expectations for the number of shifts or weeks per year that a critical care physician covers the ICU vary widely from group to group. This variation leads to differences in the definition of 1.0 CFTE because groups might consider a range of anywhere from 12 to 25 weeks or more as an FTE. For this reason, internal benchmarking with intragroup physician comparisons is also critical.

The author's institution has compared the RVU imputed/reported ratio between divisions in a pediatrics department, which has allowed them to concentrate specifically and direct resources regarding productivity in certain divisions (**Fig. 1**). Of course, differences in style of practice will make comparisons difficult at times; but generally, this has been a valuable tool to enable them to concentrate resources where they are needed. At a more granular level, they have also built a framework for assessing clinical activity where the RVU imputed/reported ratio of CFTEs is also compared with the dollars imputed/reported CFTE. The dollar ratio is calculated as actual collections divided by target collections per CFTE.

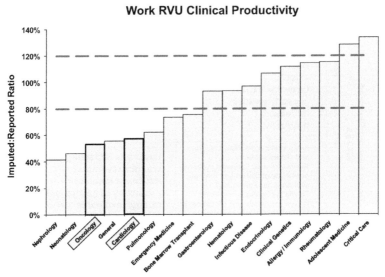

**Fig. 1.** Imputed/reported ratio of RVU on y-axis; various divisions on x-axis; RVU, relative value unit. (*Data from* Faculty Practice Solutions Center, UHC; As presented to the CHCA CMO forum on Oct 28, 2011 and SCCM annual meeting 2012 by Dr Schleien.)

Dollar imputed/reported ratio = actual collections/target collections per CFTE

Target collections per CFTE are calculated as the benchmark total RVUs per CFTE × blended contract rate as a percent of Medicare × Medicare conversion factor.

Target collections = benchmark RVUs × blended contract rate (as percentage of Medicare) × Medicare conversion factor

The FPSC designed a grid whereby the dollar ratio is plotted against the work relative value unit (WRVU) ratio to determine the financial state as it relates to revenue collection for a specific division. For example, when both the WRVU ratio and the dollar ratio are high, the division might be in the upper right quadrant or best practice (**Fig. 2**). Being associated with a lower-than-benchmark dollar ratio while maintaining a high RVU ratio could be associated with several factors that might relate to a less-than-ideal payer mix or revenue cycle problems. Citing another example, if the WRVUs are lower than the benchmark but with an acceptable dollar ratio, there could be excess capacity in the practice (too many intensivists). For other ambulatory divisions, the ability of the organization to attempt to leverage excess capacity to drive increased productivity is one possible goal. Obviously, the worst combination is a low WRVU ratio and a low dollar ratio. This situation could be caused by problems with key performance metrics, such as poor charge capture, incomplete or erroneous coding or documentation, poor collections, or major clinical productivity issues. An example of one department's efforts is seen in **Fig. 3**. Focused attempts at assessing the issue followed by a sound financial plan could lead to marked increases in productivity as seen in **Fig. 4**.

The use of more granular productivity data has been shown to improve critical care clinical revenue. Using FPSC data, units of 99292 (extra 30 minutes of critical care) have been compared with 99291 (first hour of critical care) and then compared with national benchmarks (**Fig. 5**). In one case, 13.4 units of 99292 were billed for every

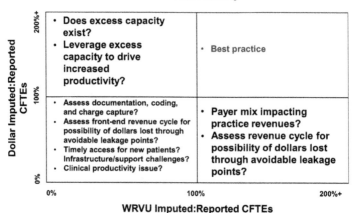

Fig. 2. Dollar Imputed/reported CFTEs on y-axis. WRVU imputed/reported CFTEs on x-axis. See text for definition of terms. (*Data from* Faculty Practice Solutions Center, UHC; As presented to the CHCA CMO forum on Oct 28, 2011 and SCCM annual meeting 2012 by Dr Schleien.)

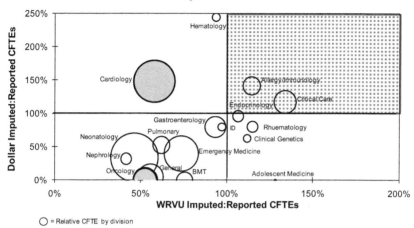

**Fig. 3.** Dollar Imputed/reported CFTEs on y-axis. WRVU imputed/reported CFTEs on x-axis. See text for definition of terms. The bubbles represent various divisions; size of bubble represents relative revenue. BMT, bone marrow transplant. (*Data from* Faculty Practice Solutions Center, UHC; As presented to the CHCA CMO forum on Oct 28, 2011 and SCCM annual meeting 2012 by Dr Schleien.)

100 units of 99291, well less than the national benchmark of 33.9. When this was shown to the group, and working with the organizational compliance officer, the ability to increase the number of 99292 codes where it was undercoded previously would theoretically increase total revenue by more than $150 000. Attention to the revenue

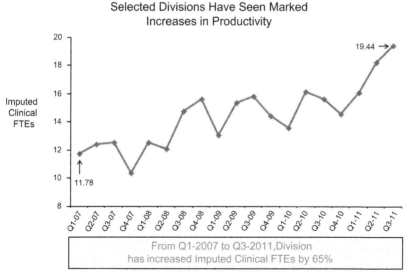

**Fig. 4.** Imputed CFTEs on y-axis; quarterly (Q) data on x-axis showing improvement over time. (*Data from* Faculty Practice Solutions Center, UHC; As presented to the CHCA CMO forum on Oct 28, 2011 and SCCM annual meeting 2012 by Dr Schleien.)

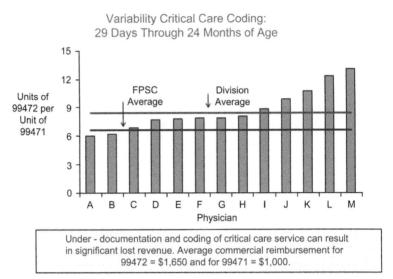

Fig. 5. Units of CPT code 99472 per unit of code 99471 for various physicians; code 99471/99472 represents critical care code for infants aged 29 days to 24 months; division average running more than FPSC average. (*Data from* Faculty Practice Solutions Center, UHC; As presented to the CHCA CMO forum on Oct 28, 2011 and SCCM annual meeting 2012 by Dr Schleien.)

cycle in one's institution, including billing lag time; management of the accounts receivable; and other key performance measures, such as the net collection rate, could greatly enhance revenue collections for an individual group.

Other efforts to improve revenue capture is seen when excellent data capture and metrics that focus on improvement coexist. Examples of this include the number of procedures billed per number of admissions for the ICU. Using FPSC illustrates how monitoring coding patterns could optimize revenue capture. Looking at initial day charge capture, which carries significantly more RVUs than a subsequent day charge, might reflect either poor documentation by an individual practitioner or an inability to capture that charge because of the lack of timely clinical care by a specific practitioner (especially at night or on the weekend) (see **Fig. 5**).

The author's institution has begun to use data like this at both a divisional and individual level. Individual intensivists (as well as other subspecialists) receive a quarterly dashboard that includes their RVU data compared with a national benchmark for their subspecialty and a blinded comparison with the rest of the group. It might also include Press Ganey satisfaction scores for the divisional practice, their personal grant portfolio, and patient complaint ledger (**Fig. 6**).

## THE FUTURE

Clearly, this is an important moment in time for the health care industry that will affect all subspecialists, including critical care physicians. As insurance coverage begins to evolve from a fee-for-service to a capitated/bundled payment system, incentives for ICU physicians and those responsible for ICU budgets may be different than seen at present. Performing ICU tasks and caring for patients in this new environment will bring up new questions for ICU physicians and administrators. If, in fact, we do become fully capitated, how will we fare in this new world? Can we use evidence-based medicine to cut costs and limit the use of wasteful resources,

Name of practitioner_____
Division_____

- RVU's
  - RVU's to date _____
  - Imputed RVUs_____
  - Benchmark_____
  - Division ave_____

- Press Ganey
  - Division_____
  - Target_____
- Grants
  - Direct $_____
  - Last year_____

Fig. 6. Individual critical care physician scorecard.

including technologies that prolong but do not alter ultimate outcomes? Does the realignment between hospitals and physicians pit the health system against our own patients in their perception of rationing care? Limitations on the use of expensive technologies and high-priced medications, when these services and products would have been made available previously, will present problems for physician groups and the relationship to their patients. Given the price bundling between hospitals and physician groups with increased competition for the dollar between surgeons, intensivists, anesthesiologists, cognitive medical specialists, and others, are critical care physicians poised to get their fair share of the pie? Will intensivists, typically independent thinkers and not usually supporters of clinical pathways, be able to exist in an economic world where the demands on standardization of care are large? Can hospitals and ICUs remain profitable or even solvent in a system where capitation and bundled payments coexist with fee-for-service payments when the incentives are totally different? All of these questions will be answered in the near future as our health system evolves. The demands on critical care administrators and physicians, from a financial and administrative point of view, are becoming more intense and complicated. It is hoped that understanding these challenges and the financial principles that form the underpinning of these decisions will assist these physicians and administrators in dealing with a rapidly changing health care environment.

## ACKNOWLEDGMENTS

Thanks to Bob Browne and his staff who prepared the data for the table and figures.

## REFERENCES

1. Isaacson W. Steve Jobs. New York: Simon & Schuster; 2011.
2. Department of Federal Affairs. Q&A on final rule: Medicaid payment for services furnished by certain physicians and charges for immunization administration under the Vaccines for Children Program. Available at: www.tnaap.org/Files/News/PaymentforServicesFurnishedbyCertainPhysiciansandChargesforImmunizationAdministrationundertheVaccinesforChildrenProgram/pdf. Accessed November 22, 2012.
3. Averill RF, Goldfield N, Hughes JS, et al. All patient refined diagnosis related groups (APR-DRGs) version 20.0: methodology overview. 3M Health Information System. 2003.
4. Iezzoni L. Examining the validity of severity measures in today's health policy context. J Gen Intern Med 1995;10(7):406–8.

5. Witcher R, Harbin K, Moody M. Adequate physician documentation can help prevent payment errors. Doctors, hospital coders can partner to reduce mistakes. J Ark Med Soc 2000;96(12):432–4.
6. Ackerman AD, Harrison JM. Practice management: the business of pediatric critical care. In: Nicholas PG, editor. Rogers textbook of Pediatric Intensive Care. 4th edition. Philadelphia: Lippincott Williams and Wilkins; 2008. p. 56–76.
7. Available at: www.economist.com/debate/days/view/863.

# Advances in Recognition, Resuscitation, and Stabilization of the Critically Ill Child

Alexis A. Topjian, MD, Robert A. Berg, MD,
Vinay M. Nadkarni, MD, MS*

## KEYWORDS

- Cardiopulmonary resuscitation • Cardiac arrest
- Extracorporeal membrane oxygenation • Pediatric • Pediatric advance life support
- Therapies

## KEY POINTS

- Advances in early recognition, effective response, and high-quality resuscitation before, during, and after cardiac arrest have resulted in improved survival for infants and children over the past 10 years.
- Several key factors can make a difference in survival outcomes, including the etiology of pediatric cardiac arrests in and out of hospital, mechanisms and techniques of circulation of blood flow during cardiopulmonary resuscitation (CPR), quality of CPR, meticulous postresuscitative care, and emphasis on effective training.
- Early warning scores with implementation of the rapid response team, and training strategies that include simulation and debriefing of events, have been shown to improve implementation of guidelines and protocols that improve outcome.
- Monitoring and quality improvement of each element in the system of resuscitation care are increasingly recognized as key factors in saving lives.
- By strategically focusing therapies on specific phases of cardiac arrest and resuscitation and on evolving pathophysiology, there is great promise that critical care interventions will lead the way to more successful cardiopulmonary and cerebral resuscitation in children.

Potential Conflicts of Interest: V.M. Nadkarni, A.A. Topjian, R.A. Berg: Receive research grant support from the National Institutes of Health. V.M. Nadkarni: Receives unrestricted research grant support from the Laerdal Foundation for Acute Care Medicine.
Department of Anesthesia and Critical Care Medicine, The Children's Hospital of Philadelphia, The University of Pennsylvania, 3401 Civic Center Boulevard, Philadelphia, PA 19063, USA
* Corresponding author. Department of Anesthesia, Critical Care and Pediatrics, University of Pennsylvania Perelman School of Medicine, The Children's Hospital of Philadelphia, University of Pennsylvania, 3401 Civic Center Boulevard, Philadelphia, PA 19104.
E-mail address: Nadkarni@email.chop.edu

## INTRODUCTION

Advances in resuscitation science and the science of education and implementation have substantially improved survival outcomes for cardiac arrest over the past 10 years, particularly for pediatric in-hospital cardiac arrest.[1–5] Cardiac arrests occur in 0.7% to 3% of pediatric hospital admissions and 1.8% to 5.5% of pediatric intensive care unit (PICU) admissions.[4,6–9] Survival rates following in-hospital cardiac arrests have improved from 9% in 1987 to 16% to 30% over the past 10 years.[2,3,6,10–12] Select inpatients, such as children who undergo cardiac surgery, are at greater risk for cardiac arrest but also have improved potential for good survival outcome.[13–15] Unfortunately, good neurologic outcome and quality of life is not universal, especially following pediatric out-of-hospital cardiac arrest.[4,16,17] This review addresses key factors that affect outcome: early recognition of warning signs before cardiac arrest, rapid response and initiation of resuscitation, adjusting the resuscitation interventions to the cause of the cardiac arrest, mechanisms of circulation of blood flow during cardiopulmonary resuscitation (CPR), focus on the quality of CPR, meticulous postresuscitative care, and emphasis on effective training techniques that can save lives and improve the quality of life for survivors.

## EARLY RECOGNITION AND RAPID RESPONSE TO WARNING SIGNS BEFORE CARDIAC ARREST

More than 4000 children in the United States receive in-hospital CPR each year, mostly in PICUs.[3,7,18–20] Many of these events are a result of progressive respiratory failure and circulatory shock. There are at least 4 phases of cardiac arrest: (1) prearrest, (2) no flow (untreated cardiac arrest), (3) low flow (CPR), and (4) postresuscitation. The prearrest phase represents the greatest opportunity to affect patient survival by preventing pulseless cardiopulmonary arrest. Preventing common childhood accidents by using car restraint devices and pool safety can decrease the incidence of cardiac arrest. Patients often have abnormal physiologic parameters associated with acute respiratory insufficiency and circulatory shock in the hours before their event.[21–24] In hospital, early warning and rapid response systems have affected early recognition, treatment, and transfer to PICUs.[24–29] Several nonrandomized adult studies have shown improvement in outcomes with the presence of rapid response teams,[30,31] although a cluster randomized trial in adults did not show a decrease in cardiac arrests or mortality.[32] Prospective randomized trials confirming that rapid response teams truly improve patient outcome are lacking. However, several pediatric studies suggest that rapid response systems decrease the incidence of cardiac arrests in comparison with retrospective control periods.[24,25,33] Reports from the American Heart Association's Get With The Guidelines—Resuscitation national database show that 93% of all inpatient CPR events from 2000 to 2010 in reporting hospitals occurred in the PICU setting.[34] The ratio of ICU-to-ward CPR has increased substantially over the past 10 years, with 9% to 13% occurring on wards from 2000 to 2003 and 4% to 6% occurring on wards from 2004 to 2010. The rates of successful initial resuscitation from these PICU and ward CPR events (ie, return of spontaneous circulation [ROSC]) increased in 2004 to 2010 compared with 2000 to 2003, concurrent with the increase in ratio of PICU-to-ward CPR events.

Rapid response systems can identify and transfer critically ill children to the PICU for intensive monitoring and aggressive interventions that might prevent cardiac arrest or provide prompt advanced life support by experienced providers. Many organizations, including the Institute for Healthcare Improvement (www.ihi.org) and the Child

Healthcare Corporation of America (www.chca.com), consider pediatric CPR events on general wards as "never" events.

## OUTCOMES AND ETIOLOGY OF PEDIATRIC CARDIAC ARREST

In most reports, 60% to 80% of in-hospital pediatric cardiac arrest patients achieve ROSC, approximately 20% to 38% survive to hospital discharge, and approximately 15% to 25% have a good neurologic outcome.[1–3,6–8,10,11,14,35–42] Outcomes following pediatric out-of-hospital cardiac arrests are much worse, typically with approximately 5% to 10% survival to hospital discharge and approximately 2% to 5% with good neurologic outcome.[4,16,17,40,43–51] Many out-of-hospital cardiac arrests are not witnessed, and only 30% of children are provided with bystander CPR.[17] In all cardiac arrests, delayed CPR initiation, unwitnessed arrests, prolonged periods of "no flow," and first documented electrocardiograph rhythm of asystole are associated with poor outcome.

Most pediatric cardiac arrests, whether in or out of hospital, are the result of respiratory failure leading to shock, bradycardia progressing to pulseless electrical activity, and loss of circulation. Interventions to improve outcome from pediatric cardiac arrest should ideally be targeted to address the presumed cause, duration, and "phase" of resuscitation. For cardiac arrests caused by asphyxia and/or ischemia, provision of adequate myocardial perfusion and myocardial oxygen delivery with ventilation titrated to blood flow is important. For ventricular fibrillation (VF) and pulseless ventricular tachycardia, rapid identification of shockable rhythms and prompt defibrillation are critical. In animal models of sudden VF cardiac arrest, acceptable partial pressures of arterial oxygen ($Pao_2$) and carbon dioxide ($Paco_2$) persist for 4 to 8 minutes during chest compressions without rescue breathing, because there is no blood flow and aortic oxygen consumption is minimal. The lungs serve as a reservoir for oxygen during the low-flow state of CPR. By contrast, animal studies of asphyxia-precipitated cardiac arrests have established that rescue breathing is a critical component of successful CPR.[52,53] During asphyxia, blood continues to flow to tissues; therefore, arterial and venous oxygen saturations decrease while carbon dioxide and lactate increase. In addition, continued pulmonary blood flow before the cardiac arrest depletes the pulmonary oxygen reservoir. Therefore, asphyxia results in significant arterial hypoxemia and acidemia before resuscitation, in contrast to VF. In this circumstance, rescue breathing can be life-saving.

Interventions during the no-flow phase of pulseless cardiac arrest focus on early recognition of cardiac arrest and prompt initiation of CPR, restoring blood flow to the brain and heart while activating emergency response and accessing equipment. Effective CPR initiates a low-flow phase, with an effort to optimize coronary and cerebral perfusion, while matching blood flow with oxygenation and ventilation needs. Basic life support with near continuous effective chest compressions (eg, push hard, push fast, allow full chest recoil, minimize interruptions, and do not overventilate) is recommended.

## MECHANISMS OF BLOOD FLOW DURING CPR

During CPR, cardiac and pulmonary blood flow is approximately 10% to 25% of that during normal sinus rhythm. The spontaneously beating heart receives the majority of its perfusion during diastole, with coronary artery blood flow linearly dependent on aortic diastolic pressure. During chest compressions, aortic pressure rises concurrently with right atrial pressure. During chest decompression, the right atrial pressure falls faster and lower than the aortic pressure, generating a pressure gradient that perfuses the heart. Thus coronary perfusion occurs during diastole or the "release" of chest compression. Coronary perfusion pressure that is lower than 15 mm Hg during CPR is associated with lack of ROSC, and perfusion pressure higher than 30 mm Hg during CPR is associated with successful return of spontaneous circulation.[54–57]

To allow good venous return in the decompression phase of chest compressions, it is important to allow full chest recoil and to avoid overventilation. Negative intrathoracic pressure assists venous return to the heart during CPR, and improves blood flow. During the decompression phase, negative intrathoracic pressure can be enhanced by briefly impeding air flow to the lungs (eg, with an inspiratory impedance threshold device). Negative intrathoracic pressure promotes venous return, cardiac output, and mean aortic pressure.[58] This approach improves organ perfusion pressures and myocardial blood flow in humans and animals.[59–62] Despite success in animal studies and human hemodynamics, adult human studies have showed mixed results on survival outcomes, and specific studies in children are lacking.[63] Further evidence that manipulating intrathoracic pressure during CPR can improve hemodynamics is suggested by studies of active compression-decompression devices.[64,65] To date, no studies of mechanical or automated CPR have been shown to be superior to high-quality manual chest compressions in children.

Animal and adult data indicate that overventilation during CPR is common, and can substantially compromise venous return and cardiac output. Most concerning, these adverse hemodynamic effects during CPR, combined with the interruptions in chest compressions to provide airway management and rescue breathing, can contribute to worse survival outcomes.[61,66–72]

### Open-Chest CPR

Excellent open-chest CPR with direct cardiac compression can generate a cerebral blood flow that approaches normal. Although open-chest massage improves coronary perfusion pressure and increases the chance of successful defibrillation in animals and humans, surgical thoracotomy is impractical in many situations. Open-chest CPR may warrant consideration in selected special resuscitation circumstances, such as after sternotomy following cardiac surgery.

### Ratio of Compressions to Ventilation

Ideal compression-ventilation ratios for pediatric patients are unknown. Physiologic models estimate that the amount of ventilation needed during CPR is much less than the amount needed during a normal perfusing rhythm, because the cardiac output during CPR is only 25% to 40% of that during normal sinus rhythm.[73,74] The best ratio of compressions to ventilations depends on many factors including the compression rate, the tidal volume, the blood flow generated by compressions, and the time that compressions are interrupted to perform ventilations. A chest compression to ventilation ratio of 15:2 delivers the same minute ventilation as CPR with a chest compression to ventilation ratio of 5:1 in a mannequin model of pediatric CPR, but the number of chest compressions delivered was 48% higher with the 15:2 ratio.[75,76] When chest compressions cease, the aortic pressure rapidly falls, thus dropping coronary perfusion pressure. Increasing the ratio of compressions to ventilations minimizes these interruptions, thus increasing coronary blood flow.

### Medications for Cardiac Arrest

Although epinephrine and vasopressors consistently improve hemodynamics and initial ROSC following both asphyxial and VF cardiac arrests, no single medication has been shown to improve survival outcome after pediatric cardiac arrest.

Medications commonly used for CPR in children are vasopressors (eg, epinephrine), antiarrhythmics (eg, amiodarone or lidocaine), sodium bicarbonate, and calcium chloride. Routine use of bicarbonate and calcium is not recommended, but may be beneficial for specific resuscitation circumstances (eg, severe acidosis, postbypass, hyperkalemia). Nonselective administration of these medications is associated with worse survival outcomes.[1,20,77]

### Extracorporeal Membrane Oxygenation–CPR

Extracorporeal membrane oxygenation (ECMO)–CPR can establish circulation and provide controlled reperfusion following cardiac arrest. Prospective, controlled outcome studies are lacking. Case series and registry reports suggest excellent outcomes when ECMO rescue therapy is applied to selected patients, with potentially reversible acute postoperative myocardial dysfunction or arrhythmias.[14,41,78–82] It is important to emphasize that the children who survived with ECMO-CPR despite prolonged CPR had brief periods of no flow, excellent CPR during the low-flow period, and a well-controlled postresuscitation phase.

## QUALITY OF CPR

Despite evidence-based guidelines, extensive provider training, and provider credentialing in resuscitation courses, the quality of CPR is typically poor because of slow compression rates, inadequate depth of compression, frequent leaning on the chest with incomplete chest recoil, and substantial pauses in chest compressions. CPR guidelines recommend target values for key CPR parameters related to rate and depth of chest compressions and ventilations, avoidance of no-flow intervals (interruptions in chest compression), and complete release of sternal pressure between compressions.[83,84] An approach that achieves "push hard, push fast, minimize interruptions, allow full chest recoil, and do not overventilate" can result in excellent myocardial, cerebral, and systemic perfusion, and will likely improve outcomes.[66,85]

During the past decade, innovative technologies have extended the ability to monitor and provide real-time feedback on CPR quality during training on mannequins,[86–90] and to apply this to use in actual cardiac arrests.[83,85,91] Feedback on chest compression rate, depth, ventilation rate, no-flow interval (pauses), and incomplete chest wall recoil (leaning) can be tracked and fed back in real time.[92] In the setting of real in-hospital pediatric cardiac arrest, several studies have confirmed the positive effect of feedback in improving CPR quality, compliance with recommended rates for chest compression depth and rate,[93] and reduced leaning.[94] Quality of postresuscitative management has also been demonstrated to be critically important in improving resuscitation survival outcomes.[95]

## METICULOUS CARE AFTER CARDIAC ARREST

The goal of postresuscitation care is to diagnose and treat the underlying cause of the arrest, minimize secondary brain injury, and support end-organ perfusion and function. The postresuscitation phase is a high-risk period for reperfusion injuries, brain injury, and ventricular arrhythmias. Myocardial dysfunction and severe hypotension are common during the postresuscitation phase, particularly in the first 6 hours after restoration of spontaneous circulation.[96] The postarrest phase may have the most potential for innovative advances in the understanding of cell injury and death, inflammation, and apoptosis, ultimately leading to novel interventions. Specific attention should be paid to oxygenation, ventilation, temperature control, seizure control, glucose and electrolytes, and hemodynamics, with the goal of matching appropriate substrate delivery to critical end-organ tissue demands.

### Oxygenation

Following ROSC, both persistent hypoxemia (low $Pao_2$) and hyperoxemia (elevated $Pao_2$) have been associated with poor neurologic outcomes, with concerns that hyperoxia may worsen oxidative injury during reperfusion.[97] Data in children are less clear, with some studies showing association with poor outcome and others showing no difference.[98] Therefore, one goal of postresuscitative care is to deliver adequate oxygen to the patient while minimizing the risk of ongoing oxidative stress. Because many patients do not have arterial monitoring early after arrest, if a patient's saturation is 100%, practitioners should wean the supplemental oxygen to a saturation goal of between 94% and 99%.[99]

### Ventilation

Arterial $CO_2$ levels directly affect cerebral vascular tone in healthy patients. Following cardiac arrest, cerebral edema may occur and titration of arterial $CO_2$ may affect blood flow. Hyperventilating patients can undergo cerebral vasoconstriction, with concerns of cerebral hypoperfusion of the already injured brain and increasing intrathoracic pressure, thus impairing cardiac output. Likewise, hypoventilation can lead to cerebral vasodilation and can increase already elevated intracranial hypertension.

### Cardiovascular Support

Postarrest myocardial stunning and hypotensive shock occur commonly after successful resuscitation in children and adults, and are generally reversible among long-term survivors. Postarrest myocardial stunning is pathophysiologically similar to sepsis-related myocardial dysfunction and post–cardiopulmonary bypass myocardial dysfunction, including increases in production of inflammatory mediators and nitric oxide.[96,100,101] Although the optimal management of post–cardiac arrest hypotension and myocardial dysfunction have not been established, adult data suggest that early hypotension in the 6 hours after ROSC is associated with increased mortality, therefore aggressive hemodynamic support may improve outcomes.[102,103]

Initially fluid resuscitation should be provided for hypotension. If a central venous pressure is being monitored, volume should be titrated to increase the central venous pressures. Inotropic and/or vasopressor support should be provided for hypotension caused by myocardial dysfunction or vasodilation. Monitoring central venous pressure, central venous oxygen saturations, lactates, and urine output may help guide the effectiveness of therapies. General principles of critical care suggest that appropriate therapeutic goals are adequate blood pressure, adequate myocardial, cerebral, and systemic blood flows, and adequate oxygen delivery.[104] Reasonable interventions for vasodilatory shock with low central venous pressure include fluid resuscitation and vasoactive infusions. Appropriate considerations for left ventricular myocardial dysfunction include euvolemia, inotropic infusions, and afterload reduction. Echocardiograms may contribute adjunctive data to guide therapies.

### Temperature Management

Hyperthermia following cardiac arrest is common in children.[105] Animal and human data show that fever following brain injury is associated with worse outcomes, therefore fever should be aggressively treated following cardiac arrest.[106,107] Induced hypothermia (32° to 34°C) following witnessed adult VF cardiac arrest improves survival and neurologic outcomes. Induced hypothermia is the most clinically promising recent goal-directed postresuscitation therapy for adults.[108,109] Interpretation and extrapolation of these studies to children is difficult, and potential benefits and risks are currently under study.[110] Induced hypothermia[32–34] may be considered for children who remain comatose after pediatric cardiac arrest; however, to date there are no prospective pediatric data proving efficacy.[99]

Following ROSC, clinicians should continuously measure the patient's core temperature (rectal, bladder, or esophageal). It is not uncommon for small children who have had a prolonged resuscitation to be hypothermic. Clinicians should discuss temperature goals with a tertiary care center. At a minimum, hyperthermia (>38°C) should be prevented with antipyretics and a cooling blanket. Similarly, hypothermia (<32°C) should be corrected, as deep hypothermia can lead to arrhythmias and repeat cardiac arrest.

### Glucose Control

Hyperglycemia following adult cardiac arrest is associated with worse neurologic outcomes.[111] However, hypoglycemia is associated with worse outcomes as well.[112] Data on evidence-based titration of specific end points in children are not available, therefore clinicians should monitor frequent blood glucose levels and treat hypoglycemia.

### Seizures

Seizures following cardiac arrest are common, and often are undetectable without electroencephalography (EEG).[113] Postarrest seizures (clinical and subclinical) are associated with worse neurologic outcomes.[114] Clinical convulsions should be aggressively treated and evaluated for correctable causes, and should be sought (eg, hypoglycemia, hyponatremia, hypocalcemia, hypomagnesemia). Many patients exhibit electrographic seizures that are undetectable to the clinician, even when not paralyzed. Therefore, clinicians should consider EEG monitoring of the comatose postarrest patient for seizure detection. If the patient is iatrogenically paralyzed, EEG monitoring will be the only means to detect postischemic seizure.

Prediction of neurologic outcome after both adult and pediatric cardiac arrests is limited. The predictive value of clinical neurologic examinations, neurophysiologic diagnostic studies (eg, EEG or somatosensory evoked potentials), biomarkers, or imaging (computed tomography, magnetic resonance imaging, or positron emission tomography) on eventual outcome following cardiac arrest is largely unknown. A burst-suppression pattern on postarrest EEG can be sensitive and specific for poor neurologic outcome.[115,116] However, many children who suffer a cardiac arrest have substantial preexisting neurologic problems.[117,118] Thus, comparison with pre-arrest neurologic function of a child is difficult, and adds another dimension/barrier to the assessment and prediction of postarrest neurologic status.

## EMPHASIS ON EFFECTIVE EDUCATION AND IMPLEMENTATION PROGRAMS

Current training is not adequate enough to maintain basic and advanced life-support skills and behaviors for critically ill children. Pediatric advanced life-support knowledge and skills decay rapidly after training, usually within 6 months.[119,120] Frequent skill refresher training is needed to address knowledge and skill decay. Teamwork and behavioral skills are now recognized as key components of clinical skill performance.[121–125] Highly realistic in situ simulation training has been used as an effective educational tool.[126–129] However, the current translation of advanced life-support training to effective basic and advanced life-support clinical practice in real events is often less than desired.[93,130]

In selected settings, simulation-based advanced life-support educational programs have improved compliance with national resuscitation guidelines for cardiac arrest in adults.[131] Implementation of in situ simulation-based interdisciplinary pediatric mock code training has been associated with improvement of real patient survival-to-discharge following in-hospital cardiac arrest.[132] In addition, simulation-based education has translated to improved patient process of care and patient outcomes in selected clinical settings.[85,133,134] Such simulations are likely to drive resuscitation implementation in the future.

## FUTURE DIRECTIONS AND POTENTIAL CHALLENGES

Exciting new epidemiologic studies, national registries of in- and out-of-hospital cardiac arrests, and large-scale, multicenter resuscitation clinical trials funded by the National Institutes of Health are providing new data to guide our resuscitation practices and generate hypotheses for new approaches to improve outcomes. It is clear that high-quality CPR and basic life support is frequently not optimally provided in both out-of-hospital and in-hospital settings. Innovative technical advances, such as directive and corrective real-time feedback combined with debriefing and skill simulation, can increase the likelihood of effective CPR. Mechanical supports, such as ECMO, are already commonplace interventions during prolonged in-hospital cardiac arrests. In the past, the concept of evidence-based pediatric cardiac arrest recommendations seemed elusive. Recommendations were based on extrapolated animal and adult data. Clinical trials of pediatric cardiac arrest are now in progress. It is likely that the evolution of systems such as "cardiac arrest centers," similar to trauma, stroke, and myocardial infarction centers, is likely to facilitate the appropriate intensive care for children who require specialized postresuscitation care.

## SUMMARY

Advances in early recognition, effective response, and high-quality resuscitation before, during, and after cardiac arrest have resulted in improved survival for infants and children over the past 10 years. Several key factors, including the etiology of pediatric cardiac arrests in and out of hospital, mechanisms and techniques of circulation of blood flow during CPR, quality of CPR, meticulous postresuscitative care, and emphasis on effective training, can make a difference in survival outcomes. Early warning scores with implementation of the rapid response team, and training strategies that include simulation and debriefing of events, have been shown to improve implementation of guidelines and protocols that improve outcome. Monitoring and quality improvement of each element in the system of resuscitation care are increasingly recognized as key factors in saving lives. By strategically focusing therapies on specific phases of cardiac arrest and resuscitation and on evolving pathophysiology, there is great promise that critical care interventions will lead the way to more successful cardiopulmonary and cerebral resuscitation in children.

## REFERENCES

1. de Mos N, van Litsenburg RR, McCrindle B, et al. Pediatric in-intensive-care-unit cardiac arrest: incidence, survival, and predictive factors. Crit Care Med 2006; 34:1209–15.

2. Samson RA, Nadkarni VM, Meaney PA, et al. Outcomes of in-hospital ventricular fibrillation in children. N Engl J Med 2006;354:2328–39.
3. Nadkarni VM, Larkin GL, Peberdy MA, et al. First documented rhythm and clinical outcome from in-hospital cardiac arrest among children and adults. JAMA 2006;295:50–7.
4. Atkins DL, Everson-Stewart S, Sears GK, et al. Epidemiology and outcomes from out-of-hospital cardiac arrest in children: the Resuscitation Outcomes Consortium Epistry—Cardiac Arrest. Circulation 2009;119:1484–91.
5. Matos RI, Watson RS, Nadkarni VM, et al. Duration of cardiopulmonary resuscitation and illness category impact survival and neurologic outcomes for in-hospital pediatric cardiac arrests. Circulation 2013;127:442–51.
6. Reis AG, Nadkarni V, Perondi MB, et al. A prospective investigation into the epidemiology of in-hospital pediatric cardiopulmonary resuscitation using the international Utstein reporting style. Pediatrics 2002;109:200–9.
7. Slonim AD, Patel KM, Ruttimann UE, et al. Cardiopulmonary resuscitation in pediatric intensive care units. Crit Care Med 1997;25:1951–5.
8. Suominen P, Olkkola KT, Voipio V, et al. Utstein style reporting of in-hospital paediatric cardiopulmonary resuscitation. Resuscitation 2000;45:17–25.
9. Ronco R, King W, Donley DK, et al. Outcome and cost at a children's hospital following resuscitation for out-of-hospital cardiopulmonary arrest. Arch Pediatr Adolesc Med 1995;149:210–4.
10. Zaritsky A, Nadkarni V, Getson P, et al. CPR in children. Ann Emerg Med 1987; 16:1107–11.
11. Tibballs J, Kinney S. A prospective study of outcome of in-patient paediatric cardiopulmonary arrest. Resuscitation 2006;71:310–8.
12. Donoghue A, Berg RA, Hazinski MF, et al. Cardiopulmonary resuscitation for bradycardia with poor perfusion versus pulseless cardiac arrest. Pediatrics 2009;124:1541–8.
13. Ortmann L, Prodhan P, Gossett J, et al. Outcomes after in-hospital cardiac arrest in children with cardiac disease: a report from get with the guidelines-resuscitation. Circulation 2011;124:2329–37.
14. Parra DA, Totapally BR, Zahn E, et al. Outcome of cardiopulmonary resuscitation in a pediatric cardiac intensive care unit. Crit Care Med 2000;28:3296–300.
15. Rhodes JF, Blaufox AD, Seiden HS, et al. Cardiac arrest in infants after congenital heart surgery. Circulation 1999;100:II194–9.
16. Donoghue AJ, Nadkarni V, Berg RA, et al. Out-of-hospital pediatric cardiac arrest: an epidemiologic review and assessment of current knowledge. Ann Emerg Med 2005;46:512–22.
17. Kitamura T, Iwami T, Kawamura T, et al. Conventional and chest-compression-only cardiopulmonary resuscitation by bystanders for children who have out-of-hospital cardiac arrests: a prospective, nationwide, population-based cohort study. Lancet 2010;375:1347–54.
18. Randolph AG, Gonzales CA, Cortellini L, et al. Growth of pediatric intensive care units in the United States from 1995 to 2001. J Pediatr 2004;144:792–8.
19. Peddy SB, Hazinski MF, Laussen PC, et al. Cardiopulmonary resuscitation: special considerations for infants and children with cardiac disease. Cardiol Young 2007;17(Suppl 2):116–26.
20. Meert KL, Donaldson A, Nadkarni V, et al. Multicenter cohort study of in-hospital pediatric cardiac arrest. Pediatr Crit Care Med 2009;10:544–53.
21. Chaplik S, Neafsey PJ. Pre-existing variables and outcome of cardiac arrest resuscitation in hospitalized patients. Dimens Crit Care Nurs 1998;17:200–7.

22. Smith AF, Wood J. Can some in-hospital cardio-respiratory arrests be prevented? A prospective survey. Resuscitation 1998;37:133–7.
23. Buist MD, Jarmolowski E, Burton PR, et al. Recognising clinical instability in hospital patients before cardiac arrest or unplanned admission to intensive care. A pilot study in a tertiary-care hospital. Med J Aust 1999;171:22–5.
24. Sharek PJ, Parast LM, Leong K, et al. Effect of a rapid response team on hospital-wide mortality and code rates outside the ICU in a Children's Hospital. JAMA 2007;298:2267–74.
25. Brilli RJ, Gibson R, Luria JW, et al. Implementation of a medical emergency team in a large pediatric teaching hospital prevents respiratory and cardiopulmonary arrests outside the intensive care unit. Pediatr Crit Care Med 2007;8:236–46 [quiz: 247].
26. Tibballs J, Kinney S. Reduction of hospital mortality and of preventable cardiac arrest and death with increased survival on introduction of a pediatric emergency team. Pediatr Crit Care Med 2009;10:306–12.
27. Hayes LW, Dobyns EL, DiGiovine B, et al. A multicenter collaborative approach to reducing pediatric codes outside the ICU. Pediatrics 2012;129:e785–91.
28. Bonafide CP, Holmes JH, Nadkarni VM, et al. Development of a score to predict clinical deterioration in hospitalized children. J Hosp Med 2012;7:345–9.
29. Brady PW, Muething S, Kotagal U, et al. Improving situation awareness to reduce unrecognized clinical deterioration and serious safety events. Pediatrics 2013;131:e298–308.
30. Bellomo R, Goldsmith D, Uchino S, et al. Prospective controlled trial of effect of medical emergency team on postoperative morbidity and mortality rates. Crit Care Med 2004;32:916–21.
31. Jones D, Bellomo R, Bates S, et al. Long term effect of a medical emergency team on cardiac arrests in a teaching hospital. Crit Care 2005;9:R808–15.
32. Hillman K, Chen J, Cretikos M, et al. Introduction of the medical emergency team (MET) system: a cluster-randomised controlled trial. Lancet 2005;365: 2091–7.
33. Tibballs J, Kinney S, Duke T, et al. Reduction of paediatric in-patient cardiac arrest and death with a medical emergency team: preliminary results. Arch Dis Child 2005;90:1148–52.
34. Berg RA, Sutton RA, Holubkov R, et al; for the Eunice Kennedy Shriver National Institute of Child Health and Human Development Collaborative Pediatric Critical Care Research Network and for the American Heart Association's Get With the Guidelines®-Resuscitation (formerly the National Registry of Cardiopulmonary Resuscitation). Increasing Ratio of Pediatric ICU versus Ward Cardiopulmonary Resuscitation Events. Crit Care Med, in press.
35. Chamnanvanakij S, Perlman JM. Outcome following cardiopulmonary resuscitation in the neonate requiring ventilatory assistance. Resuscitation 2000;45: 173–80.
36. Hintz SR, Benitz WE, Colby CE, et al. Utilization and outcomes of neonatal cardiac extracorporeal life support: 1996-2000. Pediatr Crit Care Med 2005;6: 33–8.
37. Meaney PA, Nadkarni VM, Cook EF, et al. Higher survival rates among younger patients after pediatric intensive care unit cardiac arrests. Pediatrics 2006;118: 2424–33.
38. Torres A Jr, Pickert CB, Firestone J, et al. Long-term functional outcome of inpatient pediatric cardiopulmonary resuscitation. Pediatr Emerg Care 1997;13: 369–73.

39. Tunstall-Pedoe H, Bailey L, Chamberlain DA, et al. Survey of 3765 cardiopulmonary resuscitations in British hospitals (the BRESUS Study): methods and overall results. BMJ 1992;304:1347–51.
40. Young KD, Seidel JS. Pediatric cardiopulmonary resuscitation: a collective review. Ann Emerg Med 1999;33:195–205.
41. Thiagarajan RR, Laussen PC, Rycus PT, et al. Extracorporeal membrane oxygenation to aid cardiopulmonary resuscitation in infants and children. Circulation 2007;116:1693–700.
42. Donoghue AJ, Nadkarni VM, Elliott M, et al. Effect of hospital characteristics on outcomes from pediatric cardiopulmonary resuscitation: a report from the national registry of cardiopulmonary resuscitation. Pediatrics 2006;118:995–1001.
43. Berg MD, Samson RA, Meyer RJ, et al. Pediatric defibrillation doses often fail to terminate prolonged out-of-hospital ventricular fibrillation in children. Resuscitation 2005;67:63–7.
44. Dieckmann RA, Vardis R. High-dose epinephrine in pediatric out-of-hospital cardiopulmonary arrest. Pediatrics 1995;95:901–13.
45. Gerein RB, Osmond MH, Stiell IG, et al. What are the etiology and epidemiology of out-of-hospital pediatric cardiopulmonary arrest in Ontario, Canada? Acad Emerg Med 2006;13:653–8.
46. Kuisma M, Suominen P, Korpela R. Paediatric out-of-hospital cardiac arrests—epidemiology and outcome. Resuscitation 1995;30:141–50.
47. Lopez-Herce J, Garcia C, Dominguez P, et al. Outcome of out-of-hospital cardiorespiratory arrest in children. Pediatr Emerg Care 2005;21:807–15.
48. Schindler MB, Bohn D, Cox PN, et al. Outcome of out-of-hospital cardiac or respiratory arrest in children. N Engl J Med 1996;335:1473–9.
49. Sirbaugh PE, Pepe PE, Shook JE, et al. A prospective, population-based study of the demographics, epidemiology, management, and outcome of out-of-hospital pediatric cardiopulmonary arrest. Ann Emerg Med 1999;33:174–84.
50. Suominen P, Korpela R, Kuisma M, et al. Paediatric cardiac arrest and resuscitation provided by physician-staffed emergency care units. Acta Anaesthesiol Scand 1997;41:260–5.
51. Suominen P, Rasanen J, Kivioja A. Efficacy of cardiopulmonary resuscitation in pulseless paediatric trauma patients. Resuscitation 1998;36:9–13.
52. Berg RA, Hilwig RW, Kern KB, et al. "Bystander" chest compressions and assisted ventilation independently improve outcome from piglet asphyxial pulseless "cardiac arrest". Circulation 2000;101:1743–8.
53. Berg RA, Hilwig RW, Kern KB, et al. Simulated mouth-to-mouth ventilation and chest compressions (bystander cardiopulmonary resuscitation) improves outcome in a swine model of prehospital pediatric asphyxial cardiac arrest. Crit Care Med 1999;27:1893–9.
54. Paradis NA, Martin GB, Rivers EP, et al. Coronary perfusion pressure and the return of spontaneous circulation in human cardiopulmonary resuscitation. JAMA 1990;263:1106–13.
55. Kern KB, Ewy GA, Voorhees WD, et al. Myocardial perfusion pressure: a predictor of 24-hour survival during prolonged cardiac arrest in dogs. Resuscitation 1988;16:241–50.
56. Michael JR, Guerci AD, Koehler RC, et al. Mechanisms by which epinephrine augments cerebral and myocardial perfusion during cardiopulmonary resuscitation in dogs. Circulation 1984;69:822–35.
57. von Planta I, Weil MH, von Planta M, et al. Cardiopulmonary resuscitation in the rat. J Appl Physiol 1988;65:2641–7.

58. Plaisance P, Lurie KG, Vicaut E, et al. Evaluation of an impedance threshold device in patients receiving active compression-decompression cardiopulmonary resuscitation for out of hospital cardiac arrest. Resuscitation 2004;61: 265–71.

59. Lurie K, Zielinski T, McKnite S, et al. Improving the efficiency of cardiopulmonary resuscitation with an inspiratory impedance threshold valve. Crit Care Med 2000;28:N207–9.

60. Lurie KG, Coffeen P, Shultz J, et al. Improving active compression-decompression cardiopulmonary resuscitation with an inspiratory impedance valve. Circulation 1995;91:1629–32.

61. Yannopoulos D, Aufderheide TP, Gabrielli A, et al. Clinical and hemodynamic comparison of 15:2 and 30:2 compression-to-ventilation ratios for cardiopulmonary resuscitation. Crit Care Med 2006;34:1444–9.

62. Yannopoulos D, Metzger A, McKnite S, et al. Intrathoracic pressure regulation improves vital organ perfusion pressures in normovolemic and hypovolemic pigs. Resuscitation 2006;70:445–53.

63. Aufderheide TP, Pirrallo RG, Provo TA, et al. Clinical evaluation of an inspiratory impedance threshold device during standard cardiopulmonary resuscitation in patients with out-of-hospital cardiac arrest. Crit Care Med 2005;33:734–40.

64. Wolcke BB, Mauer DK, Schoefmann MF, et al. Comparison of standard cardiopulmonary resuscitation versus the combination of active compression-decompression cardiopulmonary resuscitation and an inspiratory impedance threshold device for out-of-hospital cardiac arrest. Circulation 2003;108:2201–5.

65. Aufderheide TP, Nichol G, Rea TD, et al. A trial of an impedance threshold device in out-of-hospital cardiac arrest. N Engl J Med 2011;365:798–806.

66. Edelson DP, Abella BS, Kramer-Johansen J, et al. Effects of compression depth and pre-shock pauses predict defibrillation failure during cardiac arrest. Resuscitation 2006;71:137–45.

67. Abella BS, Sandbo N, Vassilatos P, et al. Chest compression rates during cardiopulmonary resuscitation are suboptimal: a prospective study during in-hospital cardiac arrest. Circulation 2005;111:428–34.

68. Valenzuela TD, Kern KB, Clark LL, et al. Interruptions of chest compressions during emergency medical systems resuscitation. Circulation 2005;112: 1259–65.

69. Aufderheide TP, Sigurdsson G, Pirrallo RG, et al. Hyperventilation-induced hypotension during cardiopulmonary resuscitation. Circulation 2004;109: 1960–5.

70. Aufderheide TP, Lurie KG. Death by hyperventilation: a common and life-threatening problem during cardiopulmonary resuscitation. Crit Care Med 2004; 32:S345–51.

71. Ewy GA. Continuous-chest-compression cardiopulmonary resuscitation for cardiac arrest. Circulation 2007;116:2894–6.

72. Ewy GA, Zuercher M, Hilwig RW, et al. Improved neurological outcome with continuous chest compressions compared with 30:2 compressions-to-ventilations cardiopulmonary resuscitation in a realistic swine model of out-of-hospital cardiac arrest. Circulation 2007;116:2525–30.

73. Duggal C, Weil MH, Tang W, et al. Effect of arrest time on the hemodynamic efficacy of precordial compression. Crit Care Med 1995;23:1233–6.

74. Halperin HR, Tsitlik JE, Guerci AD, et al. Determinants of blood flow to vital organs during cardiopulmonary resuscitation in dogs. Circulation 1986;73: 539–50.

75. Kinney SB, Tibballs J. An analysis of the efficacy of bag-valve-mask ventilation and chest compression during different compression-ventilation ratios in manikin-simulated paediatric resuscitation. Resuscitation 2000;43:115–20.
76. Srikantan SK, Berg RA, Cox T, et al. Effect of one-rescuer compression/ventilation ratios on cardiopulmonary resuscitation in infant, pediatric, and adult manikins. Pediatr Crit Care Med 2005;6:293–7.
77. Srinivasan V, Morris MC, Helfaer MA, et al. Calcium use during in-hospital pediatric cardiopulmonary resuscitation: a report from the National Registry of CPR. Pediatrics 2008;121:e1144–51.
78. Dalton HJ, Siewers RD, Fuhrman BP, et al. Extracorporeal membrane oxygenation for cardiac rescue in children with severe myocardial dysfunction. Crit Care Med 1993;21:1020–8.
79. del Nido PJ, Dalton HJ, Thompson AE, et al. Extracorporeal membrane oxygenator rescue in children during cardiac arrest after cardiac surgery. Circulation 1992;86(Suppl):II300–4.
80. Tecklenburg FW, Thomas NJ, Webb SA, et al. Pediatric ECMO for severe quinidine cardiotoxicity. Pediatr Emerg Care 1997;13:111–3.
81. Thalmann M, Trampitsch E, Haberfellner N, et al. Resuscitation in near drowning with extracorporeal membrane oxygenation. Ann Thorac Surg 2001;72:607–8.
82. Morris MC, Wernovsky G, Nadkarni VM. Survival outcomes after extracorporeal cardiopulmonary resuscitation instituted during active chest compressions following refractory in-hospital pediatric cardiac arrest. Pediatr Crit Care Med 2004;5:440–6.
83. Wik L, Kramer-Johansen J, Myklebust H, et al. Quality of cardiopulmonary resuscitation during out-of-hospital cardiac arrest. JAMA 2005;293:299–304.
84. Idris AH, Guffey D, Aufderheide TP, et al. Relationship between chest compression rates and outcomes from cardiac arrest. Circulation 2012;125:3004–12.
85. Sutton RM, French B, Nishisaki A, et al. American Heart Association cardiopulmonary resuscitation quality targets are associated with improved arterial blood pressure during pediatric cardiac arrest. Resuscitation 2013;84(2):168–72.
86. Handley AJ, Handley SA. Improving CPR performance using an audible feedback system suitable for incorporation into an automated external defibrillator. Resuscitation 2003;57:57–62.
87. Sutton RM, Donoghue A, Myklebust H, et al. The voice advisory manikin (VAM): an innovative approach to pediatric lay provider basic life support skill education. Resuscitation 2007;75:161–8.
88. Wik L, Thowsen J, Steen PA. An automated voice advisory manikin system for training in basic life support without an instructor. A novel approach to CPR training. Resuscitation 2001;50:167–72.
89. Wik L, Myklebust H, Auestad BH, et al. Retention of basic life support skills 6 months after training with an automated voice advisory manikin system without instructor involvement. Resuscitation 2002;52:273–9.
90. Wik L, Myklebust H, Auestad BH, et al. Twelve-month retention of CPR skills with automatic correcting verbal feedback. Resuscitation 2005;66:27–30.
91. Abella BS, Alvarado JP, Myklebust H, et al. Quality of cardiopulmonary resuscitation during in-hospital cardiac arrest. JAMA 2005;293:305–10.
92. Meaney PA, Sutton RM, Tsima B, et al. Training hospital providers in basic CPR skills in Botswana: acquisition, retention and impact of novel training techniques. Resuscitation 2012;83:1484–90.

93. Sutton RM, Niles D, Nysaether J, et al. Quantitative analysis of CPR quality during in-hospital resuscitation of older children and adolescents. Pediatrics 2009;124:494–9.

94. Niles D, Nysaether J, Sutton R, et al. Leaning is common during in-hospital pediatric CPR, and decreased with automated corrective feedback. Resuscitation 2009;80:553–7.

95. Sunde K, Pytte M, Jacobsen D, et al. Implementation of a standardised treatment protocol for post resuscitation care after out-of-hospital cardiac arrest. Resuscitation 2007;73:29–39.

96. Laurent I, Monchi M, Chiche JD, et al. Reversible myocardial dysfunction in survivors of out-of-hospital cardiac arrest. J Am Coll Cardiol 2002;40:2110–6.

97. Kilgannon JH, Jones AE, Shapiro NI, et al. Association between arterial hyperoxia following resuscitation from cardiac arrest and in-hospital mortality. JAMA 2010;303:2165–71.

98. Bennett KS, CA, Meert KL, et al. Early oxygenation and ventilation measurements after pediatric cardiac arrest: lack of association with outcome, in place of association with outcome. Crit Care Med, in press.

99. Kleinman ME, Chameides L, Schexnayder SM, et al. Part 14: pediatric advanced life support: 2010 American Heart Association Guidelines for cardiopulmonary resuscitation and emergency cardiovascular care. Circulation 2010;122:S876–908.

100. Adrie C, Adib-Conquy M, Laurent I, et al. Successful cardiopulmonary resuscitation after cardiac arrest as a "sepsis-like" syndrome. Circulation 2002;106:562–8.

101. Checchia PA, Sehra R, Moynihan J, et al. Myocardial injury in children following resuscitation after cardiac arrest. Resuscitation 2003;57:131–7.

102. Trzeciak S, Jones AE, Kilgannon JH, et al. Significance of arterial hypotension after resuscitation from cardiac arrest. Crit Care Med 2009;37:2895–903 [quiz: 2904].

103. Kilgannon JH, Roberts BW, Reihl LR, et al. Early arterial hypotension is common in the post-cardiac arrest syndrome and associated with increased in-hospital mortality. Resuscitation 2008;79:410–6.

104. Sutton RM, Friess SH, Bhalala U, et al. Hemodynamic directed CPR improves short-term survival from asphyxia-associated cardiac arrest. Resuscitation 2012. [Epub ahead of print].

105. Hickey RW, Kochanek PM, Ferimer H, et al. Hypothermia and hyperthermia in children after resuscitation from cardiac arrest. Pediatrics 2000;106:118–22.

106. Bembea MM, Nadkarni VM, Diener-West M, et al. Temperature patterns in the early postresuscitation period after pediatric inhospital cardiac arrest. Pediatr Crit Care Med 2010;11:723–30.

107. Hickey RW, Kochanek PM, Ferimer H, et al. Induced hyperthermia exacerbates neurologic neuronal histologic damage after asphyxial cardiac arrest in rats. Crit Care Med 2003;31:531–5.

108. Hypothermia After Cardiac Arrest Study Group. Mild therapeutic hypothermia to improve the neurologic outcome after cardiac arrest. N Engl J Med 2002;346:549–56.

109. Bernard SA, Gray TW, Buist MD, et al. Treatment of comatose survivors of out-of-hospital cardiac arrest with induced hypothermia. N Engl J Med 2002;346:557–63.

110. Pemberton VL, Browning B, Webster A, et al. Therapeutic hypothermia after pediatric cardiac arrest trials: the vanguard phase experience and implications for other trials. Pediatr Crit Care Med 2013;14:19–26.

111. Langhelle A, Tyvold SS, Lexow K, et al. In-hospital factors associated with improved outcome after out-of-hospital cardiac arrest. A comparison between four regions in Norway. Resuscitation 2003;56:247–63.

112. Oksanen T, Skrifvars MB, Varpula T, et al. Strict versus moderate glucose control after resuscitation from ventricular fibrillation. Intensive Care Med 2007;33: 2093–100.

113. Abend NS, Topjian A, Ichord R, et al. Electroencephalographic monitoring during hypothermia after pediatric cardiac arrest. Neurology 2009;72: 1931–40.

114. Topjian AA, Gutierrez-Colina AM, Sanchez SM, et al. Electrographic status epilepticus is associated with modality and worse short-term outcome in critically ill children. Crit Care Med 2013;41:215–23.

115. Nishisaki A, Sullivan J 3rd, Steger B, et al. Retrospective analysis of the prognostic value of electroencephalography patterns obtained in pediatric in-hospital cardiac arrest survivors during three years. Pediatr Crit Care Med 2007;8:10–7.

116. Kessler SK, Topjian AA, Gutierrez-Colina AM, et al. Short-term outcome prediction by electroencephalographic features in children treated with therapeutic hypothermia after cardiac arrest. Neurocrit Care 2011;14:37–43.

117. Moler FW, Donaldson AE, Meert K, et al. Multicenter cohort study of out-of-hospital pediatric cardiac arrest. Crit Care Med 2011;39:141–9.

118. Lopez-Herce J, Del Castillo J, Matamoros M, et al. Factors associated with mortality in pediatric in-hospital cardiac arrest: a prospective multicenter multinational observational study. Intensive Care Med 2012;39:309–18.

119. Nadel FM, Lavelle JM, Fein JA, et al. Assessing pediatric senior residents' training in resuscitation: fund of knowledge, technical skills, and perception of confidence. Pediatr Emerg Care 2000;16:73–6.

120. Grant EC, Marczinski CA, Menon K. Using pediatric advanced life support in pediatric residency training: does the curriculum need resuscitation? Pediatr Crit Care Med 2007;8:433–9.

121. Shetty P, Cohen T, Patel B, et al. The cognitive basis of effective team performance: features of failure and success in simulated cardiac resuscitation. AMIA Annu Symp Proc 2009;2009:599–603.

122. Stead K, Kumar S, Schultz TJ, et al. Teams communicating through STEPPS. Med J Aust 2009;190:S128–32.

123. Salas E, DiazGranados D, Klein C, et al. Does team training improve team performance? A meta-analysis. Hum Factors 2008;50:903–33.

124. Steinemann S, Berg B, Skinner A, et al. In situ, multidisciplinary, simulation-based teamwork training improves early trauma care. J Surg Educ 2011;68: 472–7.

125. Theilen U, Leonard P, Jones P, et al. Regular in situ simulation training of paediatric Medical Emergency Team improves hospital response to deteriorating patients. Resuscitation 2013;84(2):218–22.

126. Rosen MA, Hunt EA, Pronovost PJ, et al. In situ simulation in continuing education for the health care professions: a systematic review. J Contin Educ Health Prof 2012;32:243–54.

127. Weinstock PH, Kappus LJ, Garden A, et al. Simulation at the point of care: reduced-cost, in situ training via a mobile cart. Pediatr Crit Care Med 2009; 10:176–81.

128. Nishisaki A, Scrattish A, Boulet J, et al. Effect of recent refresher training on in situ simulated pediatric tracheal intubation psychomotor skill performance.

In: Henriksen K, Battles JB, Keyes MA, et al, editors. Advances in Patient Safety: New Directions and Alternative Approaches (Vol. 3: Performance and Tools). Rockville (MD): Agency for Healthcare Research and Quality; 2008.

129. Miller D, Crandall C, Washington C 3rd, et al. Improving teamwork and communication in trauma care through in situ simulations. Acad Emerg Med 2012;19: 608–12.

130. Hunt EA, Walker AR, Shaffner DH, et al. Simulation of in-hospital pediatric medical emergencies and cardiopulmonary arrests: highlighting the importance of the first 5 minutes. Pediatrics 2008;121:e34–43.

131. Wayne DB, Didwania A, Feinglass J, et al. Simulation-based education improves quality of care during cardiac arrest team responses at an academic teaching hospital: a case-control study. Chest 2008;133:56–61.

132. Andreatta P, Saxton E, Thompson M, et al. Simulation-based mock codes significantly correlate with improved pediatric patient cardiopulmonary arrest survival rates. Pediatr Crit Care Med 2011;12:33–8.

133. Bruppacher HR, Alam SK, LeBlanc VR, et al. Simulation-based training improves physicians' performance in patient care in high-stakes clinical setting of cardiac surgery. Anesthesiology 2010;112:985–92.

134. Draycott TJ, Crofts JF, Ash JP, et al. Improving neonatal outcome through practical shoulder dystocia training. Obstet Gynecol 2008;112:14–20.

# Advances in Monitoring and Management of Pediatric Acute Lung Injury

Ira M. Cheifetz, MD, FCCM[a,b,c],*

## KEYWORDS

- Mechanical ventilation • Acute lung injury • Acute respiratory distress syndrome
- Gas exchange • Pediatric • Hypoxia • Hypercapnia • Capnography

## KEY POINTS

- Infants and young children are particularly prone to acute respiratory failure because of multiple physiologic factors including small airways (both natural and artificial), weak and ineffective cough clearance, high chest wall compliance, and low diaphragmatic efficiency.
- A key point in the management of the patient with acute lung injury (ALI)/acute respiratory distress syndrome (ARDS) is that increased oxygenation does not correlate with improved outcome, which has been shown in studies with low tidal volume ventilation, inhaled nitric oxide, and prone positioning.
- Low tidal volume ventilation in the adult population with 6 mL/kg ideal body weight is the only approach for ALI that has been shown to reduce mortality.
- Although various modes of ventilation are currently used in clinical practice, to date, no data exist to determine the mode that provides the greatest benefit and the least risk to an individual patient, including those with ALI/ARDS.
- Airway graphic analysis and capnography may be useful monitoring tools to assist with optimal ventilatory management, including optimizing patient-ventilator interactions.

## INTRODUCTION

Acute respiratory failure accounts for more than half of the admissions to pediatric critical care units and is a major cause of morbidity and mortality.[1] Because the causes of acute respiratory failure in the pediatric population are diverse, this article focuses on the respiratory management and monitoring of pediatric acute lung injury (ALI) as a specific cause for respiratory failure. It should be noted from the start that definitive, randomized, controlled trials in pediatrics to guide the intensivist in the optimal

[a] Pediatric Critical Care Medicine, Duke University Medical Center, Box 3046, Durham, NC 27710, USA; [b] Pediatric Intensive Care Unit, Pediatric Respiratory Care and ECMO, Duke Children's Hospital, Box 3046, Durham, NC 27710, USA; [c] Pediatric Critical Care Services, Duke University Health System, Box 3046, Durham, NC 27710, USA
* Pediatric Critical Care Medicine, Duke Children's Hospital, Box 3046, Durham, NC 27710.
*E-mail address:* ira.cheifetz@duke.edu

Pediatr Clin N Am 60 (2013) 621–639
http://dx.doi.org/10.1016/j.pcl.2013.02.015
0031-3955/13/$ – see front matter © 2013 Elsevier Inc. All rights reserved.

**pediatric.theclinics.com**

ventilatory approach for an individual infant or child with acute respiratory failure and ALI are lacking.

Because much of the respiratory management for this critically ill pediatric population is influenced by data from adult patients, it must be stressed that children are not simply small adults, and, similarly, infants are not simply small adolescents. It is important to stress the basic physiologic differences between these populations. Infants and young children are particularly prone to develop acute respiratory failure because of multiple physiologic factors. Overall, from a respiratory perspective, younger children have smaller airways (both natural and artificial), weaker and less effective cough clearance, greater chest wall compliance, decreased diaphragmatic efficiency, and thus are at a higher risk for airway occlusion.

More specifically, younger patients have reduced elastic alveolar recoil, which can result in increased collapse, especially in the presence of decreased pulmonary compliance. In addition, they have fewer alveoli and collateral ventilation channels to allow ventilation distal to obstructed airways.[2] An infant's chest wall has greater compliance, making it more difficult to generate a significant negative intrathoracic pressure in the presence of decreased lung compliance. The weaker cartilaginous airway support in infants and young children may lead to dynamic compression (and subsequent airway obstruction) in conditions associated with high expiratory flow rates and increased airway resistance, such as bronchiolitis and asthma. The pediatric airway is also significantly narrower than the adult airway, thus contributing to the development of increased airway resistance and, potentially, secretion-induced obstruction. Despite these potential disadvantages of the pediatric pulmonary system, the progression of acute respiratory failure to acute respiratory distress syndrome (ARDS) is less likely to occur than in adults.[3,4]

In contrast with the 1994 American-European Consensus Conference definition of ALI and ARDS,[5] the 2011 Berlin Definition (**Table 1**) specifies the timeframe for the development of ARDS, better defines the nature of infiltrates on chest radiographs,

**Table 1**
**Berlin definition of ARDS**

| | |
|---|---|
| Time of onset of respiratory symptoms | Known clinical cause within prior week or new/worsening respiratory symptoms |
| Radiological findings | Bilateral opacities (chest radiograph or CT scan) not explained by lobar collapse, pleural effusion, or nodules |
| Degree of hypoxemia | PEEP $\geq$ 5 cm $H_2O$:<br>Mild ARDS: $Pao_2/Fio_2$ 201–300 torr (maybe CPAP >5 cm $H_2O$ if noninvasively ventilated)<br>Moderate ARDS: $Pao_2/Fio_2$ $\leq$ 200 torr<br>Severe ARDS: $Pao_2/Fio_2$ $\leq$ 100 torr |
| Risk factors | Risk factors for ARDS must be present. Respiratory failure cannot be fully explained by cardiac failure or fluid overload.<br>If no ARDS risk factors are present, objective assessment of cardiac function (eg, echocardiography) is required to exclude cardiac causes |

*Abbreviations:* CPAP, continuous positive airway pressure; CT, computed tomography; $Fio_2$, fraction of inspired oxygen; PEEP, positive end-expiratory pressure.

*Data from* Ranieri VM, Rubenfeld GD, Thompson BT, et al. Acute respiratory distress syndrome: the Berlin Definition. JAMA 2012;307:2526–33; and Ferguson ND, Fan E, Camporota L, et al. The Berlin definition of ARDS: an expanded rationale, justification, and supplementary material. Intensive Care Med 2012;38(10):1573–82.

incorporates positive end-expiratory pressure (PEEP) in the definition of the severity of hypoxemia, minimizes the need for invasive pulmonary artery measurements in the presence of cardiac risk factors, and integrates ALI into a subgroup of mild ARDS.[6,7] A comprehensive pediatric ALI consensus initiative is in progress under the leadership of the Pediatric Acute Lung Injury and Sepsis Investigator (PALISI) Network.

## GAS EXCHANGE

The overall goal of the management of ALI/ARDS is to treat the underlying disease process whenever possible, achieve adequate (but not necessarily maximal) tissue and organ oxygenation, and avoid pulmonary and nonpulmonary complications. Every patient with ALI is hypoxemic by definition and thus requires supplemental oxygen and often noninvasive or invasive mechanical ventilation. An appropriate level of tissue and organ oxygen delivery is provided by ensuring adequate cardiac output and arterial oxygen content, while avoiding excessive oxygen consumption.

A key point in the management of the patient with ALI/ARDS is that increased oxygenation does not correlate with improved outcome, which is shown by the ARDS Network low tidal volume clinical investigation in which the intervention group (6 mL/kg) showed improved survival despite decreased oxygenation compared with the control group (12 mL/kg) for the initial 72 hours of ventilation.[8] This lack of association between increased oxygenation and survival has been shown in other clinical studies as well.[9–12] Timmons and colleagues[12] showed no correlation between oxygenation and survival for pediatric ALI. Dobyns and colleagues[9,10] showed that inhaled nitric oxide (iNO) improved oxygenation but did not affect mortality for pediatric acute respiratory failure during conventional or high-frequency oscillatory ventilation (HFOV). In addition, Curley and colleagues[11] showed no survival benefit with prone positioning despite improved gas exchange.

### Permissive Hypoxemia

In contrast with maximizing arterial oxygenation, the concept of permissive hypoxemia accepts lower arterial oxygenation saturation ($Sao_2$) in an attempt to avoid toxic ventilator support.[13] Although the acceptable $Sao_2$ target remains controversial, most agree with the concept that ventilatory approaches should target adequate tissue and organ oxygenation, while minimizing $O_2$ toxicity and ventilator-induced lung injury. Definitive data to determine the optimal oxygenation level for pediatric patients are not available. The minimally acceptable oxygenation level likely varies throughout the range of the pediatric population, with neonates and adolescents potentially being more vulnerable to hypoxia than others. Because long-term neurologic effects of permissive hypoxemia have not been studied, clinicians should weigh the potential benefits and risks of this approach for each individual clinical situation.

### Permissive Hypercapnia

A logical consequence of low tidal volume ventilation (as described later) is hypercapnia. The degree of respiratory acidosis that can be safely tolerated remains controversial and likely varies between patients. However, most adverse effects associated with respiratory acidosis are minor and reversible when pH is maintained greater than approximately 7.20.[14] Laboratory data from an ischemia-reperfusion model of ALI indicate that hypercapnic acidosis may be protective and that buffering attenuates its protective effects.[15] Limited evidence suggests that low-volume ventilation allowing for permissive hypercapnia may improve outcomes in adult ARDS.[16–18] However, a Cochrane Review of the multicenter ARDS low tidal volume studies was unable to conclusively determine the clinical implications of permissive hypercapnia.[19] Because these studies were not designed to answer the specific question of hypercapnia, the review stressed the many confounding variables in ALI management. Despite the lack of definitive data, permissive hypercapnia is used for the management of severe ARDS in many intensive care units (ICUs). However, permissive hypercapnia is generally not recommended for those with intracranial disorders in which increased cerebral blood flow related to hypercapnia may be detrimental, or significant pulmonary hypertension in which an increased carbon dioxide level may further increase pulmonary vascular resistance.

## MECHANICAL VENTILATION
### Noninvasive Ventilation

Pediatric noninvasive ventilation (NIV), mechanical respiratory support without an endotracheal tube (ETT), is being increasingly used for acute hypoxemic respiratory failure in an attempt to avoid the negative aspects of intubation and invasive ventilation. Unlike the adult and neonatal populations, definitive data on the success of NIV in pediatrics remain limited. NIV for adults with acute respiratory failure secondary to pneumonia has been reported to be unsuccessful.[20] However, several nonrandomized reports have suggested that NIV may improve symptoms, augment gas exchange, and reduce the need for intubation without significant adverse events for pediatric acute respiratory failure.[21–26] A high forced inspiratory oxygen ($Fio_2$) requirement or an increased $Paco_2$ early in the course of NIV seem to be the best independent predictors for failure of this approach.[27]

In pediatrics, much of the available NIV data are in relation to acute asthma exacerbations. Among children with asthma exacerbations who required mechanical respiratory support, significantly more (41% vs 25%) were treated with noninvasive than invasive ventilation.[28] Other small clinical studies have reported the successful use of NIV in children with asthma exacerbations.[29–32] These reports note that NIV was generally well tolerated without major complications and was associated with improvement in gas exchange and respiratory effort. Martinon-Torres[33] described the use of helium-oxygen (heliox) in children with increased airways resistance.[33] Other pediatric subgroups that have benefited from NIV include those with compromised immune systems,[21,22,34–37] acute chest syndrome,[22,38] and postoperative respiratory failure.[22–24,39–41] In a more limited population, NIV after liver transplantation decreased the need for reintubation and may have led to shorter ICU length of stay.[42]

One of the biggest challenges to the effective use of NIV for infants and small children is the lack of a sufficient choice of interfaces.[43] The choice of interface and the available options are largely determined by patient age and underlying pathophysiology. Patient discomfort is the most common reason for changing the interface used.[43] With recent improvements in technology and interfaces, it can be anticipated that an increased use of NIV for pediatric acute hypoxemic respiratory failure, including ALI, will occur. With this anticipated trend, it is hoped that a concomitant increase in clinical outcome data will occur as well.

### Invasive Ventilation

#### Low tidal volume ventilation
ALI is a heterogeneous entity with regions of lung that are collapsed and others that are overdistended. Thus, large tidal volume ventilation can result in regional pulmonary overdistention and progressive secondary lung injury. Preclinical studies provided

initial insight into the pathophysiology of ventilation-induced lung injury by showing that large tidal volume ventilation caused rapid pulmonary changes despite normal lungs at baseline.[44,45] Ventilator settings that resulted in excessive pulmonary stretch led to diffuse alveolar damage with resultant pulmonary edema, an inflammatory response, and leakage of immune modulators into the systemic circulation with subsequent multiorgan dysfunction.[46–50]

Many argue that the only ventilatory approach to conclusively reduce mortality for adult ALI/ARDS is low tidal volume ventilation,[8] and that the current adult ALI/ARDS strategy should be focused on a 6 mL/kg (predicted body weight) tidal volume. Although the ARDS Network study showed that 6 mL/kg improved mortality compared with 12 mL/kg, the tidal volume associated with the least mortality may be between 6 and 12 mL/kg, or possibly lower than 6 mL/kg.

The plateau pressure ($P_{plat}$) in the ARDS Network study was significantly lower in the low tidal volume intervention group.[8] Debate continues as to whether the key variable is tidal volume or $P_{plat}$, or possibly both. Based on the medical literature, it seems optimal to maintain tidal volume at 6 mL/kg and $P_{plat}$ less than 30 to 32 cm $H_2O$ for adults with ALI/ARDS.[8,51–53] The lower safe limit for plateau pressure in pediatrics may be even less.

Gajic and colleagues[54] further showed the benefits of low tidal volume ventilation. The risk of an adult with previously normal lungs developing ALI while mechanically ventilated is directly proportional to the size of the delivered breath. Adults with previously normal lungs ventilated with tidal volumes less than or equal to 9 mL/kg were less likely to develop ALI while ventilated than those with larger volumes. It is not known whether the less injurious effects of lower tidal volumes are linear at less than 9 mL/kg or whether a plateau effect occurs. These investigators suggest that most (and possibly all) mechanically ventilated adults should be managed with a low tidal volume strategy to avoid excessive pulmonary stretch.

Until a definitive randomized, controlled pediatric trial occurs, it is reasonable to ventilate infants and children with ALI/ARDS with 6 mL/kg predicted body weight. This approach is supported by some pediatric data[55] because mortality for pediatric ALI decreased by 40% with lower tidal volumes, although this conclusion is weakened by the retrospective study design. Two mechanically ventilated cohorts were studied based on year: 1988 to 1992 versus 2000 to 2004. Patients from the earlier period were ventilated with larger tidal volume, lower PEEP, and higher peak inspiratory pressure (PIP) than in the more recent period. Mortality was lower (21% vs 35%, $P = .04$) and ventilator-free days increased (16.0 ± 9.0 vs 12.6 ± 9.9 days, $P = .03$) in the more recent time period. Significant study limitations include the retrospective design, tidal volume measurement at the expiratory valve without consideration of the volume lost because of the distensibility of the circuit, and tidal volume calculations as measured per actual (rather than predicted) body weight. Beyond the tidal volume differences, PEEP and PIP management varied between the two cohorts of patients.

As previously noted, definitive low tidal volume ventilation data are lacking for pediatric patients with injured, or normal, lungs. Thus, the pediatric clinician can extrapolate from adult data and/or rely on clinical experience plus the limited, nondefinitive pediatric data. Some may argue that infants and children are different than adults, and, thus, the available tidal volume data do not apply. However, the counter argument is that the potential benefits of low tidal volume ventilation for infants and children seem real and the risks, if any, are theoretic. Thus, many intensivists have adopted a low tidal volume ventilation approach for pediatric ALI/ARDS. For infants and children with normal lungs, extrapolation of the adult data suggests ventilation with a tidal volume less than or equal to 9 mL/kg; whereas the tidal volume should likely be 6 mL/kg for injured lungs. It seems that the critical limit for $P_{plat}$ in pediatrics is less than 30 to 32 cm $H_2O$ and may vary with patient age and size.

An important issue directly related to low tidal volume ventilation is the increasing incidence of pediatric obesity. When determining the appropriate tidal volume, the clinician must use predicted (ideal) body weight. Several Internet programs provide calculators for pediatric ideal body weight for children as young as 12 months old. As an alternative, the predicted body weight for a child can be calculated by using the 50th percentile weight for height on the appropriate growth chart based on gender and age.

### Modes of mechanical ventilation

Various modes of ventilation are currently used in clinical practice. Most patients in pediatric ICUs (PICUs) who require conventional mechanical ventilation are managed with a traditional volume-limited or pressure-limited mode with a synchronized intermittent mechanical ventilation (SIMV) or an assist control approach. To date, no data exist to determine the mode that provides the greatest benefit and the least risk to an individual patient, including those with ALI/ARDS.[56–62] The lack of definitive evidence to support a single ventilatory approach in combination with efforts to improve clinical outcome have led to the development of several innovative modes of ventilation.

One important area of emphasis for many of these novel modes is the maintenance of spontaneous respiration and improved patient-ventilator synchrony. Neurally adjusted ventilatory assist (NAVA), proportional assist ventilation (PAV), and airway pressure release ventilation (APRV) represent nontraditional modes that are the subject of investigation and much discussion. However, the impact of these novel approaches on clinical outcome remains uncertain.[63–68] It remains unclear whether these new ventilatory modes provide an outcome advantage compared with the more traditional approaches. Until definitive data become available, practitioners must carefully consider the clinical circumstances of each clinical situation as well as the potential advantages and disadvantages of the available ventilatory methodologies and use their best clinical judgment. In most pediatric ICUs, the mode of ventilation chosen for a patient is often determined by institutional purchasing decisions and individual clinician preference.

As ventilator technology advances, pediatric clinicians will continue to see the development of novel modes and ventilatory techniques. Despite considerable advancements in technology, no mode of ventilation has been shown to be superior to any other. Despite the lack of convincing evidence, there are likely circumstances in which a specific mode may be assumed to be optimal based on evaluation of airway graphic analysis and assessment of the pathophysiology. The challenge becomes one of matching a patient's pathophysiology to the presumed optimal approach to ventilation.

Additional clinical investigation is needed to determine the impact of novel techniques and ventilatory modes but, until additional data are available, practitioners must carefully consider individual clinical circumstances and the potential implementation of the available ventilatory methodologies while using their best clinical judgment. Regardless of the ventilator strategy/modality used, airway graphic analysis should be remembered in an attempt to optimize patient and ventilator interactions and minimize ventilator-induced lung injury while promoting patient comfort.

**HFOV** When toxic' conventional mechanical ventilation support is required to achieve the desired gas exchange goals, HFOV is often considered. In 1994, a randomized, controlled pediatric HFOV clinical trial showed improved oxygenation and reduced supplementation oxygen requirements at 30 days with HFOV.[69] However, the control group used a high tidal volume approach, and, thus, the application of these results in the current era of low tidal volume ventilation remains uncertain. Despite the paucity of definitive data, the use HFOV for pediatric ALI/ARDS remains common.[70–73]

In the adult population, HFOV has been shown to be equivalent to lung-protective, low tidal volume conventional ventilation.[74–78] The use of HFOV in the adult population has steadily increased but remains controversial. A meta-analysis concluded that HFOV might improve survival and is unlikely to cause harm.[78] This may be the best conclusion for HFOV in the pediatric and adult populations until new outcome data become available. It should be noted that an adult HFOV clinical trial has recently been completed.

**PEEP** Determining optimal PEEP remains an essential component of ALI/ARDS ventilator management. PEEP maintains alveolar patency, restores functional residual capacity, and maintains transthoracic pressure at greater than the level at which additional alveoli collapse during expiration. During the initial phase of inspiration, reexpansion of collapsed alveoli (if present) occurs. In alveolar collapse, airway pressure must substantially increase before a volume of gas is delivered (ie, the recruitment interval). Poor pulmonary compliance with alveolar collapse results an increased risk of barotrauma and secondary lung injury caused by the resultant increased PIP for the same tidal volume delivery and inspiratory time. Although multicenter, randomized studies of adult ALI/ARDS have addressed this important clinical issue of PEEP titration, definitive data in pediatrics are limited.[79–82]

A randomized, multicenter study by the ARDS Network,[79] in follow-up to the low tidal volume investigation, showed that an aggressive PEEP strategy resulted in similar survival compared with a more conservative approach, although arterial oxygenation and pulmonary compliance were improved with higher PEEP. The conservative PEEP group was not a low-PEEP approach but one of adequate PEEP. In addition, all patients were ventilated with 6 mL/kg and an end-inspiratory pressure limit of 30 cm $H_2O$. Safety concerns were not raised regardless of PEEP group assignment. Follow-up studies have revealed similar findings.[80,81] The implication of these data is that, once appropriate PEEP is applied to maintain the lungs at an ideal lung volume, further increases in PEEP do not improve outcome.

Briel and colleagues[82] subsequently analyzed data from the 2299 patients enrolled in the PEEP trials by Brower and colleagues,[79] Meade and colleagues,[80] and Mercat and colleagues.[81] A higher PEEP strategy benefited those with more severe lung injury.[82] The study also concluded that higher PEEP may be associated with a shorter length of ventilation and lower hospital mortality in adults with ARDS. This improvement was not seen in those who did not meet the accepted criteria for ARDS.[82] Furthermore, this study suggests that increased PEEP may be associated with a longer duration of ventilation in those with less severe lung injury.

Without definitive pediatric data, PEEP is generally increased to a level that allows adequate oxygenation at an acceptable $Fio_2$ (generally defined as <0.60). The minimal acceptable arterial oxygen saturation remains controversial, as previously described.[13] In severe ARDS, a PEEP of 10 to 15 cm $H_2O$, or more, may be required to achieve adequate oxygenation. In pediatrics, high levels of PEEP are not often used given the general approach of transitioning to HFOV.[73] Excessive PEEP, and the resultant increase in mean airway pressure, can adversely affect cardiac output by impeding systemic venous return via an increased intrathoracic pressure and/or adversely affect gas exchange by overdistending healthy lung units with redistribution of blood flow to more diseased alveoli.[83] As PEEP is increased, it is essential to monitor for clinical signs of decreased cardiac output,[84,85] which can often be corrected by intravascular volume loading and/or inotropic support.[86,87]

Although extrapolation of adult-based data to children can be helpful, the pediatric critical care clinician is again left without definitive data regarding the optimal approach to PEEP management. When managing an infant or child with ALI/ARDS, the physiology and pathophysiology must be assessed before applying the available adult data. Infants and children may react differently than adults to aggressive PEEP strategies because of differences in chest wall compliance, cardiac reserve, and sedation requirements. It is reasonable to apply the adult PEEP data to an otherwise normal older child or adolescent, but probably not to an infant with congenital heart disease. Pediatric clinicians must often rely on individual and institutional experience and a careful assessment of the specific physiology and pathophysiology involved.

**PEEP titration** PEEP should be titrated until the best possible balance of the following is achieved: lowest PIP to deliver the desired tidal volume, highest pulmonary compliance, and optimal $O_2$ delivery (requires a determination/estimation of cardiac output). There are 2 approaches to finding the optimal PEEP. In the first, PEEP is gradually increased while assessing the resultant cardiorespiratory parameters (ie, incremental PEEP strategy). The second option involves a significant and rapid increase in PEEP with a gradual reduction until optimal PEEP is determined (ie, decremental PEEP strategy). There are no conclusive data to show that either approach is optimal.

As lung is recruited and an appropriate PEEP is set, a lower PIP is required to deliver the same tidal volume given improved pulmonary compliance. Thus, optimizing PEEP results in improved pulmonary compliance and a subsequent decrease in PIP during volume-limited ventilation (or a higher tidal volume for a set PIP during pressure-limited ventilation). These effects may be seen over time as collapsed alveoli are gradually recruited. Continuous evaluation of the cardiorespiratory effects of ventilator manipulations is essential. If refractory hypoxia persists despite escalation of PEEP, high-frequency ventilation or extracorporeal life support may be considered.

### Adjunct Therapies

#### Prone positioning

Prone positioning has been shown to improve oxygenation in pediatric and adult patients with ALI. The mechanisms are theorized to be related to improvements in ventilation-perfusion matching, chest wall mechanics, and secretion clearance.[88] However, risks exist, including ETT obstruction and accidental catheter or tube dislodgment. A meta-analysis has shown that proning improves survival in adults with severe ARDS.[89] However, the only randomized clinical trial on proning in children with ALI was closed because of futility.[11]

#### Exogenous surfactant

Despite being the standard of care for infants with neonatal respiratory distress syndrome,[90–92] exogenous surfactant administration for nonneonatal lung injury is uncertain. Results of early exogenous surfactant administration trials for pediatric ALI were promising[93–95]; however, follow-up studies have been less supportive.[96–98] Willson and colleagues[96] reported that exogenous surfactant improved oxygenation and significantly decreased mortality in infants and children with ALI; however, no significant decreases in length of mechanical ventilation, PICU admission, or hospital stay were seen. The control group had a greater percentage of high-risk, immune-incompetent patients. Disappointing results have also been seen in the adult population, because exogenous surfactant administration did not improve outcome and showed a trend toward increased mortality and adverse effects.[98]

It could be speculated that alternative exogenous surfactant preparations and/or dosing regimens may lead to different results.[93,99–104] For now, surfactant administration for nonneonatal ALI remains uncertain. Although many hoped that the international Collaborative Atorvastatin Diabetes Study (CARDS) would yield definitive conclusions for the management of direct lung injury, this combined adult-pediatric study was stopped for futility.[99]

### iNO

iNO is an essential therapy for the management of newborns with persistent pulmonary hypertension, older children and adults with primary or secondary pulmonary hypertension, and a subset of patients with congenital heart disease. Many have hypothesized that iNO should benefit patients with ALI by improving oxygenation, allowing ventilatory support to be weaned, and, thus, minimizing the occurrence of ventilator-induced lung injury. However, this theory has not been proved.

Similar to proning, studies of iNO for pediatric ALI/ARDS have shown acute improvements in gas exchange[105–108]; however, this has not correlated with improved survival.[9,10,107,109,110] These studies have failed to show a statistically significant effect of iNO on length of ventilation, ventilator-free days, or ICU or hospital length of stay. In addition, in a large meta-analysis, iNO did not improve mortality.[109,110] The investigators concluded that iNO cannot be recommended for patients with acute hypoxemic respiratory failure. Based on the currently available data, this conclusion is applicable to pediatric ALI/ARDS, except in the presence of clinically significant pulmonary hypertension. The use of iNO in the pediatric ALI population may best be guided by the use of echocardiography.

### Extracorporeal Membrane Oxygenation

Extracorporeal membrane oxygenation (ECMO) uses an extracorporeal circuit with a pump and an oxygenator to support life in cases of refractory cardiac and/or respiratory failure. Venoarterial ECMO bypasses the heart and lungs to provide cardiac and/or respiratory support. Venovenous ECMO serves as an additional lung to augment gas exchange, thus allowing ventilator settings to be weaned to less than toxic levels. ECMO does not heal or treat the underlying condition(s) but it provides cardiac and/or respiratory support to allow the pathophysiology to resolve without toxic ventilator or vasoactive agent/inotrope support.

Venovenous ECMO can be used in infants, children, and adults with refractory ARDS who cannot achieve acceptable gas exchange goals without potentially injurious cardiorespiratory support. In those with severe ARDS and preserved cardiac function, venovenous ECMO can be used to minimize $O_2$ toxicity, minimize ventilator-induced lung injury, and achieve acceptable gas exchange. Although ECMO is generally used for those with high mortality, survival for respiratory failure requiring ECMO support is good at approximately 65% for children and 75% for neonates.[111] Experience with the H1N1 influenza pandemic suggests that ECMO may be an important management strategy in future viral epidemics/pandemics with reported survival rates of greater than 70%.[112,113] A more comprehensive review of ECMO is beyond the scope of this article.

## MONITORING
### Tidal Volume Measurements

An important difference between adult and neonatal-pediatric patients involving mechanical ventilation and tidal volume delivery is the location of the volume measurements. For adolescents and adults, tidal volume may be measured at the ventilator's expiratory valve because the volume of gas lost because of the distensibility of the circuit is minimal when expressed as a percentage of total tidal volume. However, for infants and small children, a significant percentage of the delivered volume may be lost because of the distensibility of the circuit. Cannon and colleagues[114] showed that the expiratory tidal volume as measured with a pneumotachometer at the ETT is only 56%, on average, of that measured at the ventilator for neonatal circuits. Correlation was slightly better for pediatric circuits, with an average tidal volume at the ETT being 73% of that measured at the expiratory valve. Similar findings have been reported by others.[115–117]

In general, when determining tidal volume delivery for small pediatric patients, a pneumotachometer placed at the ETT seems an optimal approach. The current generation of ventilators includes software algorithms to estimate the delivered tidal volume based on calculations using ventilator circuit compliance; however, a review of the medical literature indicates that these algorithms have not been systematically studied. In addition, these algorithms use the circuit compliance as determined during initial circuit setup. A key confounding variable is the potential change in the compliance of the ventilator circuit over time caused by temperature alterations, secretions, condensation, and addition of external connectors/adaptors.

### Capnography

Noninvasive carbon dioxide monitoring can provide valuable clinical information for mechanically ventilated patients regardless of age. Capnometry is the digital display of data, whereas capnography is a graphical display that can be presented as time or volume based. Time-based capnography is generally referred to as end-tidal carbon dioxide ($Etco_2$) monitoring.

A time-based capnogram provides a quantitative measurement of the $Paco_2$ in the exhaled gas. Volumetric capnography uses a combined $CO_2$ sensor and pneumotachometer to measure the net $CO_2$ expired as a volume exhaled over time (eg, mL/min). Volumetric capnography allows the calculation of airway dead space, including the dead space to tidal volume ratio ($V_d/V_T$). Volumetric capnography responds to changes in ventilation, pulmonary blood flow, and, to a lesser degree, diffusion as $CO_2$ diffuses rapidly across the epithelial-endothelial junction. Thus, volumetric capnography should be an improved indicator of dynamic changes in gas exchange compared with time-based capnography.[118,119] Carbon dioxide elimination ($Vco_2$) can be a useful clinical tool reflecting acute changes in cardiorespiratory status during invasive ventilation, because $Vco_2$ reflects changes in $Paco_2$.

Volumetric capnography is often referred to as single-breath carbon dioxide ($SBco_2$) elimination because the quantity of $CO_2$ eliminated per breath is used for most of the calculations. The $SBco_2$ waveform includes 3 distinct phases (**Fig. 1**). Phase I depicts gas exhaled from the upper airways, generally void of $CO_2$. A prolongation of phase I is consistent with an increased anatomic/apparatus/airway dead space, as can be seen with excessive PEEP leading to upper airway distension. Phase II represents a transitional phase from upper to lower airways and tends to reflect alterations in perfusion. Phase III represents alveolar gas exchange and may indicate abnormalities in gas distribution caused by heterogeneous lower airway and/or alveolar disease. An upward slope of phase III indicates significant maldistribution of gas throughout the lung regions (eg, bronchospasm). $SBco_2$ technology provides measurements of anatomic dead space, pulmonary capillary blood flow, global cardiac output, and effective ventilation.[120,121]

### Clinical applications of capnography

$Etco_2$ monitoring is standard of care for determining successful endotracheal intubation[122–125]; however, a false-positive can occur when gastric $CO_2$ is present.

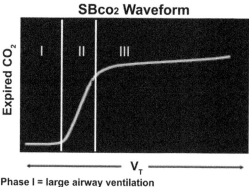

**SBco2 Waveform**

Phase I = large airway ventilation
Phase II = mixed large airway and alveolar ventilation
Phase III = alveolar ventilation

**Fig. 1.** SBco$_2$ waveform. V$_T$, tidal volume.

Volumetric capnography may be a preferred approach because it provides evidence for CO$_2$ elimination as well as gas flow in and out of the airways.[126,127]

Volumetric capnography may assist with ventilation management because changes in Vco$_2$ predict changes in Paco$_2$. As a patient exhales a greater quantity of CO$_2$ (increased Vco$_2$), Paco$_2$ must decrease, with the reverse being true as well. Because Paco$_2$ cannot increase to infinity or decrease to zero, changes in Vco$_2$ and Paco$_2$ must be transient until CO$_2$ elimination reequilibrates with production. The variable of time is a challenging aspect of the clinical use of Vco$_2$ because it varies with clinical status and the degree and timing of ventilator and clinical changes, including baseline lung volume and alterations in lung volume with ventilator manipulation.

Based on physiology, changes in pulmonary blood flow alter Vco$_2$. Decreased pulmonary perfusion regardless of cause results in decreased Vco$_2$, assuming that minute ventilation is not also increasing. Such conditions include decreased cardiac output, pulmonary hypertension, and pulmonary embolus. Vco$_2$ can be an effective monitor of pulmonary blood flow if minute ventilation remains stable. A key difficulty of volumetric capnography occurs with competing cardiorespiratory variables that drive Vco$_2$ in opposite directions. If so, the clinician must determine the primary pathophysiology.

One of the most important applications of volumetric capnography is the calculation of physiologic dead space and the V$_d$/V$_T$ ratio. V$_d$/V$_T$ has been successfully used to predict extubation readiness in a heterogeneous pediatric population as well as outcome for ARDS in adults.[128–131]

### Airway Graphic Analysis

Most clinicians agree that passive mechanical ventilation (ie, mechanical ventilation without patient effort) generally leads to respiratory muscle dysfunction and atrophy, thus potentially prolonging length of ventilation and predisposing to adverse outcome. However, when a mechanically ventilated patient spontaneously breaths during acute respiratory failure, patient-ventilator synchrony becomes essential. Dyssynchrony between ventilator and patient is recognized as a cause of ineffective ventilation, impaired gas exchange, pulmonary overdistention, increased work of breathing, and patient discomfort. Continuous analysis of airway graphics provides a comprehensive assessment of patient-ventilator interactions. The ventilator can be titrated using airway waveforms to improve patient-ventilator synchrony, reduce patient work of breathing, and calculate physiologic parameters related to respiratory mechanics.

Patient-ventilator dyssynchrony occurs when spontaneous inspiratory effort is out of phase with mechanical ventilator breaths, resulting in the patient fighting the ventilator. When ventilatory support is dyssynchronous, $O_2$ consumption may be excessive, resulting in an imbalance between delivery and consumption, and/or effective tidal volume delivery may be reduced, resulting in respiratory acidosis. Patient-ventilator dyssynchrony is diagnosed by careful observation of the patient and a comprehensive assessment of the ventilator's airway graphical display. Altering the mode of ventilation, increasing ventilator support, adjusting inspiratory flow, improving trigger sensitivity, and/or administering pharmacologic sedation (preferably as a later intervention) generally improve synchrony.

Airway graphic analysis should be used to continually assess respiratory pathophysiology by evaluating inspiratory flow, tidal volume, airway pressures, compliance, airways resistance, and pressure-volume and flow-volume relationships. Airway graphic analysis can assist with determining the effectiveness of respiratory interventions and changes in a patient's respiratory status over time. In addition to patient-ventilator dyssynchrony (including excessive patient work of breathing), abnormalities frequently diagnosed by airway graphic analysis include pulmonary overdistension, excessive air leak, premature termination of exhalation/dynamic hyperexpansion (gas trapping)/intrinsic PEEP, inspiratory and expiratory airway obstruction, and increased airways resistance.

## SUMMARY AND THOUGHTS FOR THE FUTURE

Although much has been learned about the pathophysiology of ALI and ARDS in the past 2 decades and ventilatory technology has greatly advanced, the only treatment approach that has been proved to improve clinical outcome is low tidal volume ventilation. However, definitive tidal volume data are limited to the adult population. Furthermore, the optimal tidal volume for any population remains unclear; it may not be 6 mL/kg.

In the years before publication of the low tidal volume ventilation findings, overall survival rates for adult and pediatric patients with ALI/ARDS had been gradually increasing, and this trend continues. It is reasonable to speculate that this positive trend is related to a combination of low tidal volume ventilation; improved overall attention to lung protective, open lung ventilatory strategies; increased use of respiratory monitoring techniques such as capnography and airway graphic analysis; and overall improved ICU management, including a reduction in nosocomial infections and increased attention to nutrition and muscle conditioning. It is hoped that, with time, additional definitive data in the pediatric population will become available to assist the pediatric clinician in the care of infants, children, and adolescents with ALI to further improve survival and functional outcome.

## REFERENCES

1. Farias JA, Fernandez A, Monteverde E, et al. Mechanical ventilation in pediatric intensive care units during the season for acute lower respiratory infection. A multicenter study. Pediatr Crit Care Med 2012;13(2):158–64.
2. Hoyert DL, Kung HC, Smith BL. Deaths: preliminary data for 2003. Natl Vital Stat Rep 2005;53(15):1–48.
3. Rubenfeld GD, Caldwell E, Peabody E, et al. Incidence and outcomes of acute lung injury. N Engl J Med 2005;353:1685–93.
4. Zimmerman JJ, Akhtar SR, Caldwell E, et al. Incidence and outcomes of pediatric acute lung injury. Pediatrics 2009;124:87–95.

5. Bernard GR, Artigas A, Brigham KL, et al. The American-European Consensus Conference on ARDS. Definitions, mechanisms, relevant outcomes, and clinical trial coordination. Am J Respir Crit Care Med 1994;149:818–24.

6. Ranieri VM, Rubenfeld GD, Thompson BT, et al. Acute respiratory distress syndrome: the Berlin Definition. JAMA 2012;307:2526–33.

7. Ferguson ND, Fan E, Camporota L, et al. The Berlin Definition of ARDS: an expanded rationale, justification, and supplementary material. Intensive Care Med 2012;38(10):1573–82.

8. The Acute Respiratory Distress Syndrome Network. Ventilation with lower tidal volumes as compared with traditional tidal volumes for acute lung injury and the acute respiratory distress syndrome. N Engl J Med 2000;342(18): 1301–8.

9. Dobyns EL, Cornfield DN, Anas NG, et al. Multicenter randomized controlled trial of the effects of inhaled nitric oxide therapy on gas exchange in children with acute hypoxemic respiratory failure. J Pediatr 1999;134:406–12.

10. Dobyns EL, Anas NG, Fortenberry JD, et al. Interactive effects of high-frequency oscillatory ventilation and inhaled nitric oxide in acute hypoxemic respiratory failure in pediatrics. Crit Care Med 2002;30:2425–9.

11. Curley MA, Hibberd PL, Fineman LD, et al. Effect of prone positioning on clinical outcomes in children with acute lung injury: a randomized controlled trial. JAMA 2005;294:229–37.

12. Timmons OD, Havens PL, Fackler JC. Predicting death in pediatric patients with acute respiratory failure. Pediatric Critical Care Study Group. Extracorporeal Life Support Organization. Chest 1995;108:789–97.

13. Abdelsalam M, Cheifetz IM. Goal-directed therapy for severely hypoxic patients with acute respiratory distress syndrome: permissive hypoxemia. Respir Care 2010;55:1483–90.

14. Feihl F, Perret C. Permissive hypercapnia. How permissive should we be? Am J Respir Crit Care Med 1994;150:1722–37.

15. Laffey JG, Engelberts D, Kavanagh BP. Buffering hypercapnic acidosis worsens acute lung injury. Am J Respir Crit Care Med 2000;161:141–6.

16. Hickling KG, Henderson SJ, Jackson R. Low mortality associated with low volume pressure limited ventilation with permissive hypercapnia in severe adult respiratory distress syndrome. Intensive Care Med 1990;16:372–7.

17. Hickling KG, Walsh J, Henderson S, et al. Low mortality rate in adult respiratory distress syndrome using low-volume, pressure-limited ventilation with permissive hypercapnia: a prospective study. Crit Care Med 1994;22:1568–78.

18. Milberg JA, Davis DR, Steinberg KP, et al. Improved survival of patients with acute respiratory distress syndrome (ARDS): 1983-1993. JAMA 1995;273: 306–9.

19. Petrucci N, Iacovelli W. Ventilation with lower tidal volumes versus traditional tidal volumes in adults for acute lung injury and acute respiratory distress syndrome. Cochrane Database Syst Rev 2004;(2):CD003844.

20. Ambrosino N, Vagheggini G. Noninvasive positive pressure ventilation in the acute care setting: where are we? Eur Respir J 2008;31:874–86.

21. Munoz-Bonet JI, Flor-Macian EM, Rosello PM, et al. Noninvasive ventilation in pediatric acute respiratory failure by means of a conventional volumetric ventilator. World J Pediatr 2010;6:323–30.

22. Essouri S, Chevret L, Durand P, et al. Noninvasive positive pressure ventilation: five years of experience in a pediatric intensive care unit. Pediatr Crit Care Med 2006;7:329–34.

23. Bernet V, Hug MI, Frey B. Predictive factors for the success of noninvasive mask ventilation in infants and children with acute respiratory failure. Pediatr Crit Care Med 2005;6:660–4.

24. Joshi G, Tobias JD. A five-year experience with the use of BiPAP in a pediatric intensive care unit population. J Intensive Care Med 2007;22:38–43.

25. Padman R, Lawless ST, Kettrick RG. Noninvasive ventilation via bilevel positive airway pressure support in pediatric practice. Crit Care Med 1998;26:169–73.

26. Fortenberry JD, Del Toro J, Jefferson LS, et al. Management of pediatric acute hypoxemic respiratory insufficiency with bilevel positive pressure (BiPAP) nasal mask ventilation. Chest 1995;108:1059–64.

27. Najaf-Zadeh A, Leclerc F. Noninvasive positive pressure ventilation for acute respiratory failure in children: a concise review. Ann Intensive Care 2011;1(1): 1–15.

28. Bratton SL, Newth CJ, Zuppa AF, et al, for the Eunice Kennedy Shriver National Institute of Child Health and Human Development Collaborative Pediatric Critical Care Research Network. Critical care for pediatric asthma: wide care variability and challenges for study. Pediatr Crit Care Med 2012;13(4):407–14.

29. Beers SL, Abramo TJ, Bracken A, et al. Bilevel positive airway pressure in the treatment of status asthmaticus in pediatrics. Am J Emerg Med 2007;25:6–9.

30. Carroll CL, Schramm CM. Noninvasive positive pressure ventilation for the treatment of status asthmaticus in children. Ann Allergy Asthma Immunol 2006;96: 454–9.

31. Akingbola OA, Simakajornboon N, Hadley EF Jr, et al. Noninvasive positive-pressure ventilation in pediatric status asthmaticus. Pediatr Crit Care Med 2002;3:181–4.

32. Thill PJ, McGuire JK, Baden HP, et al. Noninvasive positive-pressure ventilation in children with lower airway obstruction. Pediatr Crit Care Med 2004;5:337–42.

33. Martinon-Torres F. Noninvasive ventilation with helium-oxygen in children. J Crit Care 2012;27(2):220.e1–9.

34. Schiller O, Schonfeld T, Yaniv I, et al. Bi-level positive airway pressure ventilation in pediatric oncology patients with acute respiratory failure. J Intensive Care Med 2009;24:383–8.

35. Piastra M, De Luca D, Pietrini D, et al. Noninvasive pressure-support ventilation in immunocompromised children with ARDS: a feasibility study. Intensive Care Med 2009;35:1420–7.

36. Desprez P, Ribstein AL, Didier C, et al. Noninvasive ventilation for acute respiratory distress with febrile aplastic anemia. Arch Pediatr 2009;16:750–1.

37. Pancera CF, Hayashi M, Fregnani JH, et al. Noninvasive ventilation in immuno-compromised pediatric patients: eight years of experience in a pediatric oncology intensive care unit. J Pediatr Hematol Oncol 2008;30:533–8.

38. Padman R, Henry M. The use of bilevel positive airway pressure for the treatment of acute chest syndrome of sickle cell disease. Del Med J 2004;76:199–203.

39. Stucki P, Perez MH, Scalfaro P, et al. Feasibility of non-invasive pressure support ventilation in infants with respiratory failure after extubation: a pilot study. Intensive Care Med 2009;35:1623–7.

40. Kovacikova L, Dobos D, Zahorec M. Non-invasive positive pressure ventilation for bilateral diaphragm paralysis after pediatric cardiac surgery. Interact Cardiovasc Thorac Surg 2009;8:171–2.

41. Chin K, Uemoto S, Takahashi K, et al. Noninvasive ventilation for pediatric patients including those under 1-year-old undergoing liver transplantation. Liver Transpl 2005;11:188–95.

42. Murase K, Chihara Y, Takahashi K, et al. Use of noninvasive ventilation for pediatric patients after liver transplantation: decrease in the need for reintubation. Liver Transpl 2012;18(10):1217–25.

43. Ramirez A, Delord V, Khirani S, et al. Interfaces for long-term noninvasive positive pressure ventilation in children. Intensive Care Med 2012;38: 655–62.

44. Villar J. Ventilator or physician-induced lung injury? Minerva Anestesiol 2005; 71(6):255–8.

45. Dreyfuss D, Saumon G. Ventilator-induced lung injury: lessons from experimental studies. Am J Respir Crit Care Med 1998;157(1):294–323.

46. Sugiura M, McCulloch PR, Wren S, et al. Ventilator pattern influences neutrophil influx and activation in atelectasis-prone rabbit lung. J Appl Physiol 1994;77(3): 1355–65.

47. Ricard JD, Dreyfuss D, Saumon G. Production of inflammatory cytokines in ventilator-induced lung injury: a reappraisal. Am J Respir Crit Care Med 2001; 163(5):1176–80.

48. Tremblay L, Valenza F, Ribeiro SP, et al. Injurious ventilatory strategies increase cytokines and c-fos m-RNA expression in an isolated rat lung model. J Clin Invest 1997;99(5):944–52.

49. Haitsma JJ, Uhlig S, Goggel R, et al. Ventilator-induced lung injury leads to loss of alveolar and systemic compartmentalization of tumor necrosis factor-alpha. Intensive Care Med 2000;26(10):1515–22.

50. Haitsma JJ, Uhlig S, Lachmann U, et al. Exogenous surfactant reduces ventilator-induced decompartmentalization of tumor necrosis factor alpha in absence of positive end-expiratory pressure. Intensive Care Med 2002;28(8): 1131–7.

51. Amato MB, Barbas CS, Medeiros DM, et al. Effect of a protective-ventilation strategy on mortality in the acute respiratory distress syndrome. N Engl J Med 1998;338:347–54.

52. Stewart TE, Meade MO, Cook DJ, et al. Evaluation of a ventilation strategy to prevent barotrauma in patients at high risk for acute respiratory distress syndrome. Pressure- and Volume-Limited Ventilation Strategy Group. N Engl J Med 1998;338:355–61.

53. Brochard L, Roudot-Thoraval F, Roupie E, et al. Tidal volume reduction for prevention of ventilator-induced lung injury in acute respiratory distress syndrome. The Multicenter Trail Group on Tidal Volume reduction in ARDS. Am J Respir Crit Care Med 1998;158:1831–8.

54. Gajic O, Dara SI, Mendez JL, et al. Ventilator-associated lung injury in patients without acute lung injury at the onset of mechanical ventilation. Crit Care Med 2004;32(9):1817–24.

55. Albuali WH, Singh RN, Fraser DD, et al. Have changes in ventilation practice improved outcome in children with acute lung injury? Pediatr Crit Care Med 2007;8(4):324–30.

56. Branson RD, Johannigman JA. What is the evidence base for the newer ventilation modes? Respir Care 2004;49(7):742–60.

57. Duyndam A, Ista E, Houmes RJ, et al. Invasive ventilation modes in children: a systematic review and meta-analysis. Crit Care 2011;15:R24.

58. Fan E, Needham DM, Stewart TE. Ventilatory management of acute lung injury and acute respiratory distress syndrome. JAMA 2005;294:2889–96.

59. Campbell RS, Davis BR. Pressure-controlled versus volume-controlled ventilation: does it matter? Respir Care 2002;47:416–24.

60. Ortiz G. Outcomes of patients ventilated with synchronized intermittent mandatory ventilation with pressure support: a comparative propensity score study. Chest 2010;137:1265–77.

61. Maxwell RA, Green JM, Waldrop J, et al. A randomized prospective trial of airway pressure release ventilation and low tidal volume ventilation in adult trauma patients with acute respiratory failure. J Trauma 2010;69:501–10.

62. González M, Arroliga AC, Frutos-Vivar F, et al. Airway pressure release ventilation versus assist-control ventilation: a comparative propensity score and international cohort study. Intensive Care Med 2010;36:817–27.

63. Dreher M, Kabitz HJ, Burgardt V, et al. Proportional assist ventilation improves exercise capacity in patients with obesity. Respiration 2010;80(2):106–11.

64. Kacmarek RM. Proportional assist ventilation and neurally adjusted ventilatory assist. Respir Care 2011;56(2):140–8 [discussion: 149–52].

65. Kallet RH. Patient-ventilator interaction during acute lung injury, and the role of spontaneous breathing: part 2: airway pressure release ventilation. Respir Care 2011;56(2):190–203 [discussion: 203–6].

66. Kamath SS, Super DM, Mhanna MJ. Effects of airway pressure release ventilation on blood pressure and urine output in children. Pediatr Pulmonol 2010; 45(1):48–54.

67. Piquilloud L, Vignaux L, Bialais E, et al. Neurally adjusted ventilatory assist improves patient-ventilator interaction. Intensive Care Med 2011;37(2):263–71.

68. Verbrugghe W, Jorens PG. Neurally adjusted ventilatory assist: a ventilation tool or a ventilation toy? Respir Care 2011;56(3):327–35.

69. Arnold JH, Hanson JH, Toro-Figuero LO, et al. Prospective, randomized comparison of high-frequency oscillatory ventilation and conventional mechanical ventilation in pediatric respiratory failure. Crit Care Med 1994;22(10): 1530–9.

70. Randolph AG, Meert KL, O'Neil ME, et al. The feasibility of conducting clinical trials in infants and children with acute respiratory failure. Am J Respir Crit Care Med 2003;167:1334–40.

71. Ten IS, Anderson MR. Is high-frequency ventilation more beneficial than low-tidal volume conventional ventilation? Respir Care Clin N Am 2006;12(3):437–51.

72. Ventre KM, Arnold JH. High frequency oscillatory ventilation in acute respiratory failure. Paediatr Respir Rev 2004;5(4):323–32.

73. Arnold JH, Anas NG, Luckett P, et al. High-frequency oscillatory ventilation in pediatric respiratory failure: a multicenter experience. Crit Care Med 2000; 28(12):3913–9.

74. Chan KP, Stewart TE, Mehta S. High-frequency oscillatory ventilation for adult patients with ARDS. Chest 2007;131(6):1907–16.

75. Derdak S, Mehta S, Stewart T, et al. High frequency oscillatory ventilation for acute respiratory distress syndrome: a randomized, controlled trial. Am J Respir Crit Care Med 2002;166:801–8.

76. Derdak S. High-frequency oscillatory ventilation for acute respiratory distress syndrome in adult patients. Crit Care Med 2003;31(Suppl 4):S317–23.

77. Fessler HE, Hess DR. Respiratory controversies in the critical care setting. Does high-frequency ventilation offer benefits over conventional ventilation in adult patients with acute respiratory distress syndrome? Respir Care 2007;52(5): 595–605 [discussion: 606–8].

78. Sud S, Sud M, Friedrich JO, et al. High frequency oscillation in patients with acute lung injury and acute respiratory distress syndrome (ARDS): systematic review and meta-analysis. BMJ 2010;340:c2327.

79. Brower RG, Lanken PN, MacIntyre N, et al, on behalf of the National Heart, Lung, and Blood Institute ARDS Clinical Trials Network. Higher versus lower positive end-expiratory pressures in patients with the acute respiratory distress syndrome. N Engl J Med 2004;351(4):327–36.

80. Meade MO, Cook DJ, Guyatt GH, et al. Ventilation strategy using low tidal volumes, recruitment maneuvers, and high positive end-expiratory pressure for acute lung injury and acute respiratory distress syndrome. JAMA 2008; 299(6):637–45.

81. Mercat A, Richard JC, Vielle B, et al, on behalf of the Expiratory Pressure (Express) Study Group. Positive end-expiratory pressure setting in adults with acute lung injury and acute respiratory distress syndrome: a randomized controlled trial. JAMA 2008;299(6):646–55.

82. Briel M, Meade M, Mercat A, et al. Higher vs. lower positive end-expiratory pressure in patients with acute lung injury and acute respiratory distress syndrome: systematic review and meta-analysis. JAMA 2010;303(9):865–73.

83. Mitaka C, Nagura T, Sakanishi N, et al. Two-dimensional echocardiographic evaluation of inferior vena cava, right ventricle, and left ventricle during positive-pressure ventilation with varying levels of positive end-expiratory pressure. Crit Care Med 1989;17:205–10.

84. Cheifetz IM, Craig DM, Quick G, et al. Increasing tidal volumes and pulmonary overdistention adversely affect pulmonary vascular mechanics and cardiac output in a pediatric swine model. Crit Care Med 1998;26:710–6.

85. da Silva Almeida JR, Machado FS, Schettino GP, et al. Cardiopulmonary effects of matching positive end-expiratory pressure to abdominal pressure in concomitant abdominal hypertension and acute lung injury. J Trauma 2010;69(2):375–83.

86. Mohsenifar Z, Goldbach P, Tashkin DP, et al. Relationship between $O_2$ delivery and $O_2$ consumption in the adult respiratory distress syndrome. Chest 1983;84: 267–71.

87. Pollack MM, Fields AI, Holbrook RP. Cardiopulmonary parameters during high PEEP in children. Crit Care Med 1980;8:372–6.

88. Gattinoni L, Tognoni G, Pesenti A, et al. Effect of prone positioning on the survival of patients with acute respiratory failure. N Engl J Med 2001;345:568–73.

89. Sud S, Friedrich JO, Taccone P, et al. Prone ventilation reduces mortality in patients with acute respiratory failure and severe hypoxemia: systematic review and meta-analysis. Intensive Care Med 2010;36:585–99.

90. Jobe AH. Pulmonary surfactant therapy. N Engl J Med 1993;328(12):861–8.

91. Findlay RD, Taeusch HW, Walther FJ. Surfactant replacement therapy for meconium aspiration syndrome. Pediatrics 1996;97(1):48–52.

92. Lotze A, Mitchell BR, Bulas DI, et al. Multicenter study of surfactant (beractant) use in the treatment of term infants with severe respiratory failure. J Pediatr 1998;132(1):40–7.

93. Willson DF, Chess PR, Notter RH. Surfactant for pediatric acute lung injury. Pediatr Clin North Am 2008;55(3):545–75.

94. Willson DF, Zaritsky A, Bauman LA, et al. Instillation of calf lung surfactant extract (calfactant) is beneficial in pediatric acute hypoxemic respiratory failure. Members of the Mid-Atlantic Pediatric Critical Care Network. Crit Care Med 1999;27(1):188–95.

95. Willson DF, Jiao JH, Bauman LA, et al. Calf's lung surfactant extract in acute hypoxemic respiratory failure in children. Crit Care Med 1996;24(8):1316–22.

96. Willson DF, Thomas NJ, Markovitz BP, et al, on behalf of the Pediatric Acute Lung Injury and Sepsis Investigators (PALISI) Network. Effect of exogenous

surfactant (calfactant) in pediatric acute lung injury: a randomized controlled trial. JAMA 2005;293(4):470–6.

97. Czaja AS. A critical appraisal of a randomized controlled trial. Willson et al: effect of exogenous surfactant (calfactant) in pediatric acute lung injury (JAMA 2005, 293: 470-476). Pediatr Crit Care Med 2007;8(1):50–3.

98. Kesecioglu J, Beale R, Stewart TE, et al. Exogenous natural surfactant for treatment of acute lung injury and the acute respiratory distress syndrome. Am J Respir Crit Care Med 2009;180(10):989–94.

99. Willson DF, Notter RH. The future of exogenous surfactant therapy. Respir Care 2011;56(9):1369–86 [discussion: 1386–8].

100. Raghavendran K, Pryhuber GS, Chess PR, et al. Pharmacotherapy of acute lung injury and acute respiratory distress syndrome. Curr Med Chem 2008;15(19):1911–24.

101. Notter RH, Schwan AL, Wang Z, et al. Novel phospholipase-resistant lipid/peptide synthetic lung surfactants. Mini Rev Med Chem 2007;7(9):932–44.

102. Walther FJ, Waring AJ, Sherman MA, et al. Hydrophobic surfactant proteins and their analogues. Neonatology 2007;91(4):303–10.

103. Wang Z, Chang Y, Schwan AL, et al. Activity and inhibition resistance of a phospholipase resistant synthetic exogenous surfactant in excised rat lungs. Am J Respir Cell Mol Biol 2007;37(4):387–94.

104. Mingarro I, Lukovic D, Vilar M, et al. Synthetic pulmonary surfactant preparations: new developments and future trends. Curr Med Chem 2008;15(4):303–403.

105. Gerlach H, Keh D, Semmerow A, et al. Dose response characteristics during long-term inhalation of nitric oxide in patients with severe acute respiratory distress syndrome: a prospective, randomized, controlled study. Am J Respir Crit Care Med 2003;167(7):1008–15.

106. Dellinger RP, Zimmerman JL, Taylor RW, et al, on behalf of the Inhaled Nitric Oxide in ARDS Study Group. Effects of inhaled nitric oxide in patients with acute respiratory distress syndrome: results of a randomized phase II trial. Crit Care Med 1998;26(1):15–23.

107. Taylor RW, Zimmerman JL, Dellinger RP, et al, on behalf of the Inhaled Nitric Oxide in ARDS Study Group. Low-dose inhaled nitric oxide in patients with acute lung injury: a randomized controlled trial. JAMA 2004;291(13):1603–9.

108. Adhikari NK, Burns KE, Friedrich JO, et al. Effect of nitric oxide on oxygenation and mortality in acute lung injury: systematic review and meta-analysis. BMJ 2007;334(7597):779.

109. Afshari A, Brok J, Møller AM, et al. Inhaled nitric oxide for acute respiratory distress syndrome and acute lung injury in adults and children: a systematic review with meta-analysis and trial sequential analysis. Anesth Analg 2011;112(6):1411–21.

110. Afshari A, Brok J, Møller AM, et al. Inhaled nitric oxide for acute respiratory distress syndrome (ARDS) and acute lung injury in children and adults. Cochrane Database Syst Rev 2010;(7):CD002787.

111. Domico MB, Ridout DA, et al. The impact of mechanical ventilation time before initiation of extracorporeal life support on survival in pediatric respiratory failure: a review of the Extracorporeal Life Support Registry. Pediatr Crit Care Med 2012;13:16–21.

112. Norfolk SG, Hollingsworth CL, Wolfe CR, et al. Rescue therapy in adult and pediatric patients with pH1N1 influenza infection: a tertiary center intensive care unit experience from April to October 2009. Crit Care Med 2010;38:2103–7.

113. Turner DA, Rehder KJ, Peterson-Carmichael SL, et al. Extracorporeal membrane oxygenation for severe refractory respiratory failure secondary to 2009 H1N1 influenza A. Respir Care 2011;56:941–6.
114. Cannon ML, Cornell J, Tripp DS, et al. Tidal volumes for ventilated infants should be determined with a pneumotachometer placed at the endotracheal tube. Am J Respir Crit Care Med 2000;162(6):2109–12.
115. Castle RA, Dunne CJ, Mok Q, et al. Accuracy of displayed tidal volume in the pediatric intensive care unit. Crit Care Med 2002;39(11):2566–74.
116. Chow LC, Vanderhal A, Raber J, et al. Are tidal volume measurements in neonatal pressure-controlled ventilation accurate? Pediatr Pulmonol 2002; 34(3):196–202.
117. Heulitt MJ, Thurman TL, Holt SJ, et al. Reliability of displayed tidal volume in infants and children during dual-controlled ventilation. Pediatr Crit Care Med 2009;10(6):661–7.
118. Proquitte H, Krause S, Rudiger M, et al. Current limitations of volumetric capnography in surfactant-depleted small lungs. Pediatr Crit Care Med 2004;5:75–80.
119. Schmalisch G. Time and volumetric capnography in the neonate. In: Gravenstein JS, Jaffe MB, Paulus DA, editors. Capnography, clinical aspects. Cambridge (England): Cambridge University Press; 2004. p. 81–100.
120. Arnold JH, Thompson JE, Benjamin PK. Respiratory deadspace measurements in neonates during extracorporeal membrane oxygenation. Crit Care Med 1993; 21:1895–900.
121. Blanch L, Romero PV, Lucangelo U. Volumetric capnography in the mechanically ventilated patient. Minerva Anestesiol 2006;72:577–85.
122. Holland R, Webb RK, Runciman WB. The Australian Incident Monitoring Study. Oesophageal intubation: an analysis of 2000 incident reports. Anaesth Intensive Care 1993;21:608–10.
123. Birmingham PK, Cheney FW, Ward RJ. Esophageal intubation: a review of detection techniques. Anesth Analg 1986;65:886–91.
124. Knapp S, Kofler J, Stoiser B, et al. The assessment of four different methods to verify tracheal tube placement in the critical care setting. Anesth Analg 1999;88:766–70.
125. American Heart Association. 2005 American Heart Association (AHA) guidelines for cardiopulmonary resuscitation (CPR) and emergency cardiovascular care (ECC) of pediatric and neonatal patients: pediatric advanced life support. Pediatrics 2006;117:e1005–28.
126. Sum-Ping ST, Mehta MP, Anderton JM. A comparative study of methods of detection of esophageal intubation. Anesth Analg 1989;69:627–32.
127. Grmec S. Comparison of three different methods to confirm tracheal tube placement in emergency intubation. Intensive Care Med 2002;28:701–4.
128. Hubble CL, Gentile MA, Tripp DS, et al. Deadspace to tidal volume ratio predicts successful extubation in infants and children. Crit Care Med 2000;28:2034–40.
129. Kallet RH, Alonso JA, Pittet JF, et al. Prognostic value of the pulmonary deadspace fraction during the first 6 days of acute respiratory distress syndrome. Respir Care 2004;49:1008–14.
130. Nuckton TJ, Alonso JA, Kallet RH, et al. Pulmonary dead-space fraction as a risk factor for death in the acute respiratory distress syndrome. N Engl J Med 2002; 346:1281–6.
131. Cepkova M, Kapur V, Ren X, et al. Pulmonary dead space fraction and pulmonary artery systolic pressure as early predictors of clinical outcome in acute lung injury. Chest 2007;132(3):836–42.

# Advances in Monitoring and Management of Shock

Haifa Mtaweh, MD[a,b], Erin V. Trakas, MD[a,b], Erik Su, MD[c],
Joseph A. Carcillo, MD[a,b], Rajesh K. Aneja, MD[a,b,*]

## KEYWORDS

- Pediatric sepsis • Septic shock • Cardiac output monitoring

## KEY POINTS

- Shock is the proximate cause of death for many childhood diseases that cause significant mortality worldwide.
- Clinicians have always targeted vital signs to treat shock but new biomarkers and noninvasive cardiac output monitors are being increasingly used to diagnose, monitor, and predict outcome in pediatric shock.
- Early recognition and aggressive resuscitation have been shown to improve outcomes in pediatric shock.
- The choice of inotropes or vasopressor is largely dictated by the type of shock. The role of emerging therapies like hypothermia and ventricular assist devices needs to be delineated and the patient population whom they are likely to help needs to be identified further.

## INTRODUCTION

It has been estimated that 10 million young children die in the world every year. The common diagnoses that underlie this mortality include diarrhea, pneumonia, malaria, measles, and neonatal causes (birth asphyxia, low birth weight).[1,2] The proximate cause of death in almost all of these conditions is shock caused by hypovolemia, hypoxia, ischemia, infection, and anemia. Historically, shock has been defined as a state of acute energy failure that stems from a decrease in adenosine triphosphate production, and subsequent failure to meet the metabolic demands of the body, leading to anaerobic metabolism and cytotoxic metabolite accumulation. However,

Haifa Mtaweh and Erin V. Trakas contributed equally to this article.
[a] Department of Critical Care Medicine, Children's Hospital of Pittsburgh, University of Pittsburgh School of Medicine, 3550 Terrace Street, Pittsburgh, PA 15261, USA; [b] Department of Pediatrics, Children's Hospital of Pittsburgh, University of Pittsburgh School of Medicine, 4401 Penn Avenue, Pittsburgh, PA 15224, USA; [c] Department of Anesthesia and Critical Care Medicine, Johns Hopkins Hospital, 1800 Orleans Street, Baltimore, MD 21287, USA
* Corresponding author. Department of Critical Care Medicine, Children's Hospital of Pittsburgh, Children's Hospital Drive, 45th Street, Penn Avenue, Pittsburgh, PA 15201.
*E-mail address:* anejar@upmc.edu

the clinical definition of shock relies on a constellation of signs and symptoms that include tachycardia, poor capillary perfusion, decreased urinary output, and altered mental status. Because circulatory function is dependent on blood volume, cardiac function, and vascular tone, shock can result from an alteration in any of these parameters, and a simple way to classify shock is as hypovolemic, cardiogenic, and distributive shock.

Although little has changed in the epidemiology and pathogenesis of the types of shock mentioned earlier, the emergence of multidrug resistant (MDR) organisms has changed the treatment of septic shock. In addition, the pediatric intensive care unit (PICU) patient cohort has changed in recent years. There are a growing number of complex patients with a myriad of medical and surgical conditions, thereby increasing the burden of sepsis with MDR isolates. Three MDR organisms are increasingly responsible for morbidity and mortality in the PICU: methicillin-resistant *Staphylococcus aureus*, vancomycin-resistant enterococci, and *Klebsiella* pneumoniae carbapenemases; this situation has profound implications for the choice of empirical antibiotics for patients with severe sepsis and shock.[3–5]

Our understanding of the inflammatory pathways activated in shock has increased in the last few decades; however, this understanding has not led to new successful therapies for treatment of shock. For example, recombinant activated protein C has been used as a treatment in children with severe sepsis. Pediatric patients who received drotrecogin α (Drot AA) had more central nervous system bleeding during the infusion and 28-day study period. As a result of the adverse risk/benefit ratio, the use of Drot AA is not recommended in children with sepsis. It is hoped that as our understanding of the complex pathophysiology of inflammation accelerates, the search for novel treatments to improve outcomes and decrease mortality will increase. Advances in basic science are not discussed in this article, but instead the focus is on the recent advances in monitoring and treatment of pediatric shock.

## MONITORING IN SHOCK
### Clinical and Laboratory Parameters

Frequent or continuous monitoring is of utmost importance when treating shock. Parameters that must be monitored include heart rate (HR), systolic blood pressure (SBP), mean arterial pressure (MAP), urine output (UOP), central venous pressure (CVP), central venous ($Cvo_2$) or mixed venous oxygenation saturations ($Svo_2$), lactate, and measures of cardiac output (CO). It is important to monitor the hemodynamic profile of the patient as treatment of shock is initiated. Normal HR and perfusion pressure for age should be the goals of resuscitation. The clinical effects of fluid resuscitation manifest as a decrease in the HR along with an increase in perfusion pressure (MAP – CVP). The shock index (HR/SBP) can be used to assess the effectiveness of fluid and inotrope therapy, and with resuscitation, the stroke volume (SV) along with SBP increases and the HR decreases, leading to a decrease in shock index. In patients with central venous catheters, $Cvo_2$ of more than 70% should be used as a goal. The arterial-jugular venous oxygen difference ($AVDo_2$) can also be calculated, with a hemodynamic goal of 3% to 5%. If it is wider than 5%, CO should be increased with therapy until the $AVDo_2$ returns to the normal range. The $AVDo_2$ is most accurate when the central venous catheter is located in the pulmonary artery.

In shock, the imbalance between oxygen delivery ($Do_2$) and oxygen consumption ($Vo_2$) leads to an increase in oxygen extraction. At a critical juncture, when the oxygen extraction can no longer keep up with the decreased $Do_2$, the $Vo_2$ becomes dependent on $Do_2$. Mixed venous blood oxygen saturation ($Svo_2$) or $Cvo_2$ reflects the balance between $D_{O_2}$ and $V_{O_2}$ if blood oxygen saturations ($Sa_{O_2}$) are normal (modified Fick equation: $Sv_{O_2} = Sa_{O_2} - [V_{O_2}/D_{O_2}]$). Clinically, a decrease in $Sv_{O_2}$ of 5% from normal (70%) indicates a significant decrease in $O_2$ delivery or increase in $O_2$ demand.

Another marker to assess the degree of global tissue anoxia and anaerobic metabolism is blood lactate levels. Lactate is formed by reduction of pyruvic acid and is freely mobile through cell membranes. Lactate levels can be increased by several conditions, even in the absence of shock (eg, metabolic disorders, lymphoproliferative disorders, and liver failure). Higher blood lactate levels are associated with increased severity of illness and worse outcomes in pediatric critical illness.[6,7] Lactate is most useful in the setting of preoperative and postoperative cardiogenic shock, and it has been suggested that the mortality risk increases as serum lactate levels increase higher than 2.0 mmol/L. Higher values portend an increase in mortality; therefore, when used as a hemodynamic goal, a level of less than 2.0 mmol/L is the target.

### Biomarkers

There has been considerable interest in developing biomarkers that can be used to diagnose, monitor, and predict outcome in shock. Much of the work has been performed in patients with sepsis and the following discussion relates to severe sepsis/septic shock.[8] Biomarkers have been generally defined to have characteristics that can be objectively measured and evaluated as an indicator of normal biological processes, pathogenic processes, or pharmacologic responses to a therapeutic intervention.[9]

C-reactive protein (CRP) is an acute phase protein synthesized by the liver and increases 4 to 6 hours after onset of inflammation or injury and peaks at 36 to 50 hours.[10] CRP has been widely used in children to distinguish infection from inflammation, but it has become evident that it lacks the specificity to consistently discriminate between bacterial, viral, and noninfectious inflammatory conditions.

Procalcitonin (PCT) is produced by the thyroid gland as a precursor to calcitonin, but other tissues can also produce PCT during inflammation or sepsis. PCT has been found to be superior to CRP in distinguishing children with bacterial infections from those without.[11–13] Furthermore, PCT increases with increasing severity of illness, and clearance of PCT has been associated with improved outcome.[14,15]

Ferritin is an iron storage protein that plays a significant role in regulation of iron metabolism. It is also an acute phase reactant, and its increase induces a reduction in available serum iron.[16] Serum ferritin levels are increased in children with septic shock and are associated with poor outcomes.[17] Hyperferritinemia is one of the diagnostic criteria of hemophagocytic lymphohistiocytosis (HLH) and may alert the clinician to investigate further for the possibility of primary or secondary HLH and institute appropriate therapy.[18]

B-type natriuretic peptide (BNP) was first isolated from porcine brain, and its gene is located on chromosome 1. BNP is synthesized in atrial and ventricular myocardium. Myocardial stretch resulting from an increased left ventricle end diastolic pressure or an increase in wall stress has been postulated to act as a major stimulus to increase BNP gene transcription.[19] The main properties of BNP include natriuretic and vasodilatory effects, leading to decrease in preload and afterload.[20] Serum BNP levels have been validated as a diagnostic marker for congestive heart failure in children.[21,22] BNP has also been found to be increased in pediatric patients with myocardial dysfunction from septic shock,[23] but there are no published studies that document serum BNP levels in patients with cardiogenic shock. Although the evidence is promising, more studies need to be conducted before serum BNP levels can be validated as a screening tool for myocardial dysfunction in pediatric shock.

and thereby provide an estimate of adequate $Do_2$. There is widespread interest in using NIRS to prevent or predict a cerebral catastrophic event and have a positive effect on clinical outcome. In a study by Marimon and colleagues,[47] a statistically significant correlation between NIRS cerebral studies and $Svo_2$ values measured within the superior vena cava was shown. Further study must be completed to show such a correlation in pediatric shock.

## TREATMENT OF SHOCK

Cruz and colleagues[48] showed that the institution of a protocol to identify children with sepsis in the emergency department allowed earlier recognition and treatment of shock. Furthermore, early recognition and aggressive resuscitation can reverse the clinical signs of shock and improve outcomes in children.[49] The supportive therapy for shock includes supplemental oxygen (to enhance $Do_2$ to compromised organs) and airway management. In addition, acute circulatory shock should be treated with fluids or blood, when needed, to optimize intravascular volume before addition of vasoactive agents.

### Fluid Resuscitation

Fluid resuscitation is the cornerstone of shock resuscitation in hypovolemic infants and children. Repleting the intravascular volume with fluids improves CO and has been shown to reduce mortality. Han and colleagues[49] examined early goal-directed therapy for neonatal and pediatric septic shock in community hospital emergency departments. These investigators noted that when community physicians implemented therapies that resulted in successful shock reversal (within a median time of 75 minutes), almost all of the infants and children who presented with septic shock survived. Similarly, adults and children who received early goal-directed therapy targeting MAP, CVP, UOP, and $S_{cv}O_2$ had improved survival compared with patients who received standard therapy.[50,51]

The 2007 ACCM pediatric sepsis guidelines recommend fluid resuscitation in 20-mL/kg increments up to 60 mL/kg or shock reversal if the child does not have hepatomegaly or rales on lung examination.[31] The amount of fluid needed depends on the cause of shock. Patients in septic shock often require more fluid resuscitation compared with patients with hemorrhagic shock who require more blood products. Excessive fluids can lead to worsening heart failure and subsequent deterioration in children with cardiogenic shock or severe chronic anemia with cardiac failure.[52]

The choice of fluid for resuscitation continues to be a subject of ongoing debate. The conflicting results of various meta-analyses and clinical trials have left many clinicians unsure about the effect of albumin-containing fluids on survival in critically ill patients. One of the most widely published trials is the SAFE (Saline Versus Albumin Fluid Evaluation) study in 16 intensive care units (ICUs) in Australia and New Zealand. The investigators tested the hypothesis that when 4% albumin is compared with 0.9% sodium chloride (normal saline) for intravascular-fluid resuscitation in patients in the ICU, there is no difference in the overall 28-day rate of death.[53] However, the subgroup analysis of the SAFE trial noted a treatment effect favoring albumin in patients with severe sepsis and noted that crystalloid fluids were helpful in traumatic shock. In the pediatric literature, children with dengue shock syndrome showed no difference in resuscitation efficacy with either colloid or crystalloid solutions. The investigators noticed no clear benefit to the use of a colloid in children with moderately severe shock caused by vascular-leak syndrome.[54] In addition, a recent Cochrane review[55] showed that resuscitation with colloids does not reduce the risk of death, compared with resuscitation with crystalloids in patients with trauma, burns, or after surgery.

Fluid management is different in patients with cardiogenic shock; rather than the usual resuscitation with 20 mL/kg fluid bolus, one should use a fluid bolus that is 5 to 10 mL/kg and monitor for signs of worsening heart failure (ie, worsening of hepatomegaly, jugular venous distention, and pulmonary edema). After initial stabilization, diuresis may have to be initiated in fluid-overloaded patients with cardiogenic shock.

In hemorrhagic shock, the primary cause is loss of intravascular blood volume. Depending on the degree of hemodynamic instability, fluid resuscitation can be started with crystalloids, including normal saline and lactated Ringer solution. The definitive treatment includes achieving hemostasis and blood transfusion. Packed red blood cells (pRBC) are needed, along with platelets and fresh frozen plasma to restore the blood loss.[56] In shock associated with acute-on-chronic anemia, crystalloid or colloid boluses can also be harmful, and blood resuscitation is needed. Under these circumstances, crystalloid at maintenance along with blood transfusions for hemoglobin less than 5 g/dL should be given.[52] Careful attention should be paid to signs of volume overload and heart failure.

### Blood Transfusions

The primary goal of pRBC transfusion is to increase $Do_2$, with subsequent improvement in tissue oxygen use. Although there is little debate about the role of blood transfusion in hemorrhagic shock resuscitation, there is significant variation in the practice of administering blood transfusion in other critically ill patients.[57] The ACCM guidelines for treatment of pediatric septic shock recommend blood transfusions for hemoglobin less than 10 g/dL and central venous oxygen saturation ($S_{cv}O_2$) less than 70%.[31] Lacroix and colleagues[58] compared liberal transfusion strategy (target hemoglobin level, 10.0–12.0 g/dL, with a transfusion trigger of 10.0 g/dL) with a restrictive transfusion strategy (target hemoglobin level, 7.0–9.0 g/dL, with a transfusion trigger of 7.0 g/dL) in a pediatric general medical and surgical setting. With a restrictive strategy, these investigators reported a 96% reduction in the number of patients who had any transfusion exposure and a 44% decrease in the number of red-cell transfusions administered. Furthermore, there was no increase in the incidence of new or progressive multiple organ dysfunctions in critically ill children.[59] Because of the exclusion criteria of the study, these results cannot be applied to premature infants, or children with severe hypoxemia, hemodynamic instability, active blood loss, or cyanotic heart disease, which constitutes a big cohort of the PICU population. The results of this study were different from smaller trials in pediatric subpopulations, in which complications like poor neurodevelopmental outcome, intraparenchymal brain hemorrhage, periventricular leukomalacia, and apnea were higher in the restrictive-strategy group.[60,61] These differences in outcomes were not designated a priori and were not confirmed in a subsequent larger trial.[62]

Although RBC transfusion is indicated for critically ill hemodynamically unstable with low hemoglobin concentrations, the evidence does not support the unrestricted use of red-cell transfusion in critically ill patients.

### Vasopressor and Inotropic Support

The next tier of therapy is vasopressors or inotrope administration, and is largely dictated by the cause of shock. For example, for children with septic shock, dopamine (5–9 µg/kg/min), dobutamine, or epinephrine (0.05–0.3 µg/kg/min) can be used as first-line inotropic support.[31] Recent adult data have raised the concern of increased mortality with the use of dopamine.[63] There is no clear explanation for these observations, but they may be related to the action of dopamine infusion to reduce the release of hormones from the anterior pituitary gland (prolactin-releasing and thyrotropin-releasing hormone release). Therefore, many centers are now routinely using epinephrine as a first-line inotropic agent.

Critically ill children who are normotensive with a low CO and high SVR often require a short-acting vasodilator (eg, sodium nitroprusside, nitroglycerin, or type III phosphodiesterase inhibitors) to lower SVR. In contrast, the use of low-dose norepinephrine has been recommended as a first-line agent for fluid-refractory hypotensive hyperdynamic shock (low CO, low SVR).

In cardiogenic shock, afterload reduction improves blood flow by reducing ventricular afterload and increasing ventricular emptying. In children with cardiogenic shock a combination of low-dose epinephrine and milrinone can be used for inotropy and afterload reduction.

The mechanism of action of different inotropic and vasopressor medications that are used in treatment of shock is summarized in **Table 2**.[64]

Dopamine is an endogenous catecholamine and binds $\alpha_1$, $\beta_1$, $\beta_2$, and dopaminergic ($D_1$ and $D_2$) receptors. Similar to the $\beta_1$ receptors, the $D_1$ receptors activate adenylate cyclase through $G_s$ protein coupling, resulting in vasodilation. Dopamine stimulates $\beta_1$ receptors and $\alpha_1$ receptors in the myocardium, resulting in increased inotropy, chronotropy, and vascular smooth muscle contraction.

Dobutamine is a synthetic catecholamine that acts on $\alpha$-adrenergic and $\beta$-adrenergic receptors. It increases CO and vascular smooth muscle relaxation. In the treatment of pediatric postoperative cardiac surgery patients, dobutamine increases CO by increasing HR, and significant tachycardia may prompt discontinuation of use of the drug.[65] The ACCM guidelines consider dobutamine an alternative to dopamine for patients with septic shock with adequate or increased SVR.

Epinephrine is a hormone produced in the adrenal medulla and stimulates $\alpha$, $\beta_1$, and $\beta_2$ receptors. At low infusion rates, the $\beta_1$ and $\beta_2$ receptor effects predominate, leading to myocardial contraction, increased $Vo_2$ along with a decrease in SVR. Higher infusion rates cause systemic and pulmonary vasoconstriction through $\alpha$ receptor stimulation.

Norepinephrine is a central nervous system neurotransmitter with strong $\alpha$ and $\beta_1$ agonist with little $\beta_2$ agonist activity. It is a second-line vasopressor after dopamine for warm shock in the ACCM guidelines. SV increases and CO changes little. The myocardial oxygen supply-demand relationship is neutral or favorably affected.[65] Clinical use of norepinephrine centers on treatment of hypotensive and distributive forms of shock, such as warm septic shock.

Vasopressin is a nonapeptide hormone that stimulates 3 receptor subtypes ($V_1$, $V_2$, and $V_3$), which are G-protein coupled to intracellular modulators. Vasopressin

| Table 2 | | | | | |
|---|---|---|---|---|---|
| **Receptor affinity of different inotropes and vasopressors** | | | | | |
| **Drug** | **α** | **β₁** | **β₂** | **Dopamine** | **Vasopressin** |
| Dobutamine | + | +++ | + | | |
| Dopamine | ++ | +++ | + | ++ | |
| Epinephrine | +++ | +++ | +++ | | |
| Norepinephrine | +++ | + | | | |
| Vasopressin | | | | | ++ |

*Data from* Shekerdemian L, Redington A. Cardiovascular pharmacology. In: Chang AC, editor. Pediatric cardiac intensive care, vol. xxiv. Baltimore (MD): Williams & Wilkins; 1998. p. 574.

increases SVR and blood pressure with no inotropy and reduces the need for catecholamine support in patients with shock. Vasopressin has been shown to lower CI and adversely affect outcome in cardiogenic shock.[65] The safety and efficacy of low-dose vasopressin was investigated in pediatric patients with vasodilatory shock and it did not show any beneficial effects.[66,67]

Milrinone, a bipyridine, is a nonsympathomimetic inotropic agent that is a selective inhibitor of phosphodiesterase III. It increases CO, reduces SVR, and shows no chronotropic effect. Milrinone has been the drug of choice for afterload reduction in postoperative pediatric cardiac patients and results in a slight decrease in SBP, increased CI, decreased SVR, and pulmonary vascular resistance. Milrinone has been investigated in children with nonhyperdynamic septic shock (low to normal CI and normal to high SVR), and it resulted in increased CI and $Do_2$ and decreased SVR.[65]

### Corticosteroids

Adrenal insufficiency can be classified as absolute or relative. Absolute adrenal insufficiency is baseline cortisol level less than 5 μg/dL or stressed cortisol level less than 20 μg/dL. Relative adrenal insufficiency is diagnosed if basal cortisol level is greater than 20 μg/dL and adrenocorticotropic hormone response increment increase in cortisol of 9 μg/dL or less.[68] It should be suspected in patients with refractory shock and history of trauma (head or abdominal), sepsis, central nervous system disease, Waterhouse-Friedrickson syndrome, treatment with etomidate, or steroid use in the 6 months before presentation.[69] In a cohort analysis by Zimmerman and Williams,[70] children who received corticosteroids had no improvement in mortality, days of vasoactive-inotropic infusion, days of mechanical ventilation, change in pediatric overall performance category score, or length of stay in PICU and hospital. The current recommendations are to use steroids in absolute adrenal insufficiency in presence of catecholamine-resistant shock. As for the recommended dosage, stress-shock dose has been considered to be 2 to 50 mg/kg/d.[71] Clinicians have extrapolated these recommendations to other types of shock.

### Antibiotics

Current guidelines recommend initiation of antibiotics within 1 hour of presentation of severe sepsis and septic shock.[31] In a study by Kumar and colleagues[72] examining the duration of hypotension in adult septic patients and administration of effective antimicrobial therapy, each hour delay over the first 6 hours was associated with a mean decrease in survival of 7.6%. These results were validated in another recent study by Gaieski and colleagues,[73] who noted that mortality was significantly decreased when time from triage to appropriate antibiotic administration was 1 hour or less.

### Temperature Control

In a recent multicenter randomized controlled trial, febrile patients with septic shock who needed vasopressors, mechanical ventilation, and sedation were allocated to achieve normothermia with external cooling (36.5°C–37°C) or no external cooling. The investigators reported shock reversal and decrease in early mortality with normothermia.[74]

The use of hypothermia in refractory shock and impending cardiac arrest has increased in the last few years, largely because of its role in neuroprotection. A study by Schmidt-Schweda and colleagues[75] investigated use of moderate hypothermia (33°C) in patients with cardiogenic shock (50% of patients were recovering from cardiac arrest); these investigators demonstrated a decrease in HR and increase in

SV and CI, without any major adverse effects. Further studies are warranted to identify the patient cohort that is most likely to benefit from use of hypothermia in shock.

### Extracorporeal Membrane Oxygenation/Ventricular Assist Device

Extracorporeal membrane oxygenation (ECMO) was considered the last resort in refractory shock of any cause, and its use has increased in the last few years to provide hemodynamic support. Clinicians have been encouraged by the survival data in patients who were placed on ECMO during cardiopulmonary resuscitation (ECPR). In a study drawn from the Extracorporeal Life Support Organization (ELSO) registry, 682 patients younger than 18 years received ECPR[76]; underlying cardiac disease was present in 73%, sepsis in 8%, and respiratory failure in 5%. The survival to discharge in this cohort was 38%. The neurologic outcomes of these patients were not available in this study. Similarly, a single-institution study showed a survival to discharge rate of 33%.[77] Another ELSO registry report stated that 40% of cannulated patients who had cardiogenic shock survived to discharge from the hospital. Approximately a third of the survivors had neurologic morbidity, with significant deficits in approximately 10%.[78] In shock arrest, central cannulation seems to be beneficial in cardiogenic and septic shock.[79] Therefore, although these data support the use of ECMO in shock, efforts must be made to improve survival and long-term outcome in these patients.

Historically, ECMO has been the mainstay of pediatric circulatory support after unresponsiveness to inotropic/vasopressor support. Ventricular assist device (VAD) support has been used in children for circulatory support after cardiogenic shock from myocarditis, cardiomyopathy, and congenital heart disease. A single-institution retrospective study[80] reported the use of pulsatile VADs in 14 children with refractory cardiogenic shock, with 79% survival and 29% neurologic morbidity.

### SUMMARY

Shock is the proximate cause of death for many childhood diseases that cause significant mortality worldwide. Clinicians have always targeted vital signs to treat shock, but new biomarkers and noninvasive CO monitors are being increasingly used to diagnose, monitor, and predict outcome in pediatric shock. Early recognition and aggressive resuscitation has been shown to improve outcomes in pediatric shock. The choice of inotropes or vasopressor is largely dictated by the type of shock. The role of emerging therapies like hypothermia and VADs needs to be delineated and the patient population whom they are likely to help needs to be identified further.

### REFERENCES

1. Ahmad OB, Lopez AD, Inoue M. The decline in child mortality: a reappraisal. Bull World Health Organ 2000;78:1175–91.
2. Black RE, Morris SS, Bryce J. Where and why are 10 million children dying every year? Lancet 2003;361:2226–34.
3. Aneja R, Carcillo J. Differences between adult and pediatric septic shock. Minerva Anestesiol 2011;77:986–92.
4. Aneja RK, Varughese-Aneja R, Vetterly CG, et al. Antibiotic therapy in neonatal and pediatric septic shock. Curr Infect Dis Rep 2011;13:433–41.
5. Fuhrman BP. Pediatric critical care. 4th edition. Philadelphia: Elsevier Saunders; 2011.
6. Jat KR, Jhamb U, Gupta VK. Serum lactate levels as the predictor of outcome in pediatric septic shock. Indian J Crit Care Med 2011;15:102–7.

7. Hatherill M, McIntyre AG, Wattie M, et al. Early hyperlactataemia in critically ill children. Intensive Care Med 2000;26:314–8.
8. Standage SW, Wong HR. Biomarkers for pediatric sepsis and septic shock. Expert Rev Anti Infect Ther 2011;9:71–9.
9. Biomarkers Definitions Working Group. Biomarkers and surrogate endpoints: preferred definitions and conceptual framework. Clin Pharmacol Ther 2001;69: 89–95.
10. McWilliam S, Riordan A. How to use: C-reactive protein. Arch Dis Child Educ Pract Ed 2010;95:55–8.
11. Fioretto JR, Martin JG, Kurokawa CS, et al. Comparison between procalcitonin and C-reactive protein for early diagnosis of children with sepsis or septic shock. Inflamm Res 2010;59:581–6.
12. Castelli GP, Pognani C, Meisner M, et al. Procalcitonin and C-reactive protein during systemic inflammatory response syndrome, sepsis and organ dysfunction. Crit Care 2004;8:R234–42.
13. Rey C, Los Arcos M, Concha A, et al. Procalcitonin and C-reactive protein as markers of systemic inflammatory response syndrome severity in critically ill children. Intensive Care Med 2007;33:477–84.
14. Ruiz-Rodriguez JC, Caballero J, Ruiz-Sanmartin A, et al. Usefulness of procalcitonin clearance as a prognostic biomarker in septic shock. A prospective pilot study. Med Intensiva 2012;36:475–80.
15. Lobo SM. Sequential C-reactive protein measurements in patients with serious infections: does it help? Crit Care 2012;16:130.
16. Bullen JJ, Rogers HJ, Spalding PB, et al. Iron and infection: the heart of the matter. FEMS Immunol Med Microbiol 2005;43:325–30.
17. Garcia PC, Longhi F, Branco RG, et al. Ferritin levels in children with severe sepsis and septic shock. Acta Paediatr 2007;96:1829–31.
18. Demirkol D, Yildizdas D, Bayrakci B, et al. Hyperferritinemia in the critically ill child with secondary HLH/sepsis/MODS/MAS: what is the treatment? Crit Care 2012;16:R52.
19. Tervonen V, Arjamaa O, Kokkonen K, et al. A novel cardiac hormone related to A-, B- and C-type natriuretic peptides. Endocrinology 1998;139:4021–5.
20. de Lemos JA, McGuire DK, Drazner MH. B-type natriuretic peptide in cardiovascular disease. Lancet 2003;362:316–22.
21. Cohen S, Springer C, Avital A, et al. Amino-terminal pro-brain-type natriuretic peptide: heart or lung disease in pediatric respiratory distress? Pediatrics 2005;115:1347–50.
22. Koulouri S, Acherman RJ, Wong PC, et al. Utility of B-type natriuretic peptide in differentiating congestive heart failure from lung disease in pediatric patients with respiratory distress. Pediatr Cardiol 2004;25:341–6.
23. Domico M, Liao P, Anas N, et al. Elevation of brain natriuretic peptide levels in children with septic shock. Pediatr Crit Care Med 2008;9:478–83.
24. Adams JE 3rd, Bodor GS, Davila-Roman VG, et al. Cardiac troponin I. A marker with high specificity for cardiac injury. Circulation 1993;88:101–6.
25. Carcillo JA, Pollack MM, Ruttimann UE, et al. Sequential physiologic interactions in pediatric cardiogenic and septic shock. Crit Care Med 1989;17:12–6.
26. Pollack MM, Fields AI, Ruttimann UE. Distributions of cardiopulmonary variables in pediatric survivors and nonsurvivors of septic shock. Crit Care Med 1985;13: 454–9.
27. Pollack MM, Fields AI, Ruttimann UE. Sequential cardiopulmonary variables of infants and children in septic shock. Crit Care Med 1984;12:554–9.

28. Simma B, Fritz MG, Trawoger R, et al. Changes in left ventricular function in shocked newborns. Intensive Care Med 1997;23:982–6.

29. Walther FJ, Siassi B, Ramadan NA, et al. Cardiac output in newborn infants with transient myocardial dysfunction. J Pediatr 1985;107:781–5.

30. Ceneviva G, Paschall JA, Maffei F, et al. Hemodynamic support in fluid-refractory pediatric septic shock. Pediatrics 1998;102:e19.

31. Brierley J, Carcillo JA, Choong K, et al. Clinical practice parameters for hemodynamic support of pediatric and neonatal septic shock: 2007 update from the American College of Critical Care Medicine. Crit Care Med 2009;37:666–88.

32. Kliegman R, Nelson WE. Nelson textbook of pediatrics. 19th edition. Philadelphia: Elsevier Saunders; 2011.

33. Gardner RM, Beale RJ. Pressure to perform: is cardiac output estimation from arterial waveforms good enough for routine use? Crit Care Med 2009;37: 337–8.

34. Sun JX, Reisner AT, Saeed M, et al. The cardiac output from blood pressure algorithms trial. Crit Care Med 2009;37:72–80.

35. Fakler U, Pauli C, Balling G, et al. Cardiac index monitoring by pulse contour analysis and thermodilution after pediatric cardiac surgery. J Thorac Cardiovasc Surg 2007;133:224–8.

36. Mahajan A, Shabanie A, Turner J, et al. Pulse contour analysis for cardiac output monitoring in cardiac surgery for congenital heart disease. Anesth Analg 2003; 97:1283–8.

37. Tibby SM, Hatherill M, Marsh MJ, et al. Clinical validation of cardiac output measurements using femoral artery thermodilution with direct Fick in ventilated children and infants. Intensive Care Med 1997;23:987–91.

38. McLuckie A, Murdoch IA, Marsh MJ, et al. A comparison of pulmonary and femoral artery thermodilution cardiac indices in paediatric intensive care patients. Acta Paediatr 1996;85:336–8.

39. Pauli C, Fakler U, Genz T, et al. Cardiac output determination in children: equivalence of the transpulmonary thermodilution method to the direct Fick principle. Intensive Care Med 2002;28:947–52.

40. Jaffe MB. Partial CO2 rebreathing cardiac output–operating principles of the NICO system. J Clin Monit Comput 1999;15:387–401.

41. Chong SW, Peyton PJ. A meta-analysis of the accuracy and precision of the ultrasonic cardiac output monitor (USCOM). Anaesthesia 2012;67:1266–71.

42. Marik PE. Noninvasive cardiac output monitors: a state-of the-art review. J Cardiothorac Vasc Anesth 2013;27(1):121–34.

43. Keren H, Burkhoff D, Squara P. Evaluation of a noninvasive continuous cardiac output monitoring system based on thoracic bioreactance. Am J Physiol Heart Circ Physiol 2007;293:H583–9.

44. Ballestero Y, Lopez-Herce J, Urbano J, et al. Measurement of cardiac output in children by bioreactance. Pediatr Cardiol 2011;32:469–72.

45. Weisz DE, Jain A, McNamara PJ, et al. Non-invasive cardiac output monitoring in neonates using bioreactance: a comparison with echocardiography. Neonatology 2012;102:61–7.

46. Levitov A, Marik PE. Echocardiographic assessment of preload responsiveness in critically ill patients. Cardiol Res Pract 2012;2012:819696.

47. Marimon GA, Dockery WK, Sheridan MJ, et al. Near-infrared spectroscopy cerebral and somatic (renal) oxygen saturation correlation to continuous venous oxygen saturation via intravenous oximetry catheter. J Crit Care 2012;27: 314.e13–8.

48. Cruz AT, Perry AM, Williams EA, et al. Implementation of goal-directed therapy for children with suspected sepsis in the emergency department. Pediatrics 2011; 127:e758–66.

49. Han YY, Carcillo JA, Dragotta MA, et al. Early reversal of pediatric-neonatal septic shock by community physicians is associated with improved outcome. Pediatrics 2003;112:793–9.

50. Rivers E, Nguyen B, Havstad S, et al. Early goal-directed therapy in the treatment of severe sepsis and septic shock. N Engl J Med 2001;345:1368–77.

51. de Oliveira CF, de Oliveira DS, Gottschald AF, et al. ACCM/PALS haemodynamic support guidelines for paediatric septic shock: an outcomes comparison with and without monitoring central venous oxygen saturation. Intensive Care Med 2008;34:1065–75.

52. Maitland K, Kiguli S, Opoka RO, et al. Mortality after fluid bolus in African children with severe infection. N Engl J Med 2011;364:2483–95.

53. Finfer S, Bellomo R, Boyce N, et al. A comparison of albumin and saline for fluid resuscitation in the intensive care unit. N Engl J Med 2004;350:2247–56.

54. Wills BA, Nguyen MD, Ha TL, et al. Comparison of three fluid solutions for resuscitation in dengue shock syndrome. N Engl J Med 2005;353:877–89.

55. Perel P, Roberts I. Colloids versus crystalloids for fluid resuscitation in critically ill patients. Cochrane Database Syst Rev 2012;(6):CD000567.

56. Spaniol JR, Knight AR, Zebley JL, et al. Fluid resuscitation therapy for hemorrhagic shock. J Trauma Nurs 2007;14:152–60 [quiz: 61–2].

57. Laverdiere C, Gauvin F, Hebert PC, et al. Survey on transfusion practices of pediatric intensivists. Pediatr Crit Care Med 2002;3:335–40.

58. Lacroix J, Hebert PC, Hutchison JS, et al. Transfusion strategies for patients in pediatric intensive care units. N Engl J Med 2007;356:1609–19.

59. Tyrrell CT, Bateman ST. Critically ill children: to transfuse or not to transfuse packed red blood cells, that is the question. Pediatr Crit Care Med 2012;13: 204–9.

60. Jonas RA, Wypij D, Roth SJ, et al. The influence of hemodilution on outcome after hypothermic cardiopulmonary bypass: results of a randomized trial in infants. J Thorac Cardiovasc Surg 2003;126:1765–74.

61. Bell EF, Strauss RG, Widness JA, et al. Randomized trial of liberal versus restrictive guidelines for red blood cell transfusion in preterm infants. Pediatrics 2005; 115:1685–91.

62. Kirpalani H, Whyte RK, Andersen C, et al. The Premature Infants in Need of Transfusion (PINT) study: a randomized, controlled trial of a restrictive (low) versus liberal (high) transfusion threshold for extremely low birth weight infants. J Pediatr 2006;149:301–7.

63. Beale RJ, Hollenberg SM, Vincent JL, et al. Vasopressor and inotropic support in septic shock: an evidence-based review. Crit Care Med 2004;32: S455–65.

64. Shekerdemian L, Redington A. Cardiovascular pharmacology. In: Chang AC, editor. Pediatric cardiac intensive care, vol. xxiv. Baltimore (MD): Williams & Wilkins; 1998. p. 574.

65. Kelly M, Sturgill M, Notterman D. Pharmacology of the cardiovascular system. In: Fuhrman B, Zimmerman J, editors. Pediatric critical care, vol. xxviii, 3rd edition. Philadelphia: Mosby-Elsevier; 2006. p. 1872, 10 p. of plates.

66. Choong K, Bohn D, Fraser DD, et al. Vasopressin in pediatric vasodilatory shock: a multicenter randomized controlled trial. Am J Respir Crit Care Med 2009;180: 632–9.

67. Yildizdas D, Yapicioglu H, Celik U, et al. Terlipressin as a rescue therapy for catecholamine-resistant septic shock in children. Intensive Care Med 2008;34: 511–7.
68. Pizarro CF, Troster EJ, Damiani D, et al. Absolute and relative adrenal insufficiency in children with septic shock. Crit Care Med 2005;33:855–9.
69. Smith L, Hernan L. Shock states. In: Fuhrman BP, Zimmerman JJ, editors. Pediatric critical care, vol. xxviii, 3rd edition. Philadelphia: Mosby-Elsevier; 2006. p. 1872, 10 p. of plates.
70. Zimmerman JJ, Williams MD. Adjunctive corticosteroid therapy in pediatric severe sepsis: observations from the RESOLVE study. Pediatr Crit Care Med 2011;12:2–8.
71. Aneja R, Carcillo JA. What is the rationale for hydrocortisone treatment in children with infection-related adrenal insufficiency and septic shock? Arch Dis Child 2007;92:165–9.
72. Kumar A, Roberts D, Wood KE, et al. Duration of hypotension before initiation of effective antimicrobial therapy is the critical determinant of survival in human septic shock. Crit Care Med 2006;34:1589–96.
73. Gaieski DF, Mikkelsen ME, Band RA, et al. Impact of time to antibiotics on survival in patients with severe sepsis or septic shock in whom early goal-directed therapy was initiated in the emergency department. Crit Care Med 2010;38: 1045–53.
74. Schortgen F, Clabault K, Katsahian S, et al. Fever control using external cooling in septic shock: a randomized controlled trial. Am J Respir Crit Care Med 2012;185: 1088–95.
75. Schmidt-Schweda S, Ohler A, Post H, et al. Moderate hypothermia for severe cardiogenic shock (COOL Shock Study I & II). Resuscitation 2012. http:// dx.doi.org/10.1016/j.resuscitation.2012.09.034.
76. Thiagarajan RR, Laussen PC, Rycus PT, et al. Extracorporeal membrane oxygenation to aid cardiopulmonary resuscitation in infants and children. Circulation 2007;116:1693–700.
77. Morris MC, Wernovsky G, Nadkarni VM. Survival outcomes after extracorporeal cardiopulmonary resuscitation instituted during active chest compressions following refractory in-hospital pediatric cardiac arrest. Pediatr Crit Care Med 2004;5:440–6.
78. Costello JM, Cooper DS, Jacobs JP, et al. Intermediate-term outcomes after paediatric cardiac extracorporeal membrane oxygenation–what is known (and unknown). Cardiol Young 2011;21(Suppl 2):118–23.
79. Maclaren G, Butt W, Best D, et al. Extracorporeal membrane oxygenation for refractory septic shock in children: one institution's experience. Pediatr Crit Care Med 2007;8:447–51.
80. Sharma MS, Forbess JM, Guleserian KJ. Ventricular assist device support in children and adolescents with heart failure: the Children's Medical Center of Dallas experience. Artif Organs 2012;36:635–9.

# Advances in Pediatric Cardiac Intensive Care

Ronald A. Bronicki, MD*, Paul A. Checchia, MD

## KEYWORDS

- Pediatric • Cardiac surgery • Outcomes • Monitoring
- Mechanical circulatory support

## KEY POINTS

- Prevention of neurologic injury following cardiac surgery or critical cardiac events has become one of the overarching goals of pediatric cardiac critical care.
- Advances in hemodynamic monitoring are allowing early, goal-directed therapy, thereby reducing complications and improving outcomes.
- The evolution of pediatric mechanical circulatory support represents one of the most significant advancements in pediatric critical cardiac disease.

## INTRODUCTION

Pediatric cardiac intensive care continues to evolve, which is in large part the result of collaborative efforts from anesthesia, surgery, cardiology, critical care, and other subspecialties, including neonatology and neurology. Examples include an increasing number of surgeries in very low birth weight infants; the application of advances in neuroimaging; the extension of technology such as cerebral oximetry from the operating room into the intensive care setting; and innovations in mechanical circulatory devices. Industry-sponsored studies and initiatives from the National Institutes of Health such as the Pediatric Heart Network have contributed to the evolution of pediatric cardiac critical care. These collective efforts are evident in the recently published results of the Berlin EXCOR Ventricular Assist Device trial and the Single Ventricle Reconstruction trial.

The increase in complexity of disease, innovations in technology, and evolving therapeutic strategies, as well as national quality initiatives, individually and collectively place a serious demand on the team, necessitating a focused, concerted effort by all members to challenge current practices while practicing state-of the-art care. Outcomes for pediatric cardiac diseases have improved so much in the past decades

Cardiac Intensive Care Unit, Texas Children's Hospital, Baylor College of Medicine, 6621 Fannin Street, Suite WT6-006, Houston, TX 77030, USA
* Corresponding author.
*E-mail address:* rxbronic@texaschildrens.org

Pediatr Clin N Am 60 (2013) 655–667
http://dx.doi.org/10.1016/j.pcl.2013.02.004
0031-3955/13/$ – see front matter © 2013 Elsevier Inc. All rights reserved.

that there is now the expectation of perfection and a zero tolerance for complications. Improved mortality is no longer an acceptable goal. This article presents recent advancements in the field that are designed to give improved outcomes that are meaningful, low cost, high value, and reproducible.

## NEUROLOGIC INJURY AND NEURODEVELOPMENT

Since the first intracardiac repair of congenital heart disease in 1953 (an atrial septal defect by Dr John Gibbon), the mortality in pediatric cardiac surgery has progressively declined, and is currently at less than 3%. With these successes came the appreciation that survivors displayed a high incidence of neurologic, developmental, and psychiatric disabilities. Over the last several years the focus has shifted from efforts directed at improving survival to efforts to improve neurodevelopmental outcomes. Identification of perioperative factors responsible for neurologic injury and impaired neurodevelopment may allow implementation of strategies that will lead to improved outcomes.

With advancements in magnetic resonance imaging (MRI) over the last several years, it has become clear that for some patients abnormal neurodevelopment begins in utero. Limperopoulos and colleagues[1] used three-dimensional volumetric MRI and proton magnetic resonance (MR) spectroscopy to show progressive and significant declines in gestational age-adjusted total brain volume in third-trimester fetuses with some forms of congenital heart disease compared with controls. They also found evidence of impaired neuroaxonal development and metabolism. Abnormal in utero cerebral perfusion impairs cerebral metabolism, and may contribute to impaired neurologic development.[2]

Miller and colleagues[3] used MR spectroscopy and diffusion tensor imaging in newborns with transposition of the great arteries or single-ventricle physiology and found abnormalities of brain metabolism and microstructure before surgery. These alterations were shown in areas of the brain where visible injury on MRI was unappreciated. These abnormalities were widespread and did not conform to the pattern of brain injury that is consistent with hypoxic-ischemic injury of newborns. Syndromic congenital heart disease such as Down, DiGeorge, and Williams include significant neurodevelopmental abnormalities. Additional less well-defined genetic factors may also affect neurodevelopment and recovery from neurologic insults such as ischemia-reperfusion injury.[4–6]

The advent of noninvasive monitoring of cerebral oxygenation (discussed later) has identified intraoperative and postoperative cerebral hypoxia as an additional factor responsible for neurologic injury and adverse neurodevelopmental outcomes.[6–8] Kussman and colleagues[6] found perioperative periods of diminished cerebral oxygenation in infants undergoing biventricular repair without aortic arch reconstruction to be associated with significantly lower 1-year psychomotor development index scores and brain MRI abnormalities. Dent and colleagues[7] evaluated brain MRIs before and following the Norwood procedure. Postoperative imaging showed new or worsened ischemic lesions in 73% of patients, which were associated with prolonged low postoperative cerebral oximetry.

Studies have identified the length of stay in the intensive care unit to be strongly associated with adverse neurodevelopmental outcomes, even when adjusting for perioperative events.[9,10] One factor responsible for this relationship may be the exposure of developing brains to sedatives, analgesics, and anesthetics.[11] Noxious and painful stimuli trigger an immediate neuroendocrine and metabolic stress response that has as an adverse impact in the immediate postoperative period and leads to impaired brain development and abnormalities in behavior. Sedatives and analgesics are provided to minimize the adverse affects of these stimuli; however, the use of these agents is associated with adverse neurodevelopment in newborn animals. Sedatives and analgesics that act through altering synaptic transmission at gamma-aminobutyrate type A ($GABA_A$) (benzodiazepines, propofol, chloral hydrate) and N-methyl-D-aspartate glutamate (NMDA) (ketamine) receptors may interfere with normal brain development, because GABA-mediated and NMDA-mediated neuronal activity are essential for normal brain development. Several studies in newborn animals have shown widespread neuronal death and impaired neurocognitive function associated with exposure to these agents. Opioids act through different receptors but have also been shown to have a detrimental affect on the developing brain and neuro-developmental outcomes. The extent to which these findings can be extrapolated to the clinical setting remains to be determined and is currently being evaluated.

## CARDIOPULMONARY BYPASS–INDUCED INFLAMMATION

Cardiopulmonary bypass (CPB) invariably, and to varying degrees, stimulates a systemic inflammatory response that contributes to the development of postopera-tive organ dysfunction, most notably an increase in vascular permeability, pulmonary edema, and myocardial dysfunction. Kirklin and colleagues[12] were the first to show a positive relationship between complement activation and postoperative morbidity in adults and children undergoing cardiac surgery. The primary stimuli for the inflam-matory response are exposure of the blood elements to the nonendothelialized circuit and myocardial and pulmonary reperfusion injury.[13–15] Numerous studies in animals and humans have investigated the potential role of immune-modulatory strategies for ameliorating the inflammatory response to CPB. Glucocorticoids have been the most extensively studied and are used by most pediatric cardiac centers in the United States and United Kingdom.[16]

There have been several small prospective randomized studies that have evaluated the role of glucocorticoids in suppressing the inflammatory response to CPB.[17–20] Initial studies showed an improved postoperative course and evidence of reduced myocardial injury in those patients randomized to glucocorticoids before CPB. Two recently conducted prospective randomized dose-response studies evaluated whether an additional dose of glucocorticoids was of any benefit.[21,22] Patients were randomized to receive a dose of glucocorticoid or placebo 8 hours before the intrao-perative dose. Although each study showed a significant reduction in serum inflamma-tory mediators in patients who received 2 doses of glucocorticoids, neither study showed an improved postoperative course. Checchia and colleagues[23] evaluated a novel strategy for ameliorating the inflammatory response to CPB by delivering gaseous nitric oxide to the membrane oxygenator. Nitric oxide modulates the interac-tions between platelets, neutrophils, and endothelial cells, thereby exerting an antiin-flammatory effect. There was evidence of reduced myocardial injury and an improved postoperative course in those infants randomized to therapy.

## ASSESSMENT OF CARDIOVASCULAR FUNCTION AND TISSUE OXYGENATION

The primary task in the critical care setting is to make a timely and accurate assess-ment of cardiovascular function, cardiac output, and tissue oxygenation. Studies have shown that estimations of these hemodynamic parameters based on routine or stan-dard clinical parameters, such as the physical examination, heart rate, blood pressure, and urine output, are often discordant from measured values.[24] Studies in children have shown that there is no correlation between estimations of cardiac output and systemic vascular resistance based on peripheral pulses, capillary refill, and peripheral to core body temperatures, and measured values of these parameters.[25,26] Although the physical examination and the interpretation of standard hemodynamic parameters are essential parts of the assessment of cardiovascular function, studies have shown that the adjunctive use of technology such as near-infrared spectroscopy–derived tissue oxygenation and venous oximetry are invaluable tools in this assessment.[27–29]

### Venous Oximetry

Venous oximetry relies on the measurement of mixed venous oxygen saturations to evaluate the relationship between oxygen delivery ($Do_2$) and oxygen demand ($Vo_2$), or oxygen transport balance, and in assessing the adequacy of tissue oxygenation (**Box 1**). As $Do_2$ decreases, oxygen extraction increases to maintain adequate oxygen availability. As $Do_2$ decreases further, oxygen extraction and the oxygen extraction ratio continue to increase (**Box 2, Fig. 1**); as the oxygen extraction ratio exceeds 50% to 60%, serum lactate levels begin to increase as its production exceeds its clearance, defining the onset of anaerobic metabolism and the critical oxygen extraction ratio (see **Box 2**). Thus, oxygen extraction increases and becomes critical before serum lactate levels begin to increase. The critical oxygen extraction ratio is 50% to 60%, regardless of whether the perturbation in oxygen transport balance is caused by hypoxemia, anemia, low cardiac output, or an increase in oxygen demand.

Mixed venous oxygen saturations are seldom available because the use of pulmonary artery catheters has declined significantly over the last several years. Central venous oximetry is increasingly being used and studies have shown a good correlation between central venous (right atrium or superior vena cava) and pulmonary artery saturations (in the absence of left to right cardiac shunting).[30] Studies have shown that the use of central venous oximetry to guide resuscitation in pediatric and adult septic shock and its use in managing patients following the Norwood procedure have led to improved survival.[27–29]

### Cerebral Near-infrared Spectroscopy

Cerebral near-infrared spectroscopy noninvasively measures cerebral oxygenation and, in doing so, assesses the relationship between cerebral oxygen delivery and oxygen demand or cerebral oxygen transport balance.

This technology was introduced into the clinical setting in the mid-1990s, when it was used to monitor cerebral oxygenation during cardiopulmonary bypass in adults.

---

**Box 1**
**Oxygen transport balance**

Fick equation:

$$Vo_2 = CO \times Cao_2 - Cvo_2 I$$

By ignoring the amount of oxygen dissolved in blood, the Fick equation may be simplified to:

$$Sao_2 - Smvo_2 = Vo_2/Do_2 = \text{Oxygen transport balance}$$

$Vo_2$, oxygen consumption (mL/min); CO, cardiac output (L/min); $Cao_2$, arterial oxygen content (m$Lo_2$/dL); $Cvo_2$, venous oxygen content (m$Lo_2$/dL); $Sao_2$, arterial oxygen saturation; $Smvo_2$, mixed venous oxygen saturation; $Do_2$, oxygen delivery (CO $\times$ $Cao_2$; m$LO_2$/min).

| Box 2 |
| --- |
| **Oxygen extraction ratio** |

A. Oxygen extraction ratio ($o_2ER$)

$$o_2ER = \frac{Sao_2 - Smvo_2}{Sao_2}$$

$Sao_2$, arterial oxygen saturation; $Smvo_2$, mixed venous oxygen saturation

B. Oxygen extraction ratios

   25%, normal

   30% to 40%, increased

   40 to 50%, impending shock

   >50% to 60%, shock, lactic acidosis

Based on mixed venous oxygen saturations.

It has since been applied to pediatric cardiac surgery and, over the last several years, this technology has permeated pediatric critical care and pediatric cardiac critical care units. The first cerebral oximetry device to receive US Food and Drug Administration (FDA) approval was the INVOS system (Covidien Corp., Boulder, CO) (**Fig. 2**).

Cerebral oximetry relies on the relative transparency of biologic tissue to near-infrared light, whereas oxyhemoglobin and deoxyhemoglobin have distinct absorption spectra. The proprietary algorithm monitors the nonpulsatile signal reflecting the microcirculation where 75% to 85% of the blood volume is venous. Thus, the oxygen saturation is used as an indicator of oxygen extraction for the area of the brain immediately beneath the probe (frontal cortex). Because of technical constraints, the technology is limited to relative quantitation and is thus useful for tracking changes for a given patient. Studies have shown a good correlation between cerebral oxygen saturations and jugular bulb and superior vena cava saturations.[31,32] Li and colleagues[33]

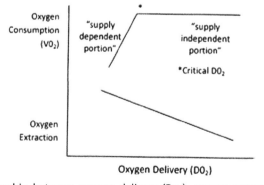

Fig. 1. The relationship between oxygen delivery ($Do_2$), oxygen consumption ($Vo_2$), and oxygen extraction. At first, as $Do_2$ decreases, $Vo_2$ remains constant as a result of an increase in oxygen extraction ($Vo_2$ is independent of $Do_2$). As $Do_2$ decreases further, oxygen extraction continues to increase but not enough to maintain a constant $Vo_2$ ($Vo_2$ becomes dependent on $Do_2$). The critical $Do_2$ is defined when $Vo_2$ begins to decrease.

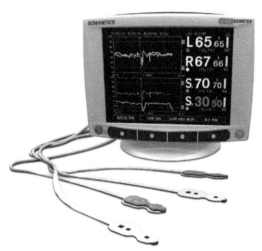

**Fig. 2.** The INVOS cerebral/somatic oximeter monitor with sensors. (*Courtesy of* Nellcor Puritan Bennett LLC, Boulder, CO, doing business as Covidien; with permission.)

found cerebral oxygen saturations to closely and negatively correlate with the oxygen extraction ratio derived from the superior vena cava in patients following the Norwood procedure.

Cerebral oximetry is also used as a surrogate for central and mixed venous oxygen; however, the correlation between these readings is marginal. In a low cardiac output state, blood flow is redistributed to maintain perfusion of vital organs. Thus, global indicators of oxygen supply/demand such as central or mixed venous oxygen saturations decrease earlier and to a greater extent than would an indicator of cerebral oxygenation. Another consideration is the effect of changes in $Paco_2$ on cerebral blood flow. Changes in $Paco_2$ uncouple cerebral blood flow from metabolism. As $Paco_2$ increases, for example, cerebral vascular resistance decreases and cerebral blood flow increases. Thus, cerebral oxygenation increases and the cerebral oxygen extraction ratio decreases without changes in cerebral oxygen demand or systemic perfusion. The converse occurs with decreases in $Paco_2$. In addition, because of the technical constraints described earlier, cerebral oximetry is useful for trend monitoring and a relative quantitation of cerebral and global oxygenation, rather than as an absolute indication. Despite these limitations, a clear understanding of the differences in pathophysiology of global and regional tissue oxygenation enables the clinician to use cerebral oximetry as an indicator of global oxygen transport balance.

### Echocardiography

Echocardiography is an essential diagnostic tool in the critical care setting, providing information about cardiopulmonary function that is not available from other monitoring modalities. Access to this information may be hampered by the limited availability of experienced sonographers and cardiologists and by the limited number of these expensive and cumbersome devices. The advent of portable and inexpensive ultrasound platforms that produce high-quality images has contributed to the evolving use of echocardiography as an acute monitoring modality, readily enabling critical care physicians to perform a timely and accurate diagnosis and to monitor responses to interventions. Studies have shown that with adequate, albeit limited, training the accuracy of limited transthoracic echocardiograms performed by noncardiologists is good. Emergency medicine resident curriculum formally includes ultrasound education, a practice that is supported by the American Society of Echocardiography.[34] With this approach, echocardiography plays an integral role in the acute management of critically ill patients.

As discussed earlier, the routine or standard clinical assessment of cardiovascular function has significant limitations. The use of technology such as echocardiography further shows the limitations of this approach and also shows the important role that additional strategies (eg, monitoring venous oximetry) and technologies (eg, cerebral oximetry and portable ultrasound platforms) play in overcoming these clinical shortfalls by establishing a timely and accurate diagnosis of cardiovascular function and tissue oxygenation. Spencer and colleagues[35] showed the limited ability of experienced clinicians to detect cardiovascular abnormalities on physical examination. Thirty-six adult patients with cardiovascular disease underwent physical examination by 4 board-certified cardiologists, the results of which were compared with findings from a complete echocardiographic study. When considering only the major cardiovascular findings, the cardiologists' physical examination failed to correctly detect 43% of these abnormalities. The use of the portable ultrasound platform by a cardiologist reduced this to 21%. Other studies have shown similar findings.[36,37]

Several hemodynamic parameters can be readily assessed with a limited transthoracic echocardiogram. Left ventricular systolic function can be evaluated by determining the fractional shortening, which is a determination of the change in left ventricular short-axis diameter based on one-dimensional wall motion analysis or M-mode echocardiography. The primary limitation of this technique is that the contraction of the left ventricle cannot be assumed to be uniform or symmetric. M-mode interrogation may not capture regional differences in wall motion and wall thickening. A flattened interventricular septum similarly nullifies the measurement. Two-dimensional imaging measures left ventricular systolic function by quantifying changes in ventricular volume during the cardiac cycle. This technique relies on the modified Simpson rule method for measuring volumes. Because of its complex geometric shape and the motion of the interventricular septum during systole, an assessment of right ventricular systolic function is most often qualitative and based on the inward motion of the right ventricular free wall toward the ventricular septum. Assessment of ventricular systolic function with either technique is sensitive to ventricular loading conditions and heart rate. The presence of tricuspid or mitral valve insufficiency allows the ventricle to eject retrograde into a low-pressure atrium while increasing ventricular operating volumes. Thus, an index of systolic function in this setting is expected to be normal if not greater than normal. In those with significant experience of reading echocardiograms, there is a good correlation between visually estimated and measured ejection fractions.[38,39] Ventricular wall thickness can be assessed, giving some indication of diastolic function, as can ventricular volume, giving some indication of operating volumes.

The use of continuous wave and color Doppler enables clinicians to estimate intracardiac and vascular pressures by measuring the velocity of blood in relation to the ultrasound beam. Based on a modified Bernoulli equation, the pressure gradient that exists across an obstructive lesion is equal to $4 V^2$, where V is the velocity of blood as is accelerates across a narrowed orifice. Pulmonary artery systolic pressure may be estimated by interrogating the tricuspid regurgitant jet. Another method for assessing pulmonary artery pressures is to evaluate the position and orientation of the interventricular septum during ventricular systole. The transseptal pressure gradient determines the position and orientation of the septum throughout the cardiac cycle. Under normal conditions, left ventricular pressures exceed right ventricular pressures. As a result, the interventricular septum bows into the right ventricle throughout the cardiac cycle. With systolic flattening of the interventricular septum, right ventricular systolic pressure is at least half systemic. In a similar way, the orientation of the septum during ventricular diastole gives some indication of biventricular filling pressures. A midline position during diastole indicates that filling pressures are similar. In this instance, the deviated septum reduces the effective compliance of the left ventricle. The modified Bernoulli equation may be used to assess the pressure gradients across valves, septum, and coarctations. A qualitative assessment may also be made on the severity of a regurgitant valve. The presence, magnitude, and physiologic consequence of a pericardial effusion can be determined. The earliest indication of tamponade physiology is collapse of the right atrium. Interrogation of the atrial and ventricular septum may used to detect right to left shunting and thus provide an explanation for refractory arterial hypoxemia. The appearance of left-sided saline contrast and the use of color Doppler may be used to detect right to left intracardiac shunting.

## MECHANICAL CIRCULATORY SUPPORT

Mechanical circulatory support devices may be used as a bridge to recovery, as in fulminant myocarditis and postcardiotomy syndrome, or as a bridge to transplantation. The mainstay of short-term pediatric mechanical circulatory support has been, and remains, extracorporeal membrane oxygenation (ECMO) and the centrifugal ventricular assist device (VAD). In general, long-term mechanical circulatory support in pediatrics has relied on ECMO with a 47% to 57% rate of survival to transplantation.[40] Over the last several years, several long-term VADs have been designed for or applied to the pediatric patient, leading to improved outcomes.[40] A study of the Pediatric Heart Transplant Study database found a survival to transplantation rate of 77% using VADs from 1993 to 2003, with an even higher success rate from 2000 to 2003 of 86%. Despite improved overall outcomes, the success rate is significantly lower in patients with congenital heart disease and in smaller, younger patients.

The Berlin Heart EXCOR (Berlin GmbH, Berlin, Germany) is the first commercially available long-term VAD designed for the pediatric population. It has specialized cannulae and a miniaturized pneumatically driven pump that produces pulsatile flow. The device is suitable for patients with a body weight of greater than 2.5 kg and there are several sizes to choose from (**Fig. 3**). The device may be implanted as a left VAD or bilateral VAD. The Berlin EXCOR has been in use in Europe since 1992. A recently published prospective, multicenter study compared children who underwent implantation of the Berlin EXCOR VAD as a bridge to transplantation with a historical control group of children from the Extracorporeal Life Support Organization (ELSO) registry who received circulatory support with ECMO.[41] A propensity-score

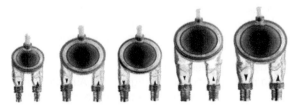

**Fig. 3.** Berlin Heart EXCOR pumps of different sizes (range 1–60 mL). (*Courtesy of* Berlin Heart, The Woodlands, TX; with permission.)

analysis was used to match each participant who received a VAD to 2 children who had received support with ECMO. VAD recipients were divided into 2 cohorts based on body surface area (BSA): cohort 1 included children with a BSA of less than 0.7 m$^2$ and cohort 2 children with a BSA between 0.7 m$^2$ and 1.5 m$^2$. At 30 days, the number of children receiving mechanical support, having undergone transplantation, or having been weaned from mechanical support was significantly higher for both VAD cohorts ($P = .048$ and $P = .007$ for cohorts 1 and 2, respectively) compared with ECMO matched groups. At the end of circulatory support, the number of children having undergone transplantation or having been weaned from the device was significantly greater for the VAD cohorts than for the ECMO matched groups ($P = .059$ and $P = .021$ for cohorts 1 and 2, respectively). Following the results of this study, the Berlin EXCOR VAD received FDA approval.

## SINGLE-VENTRICLE PHYSIOLOGY

Single-ventricle physiology is present when there is complete mixing of systemic and pulmonary venous return, and the determinant of pulmonary and systemic blood flow ($Q_p$ and $Q_s$, respectively) is the relative resistances in the pulmonary and systemic circulations (the pulmonary vascular resistance [PVR]/systemic vascular resistance [SVR] ratio). Single-ventricle–like physiology may also be present in certain neonates with biventricular anatomy, such as those with an interrupted aortic arch, critical aortic stenosis, and truncus arteriosus, with the caveat being that in some cases there may not be complete mixing of systemic and pulmonary venous return. Blood flow to the systemic and pulmonary circulations is ideally balanced, thus minimizing the ventricular volume load while maintaining $Q_s$. The ratio of systemic and pulmonary blood flow may be calculated by the following modified Fick equation: $Q_p/Q_s = (Sao_2 - Scvo_2)/(Spvo_2 - Spao_2)$, where $Sao_2$ is aortic saturation (and therefore $Spao_2$ or pulmonary artery oxygen saturation); $Scvo_2$ is central venous saturation (estimated by the superior vena cava oxygen saturation); and $Spvo_2$ is pulmonary venous oxygen saturation.

If the systemic venous and pulmonary venous oxygen saturations are unknown and if normal values are assumed for each, the calculated $Q_p/Q_s$ ratio may underestimate the $Q_p/Q_s$ ratio and therefore increasing the propensity to develop inadequate $Q_s$. Studies have shown that pulmonary venous saturations are commonly depressed following the Norwood procedure, particularly in those patients on room air[42]; clinical parameters such as systemic blood pressure and $Sao_2$ are not indicators of $Q_s$. As described earlier, the physical examination does not reliably indicate $Q_s$. Cerebral near-infrared spectroscopy and central venous oximetry (see sections on venous oximetry and cerebral near-infrared spectroscopy) may be used to provide a more robust estimation of the $Q_p/Q_s$ ratio and, more importantly, the adequacy of $Q_s$.

### Hypoplastic Left Heart Syndrome and the Norwood Procedure

The hypoplastic left heart syndrome (HLHS) is characterized by hypoplasia/atresia of left-sided structures and a dependence on a patent ductus arteriosus to maintain systemic perfusion. Surgical palliation, the Norwood procedure, includes an atrial septectomy, ensuring unrestricted pulmonary venous return to the right atrium; placement of a restrictive subclavian or innominate artery to pulmonary artery shunt (modified Blalock-Taussig [mBT] shunt) to secure pulmonary blood flow; arch reconstruction to eliminate obstruction to systemic flow; and construction of a neoaorta, which involves anastomosing the main pulmonary artery to the markedly hypoplastic ascending aorta and the use of homograft tissue. Coronary blood flow is thus provided in a retrograde manner, relying on an unobstructed neoaorta as the conduit for perfusion of coronary ostia. Mortality from the Norwood procedure has decreased dramatically from greater than 50% to 10 to 25% in the current era. Several clinical innovations are responsible for improved outcomes.

The use of intraoperative and postoperative afterload reduction has been shown to improve outcomes.[43–46] Perioperative management historically focused on manipulation of the pulmonary circulation to maintain adequate $Q_s$ (for example, altering PVR by manipulating ventilation and oxygenation). However, over the last 10 years or so, it has become increasingly clear that limiting increases in SVR has a much greater impact on $Q_s$. Systemic vascular resistance is greater than PVR and in the parallel circulation of single-ventricle physiology this increases $Q_p$ at the expense of $Q_s$. As $Q_s$ wanes, SVR increases, further increasing the $Q_p/Q_s$ ratio and a vicious cycle ensues, culminating in circulatory failure. Afterload reduction limits increases in the SVR/PVR ratio while increasing stroke volume and total cardiac output ($Q_p + Q_s$). The increase in total cardiac output and reduction in SVR and PVR leads to an increase in oxygen content, systemic perfusion, and, most importantly, an increase in systemic oxygen delivery.[45,47]

Despite a marked improvement in outcomes for the Norwood procedure since its inception some 30 years ago, the mortality remains high, ranging from 10% to 20% with interstage mortality contributing an additional 10% (following the Norwood procedure and before the bidirectional Glenn). The prevailing consensus is that coronary perfusion becomes inadequate as a result of diastolic hypotension.

The mBT shunt allows for shunting throughout the cardiac cycle, resulting in diastolic runoff, retrograde flow in the descending aorta, and diastolic hypotension. Meanwhile, myocardial and circulatory demands are increased because of the inefficiencies of the parallel circulation. These factors have led to the emergence of the right ventricle to pulmonary artery shunt (RVPA shunt) as an alternative to the mBT shunt as the source of pulmonary blood flow. With the RVPA shunt, shunting occurs only during ventricular systole. Although some degree of conduit regurgitation is present, the primary concern of the RVPA shunt is the obligatory right ventriculotomy and its effect on long-term right ventricular function.

Studies have shown that the Norwood procedure with the RVPA shunt has significantly greater diastolic blood pressures and a tendency to have a lower $Q_p/Q_s$ ratio than the classic Norwood procedure.[48–50] The Pediatric Heart Network of the National Heart, Lung and Blood Institute recently completed a study in which infants undergoing the Norwood procedure were randomized to the mBT (n = 275) or the RVPA shunt (n = 274) at 15 North American centers.[51] The primary outcome was death or cardiac transplantation 12 months after randomization. Transplantation-free survival at 12 months was higher with the RVPA shunt than with the mBT shunt (74 vs 64%, $P = .01$). In addition, the rate of composite serious adverse events (death, acute shunt failure, cardiac arrest, extracorporeal membrane oxygenation, unplanned cardiovascular reoperation, or necrotizing enterocolitis) was significantly lower in those randomized to the RVPA shunt (98 [36%] vs 133 [48%], $P = .02$) during hospitalization for the Norwood procedure. Data collected over a mean follow-up period of 32 ±11 months showed a trend toward transplantation-free survival between groups ($P = .06$).

## SUMMARY

Pediatric cardiac critical care has made, and continues to make, significant strides in improving outcomes. It is a measure of these successes that much of the discussion in this article does not focus on the reduction of mortality, but rather on perioperative management strategies intended to improve neurologic outcomes. The care of children with critical cardiac disease will continue to rely on broad and collaborative efforts by specialists and primary care practitioners to build on this foundation of success.

## REFERENCES

1. Limperopoulos C, Tworetzky W, McElhinney DB, et al. Brain volume and metabolism in fetuses with congenital heart disease: evaluation with quantitative magnetic resonance imaging and spectroscopy. Circulation 2010;121:26–33.
2. Kaltman JR, Di H, Tian Z, et al. Impact of congenital heart disease on cerebrovascular blood flow dynamics in the fetus. Ultrasound Obstet Gynecol 2005;25:32–6.
3. Miller SP, McQuillen PS, Hamrick S, et al. Abnormal brain development in newborns with congenital heart disease. N Engl J Med 2007;357:1928–38.
4. Gaynor JW, Wernovsky G, Jarvik GP, et al. Patient characteristics are important determinants of neurodevelopmental outcome at one year of age after neonatal and infant cardiac surgery. J Thorac Cardiovasc Surg 2007;133:1344–53, 1353.e1–3.
5. Gaynor JW, Nord AS, Wernovsky G, et al. Apolipoprotein e genotype modifies the risk of behavior problems after infant cardiac surgery. Pediatrics 2009;124: 241–50.
6. Kussman BD, Wypij D, DiNardo JA, et al. Cerebral oximetry during infant cardiac surgery: evaluation and relationship to early postoperative outcome. Anesth Analg 2009;108:1122–31.
7. Dent CL, Spaeth JP, Jones BV, et al. Brain magnetic resonance imaging abnormalities after the Norwood procedure using regional cerebral perfusion. J Thorac Cardiovasc Surg 2006;131:190–7.
8. McQuillen PS, Barkovich AJ, Hamrick SE, et al. Temporal and anatomic risk profile of brain injury with neonatal repair of congenital heart defects. Stroke 2007;38:736–41.
9. Newburger JW, Wypij D, Bellinger DC, et al. Length of stay after infant heart surgery is related to cognitive outcome at age 8 years. J Pediatr 2003;143:67–73.
10. Limperopoulos C, Majnemer A, Shevell MI, et al. Predictors of developmental disabilities after open heart surgery in young children with congenital heart defects. J Pediatr 2002;141:51–8.
11. Loepke AW. Developmental neurotoxicity of sedatives and anesthetics: a concern for neonatal and pediatric critical care medicine? Pediatr Crit Care Med 2010;11: 217–26.
12. Kirklin JK, Westaby S, Blackstone EH, et al. Complement and the damaging effects of cardiopulmonary bypass. J Thorac Cardiovasc Surg 1983;86:845–57.
13. Kronon MT, Allen BS, Halldorsson A, et al. Dose dependency of L-arginine in neonatal myocardial protection: the nitric oxide paradox. J Thorac Cardiovasc Surg 1999;118:655–64.
14. Fischer UM, Cox CS Jr, Laine GA, et al. Induction of cardioplegic arrest immediately activates the myocardial apoptosis signal pathway. Am J Physiol Heart Circ Physiol 2007;292:H1630–3.
15. Massoudy P, Zahler S, Becker BF, et al. Evidence for inflammatory responses of the lungs during coronary artery bypass grafting with cardiopulmonary bypass. Chest 2001;119:31–6.
16. Checchia PA, Bronicki RA, Costello JM, et al. Steroid use before pediatric cardiac operations using cardiopulmonary bypass: an international survey of 36 centers. Pediatr Crit Care Med 2005;6:441–4.

17. Bronicki RA, Backer CL, Baden HP, et al. Dexamethasone reduces the inflammatory response to cardiopulmonary bypass in children. Ann Thorac Surg 2000;69: 1490–5.

18. Checchia PA, Backer CL, Bronicki RA, et al. Dexamethasone reduces postoperative troponin levels in children undergoing cardiopulmonary bypass. Crit Care Med 2003;31:1742–5.

19. Schroeder VA, Pearl JM, Schwartz SM, et al. Combined steroid treatment for congenital heart surgery improves oxygen delivery and reduces postbypass inflammatory mediator expression. Circulation 2003;107:2823–8.

20. Malagon I, Hogenbirk K, van Pelt J, et al. Effect of dexamethasone on postoperative cardiac troponin T production in pediatric cardiac surgery. Intensive Care Med 2005;31:1420–6.

21. Bronicki RA, Checchia PA, Stuart-Killon RB, et al. The effects of multiple doses of glucocorticoids on the inflammatory response to cardiopulmonary bypass in children. World J Pediatr Congenit Heart Surg 2012;3:439–45.

22. Graham EM, Atz AM, Butts RJ, et al. Standardized preoperative corticosteroid treatment in neonates undergoing cardiac surgery: results from a randomized trial. J Thorac Cardiovasc Surg 2011;142:1523–9.

23. Checchia PA, Bronicki RA, Muenzer JT, et al. Nitric oxide delivery during cardiopulmonary bypass reduces postoperative morbidity in children - a randomized trial. J Thorac Cardiovasc Surg 2012. [Epub ahead of print].

24. Connors AF Jr, McCaffree DR, Gray BA. Evaluation of right-heart catheterization in the critically ill patient without acute myocardial infarction. N Engl J Med 1983; 308:263–7.

25. Tibby SM, Hatherill M, Murdoch IA. Capillary refill and core-peripheral temperature gap as indicators of haemodynamic status in paediatric intensive care patients. Arch Dis Child 1999;80:163–6.

26. Lobos AT, Lee S, Menon K. Capillary refill time and cardiac output in children undergoing cardiac catheterization. Pediatr Crit Care Med 2012;13:136–40.

27. Rivers E, Nguyen B, Havstad S, et al. Early goal-directed therapy in the treatment of severe sepsis and septic shock. N Engl J Med 2001;345:1368–77.

28. de Oliveira CF, de Oliveira DS, Gottschald AF, et al. ACCM/PALS haemodynamic support guidelines for paediatric septic shock: an outcomes comparison with and without monitoring central venous oxygen saturation. Intensive Care Med 2008;34:1065–75.

29. Tweddell JS, Hoffman GM, Mussatto KA, et al. Improved survival of patients undergoing palliation of hypoplastic left heart syndrome: lessons learned from 115 consecutive patients. Circulation 2002;106:I82–9.

30. Lee J, Wright F, Barber R, et al. Central venous oxygen saturation in shock: a study in man. Anesthesiology 1972;36:472–8.

31. Kirshbom PM, Forbess JM, Kogon BE, et al. Cerebral near infrared spectroscopy is a reliable marker of systemic perfusion in awake single ventricle children. Pediatr Cardiol 2007;28:42–5.

32. Nagdyman N, Fleck T, Schubert S, et al. Comparison between cerebral tissue oxygenation index measured by near-infrared spectroscopy and venous jugular bulb saturation in children. Intensive Care Med 2005;31:846–50.

33. Li J, Zhang G, Holtby H, et al. The influence of systemic hemodynamics and oxygen transport on cerebral oxygen saturation in neonates after the Norwood procedure. J Thorac Cardiovasc Surg 2008;135:83–90, 90.e1–2.

34. Labovitz AJ, Noble VE, Bierig M, et al. Focused cardiac ultrasound in the emergent setting: a consensus statement of the American Society of Echocardiography and

American College of Emergency Physicians. J Am Soc Echocardiogr 2010;23: 1225–30.

35. Spencer KT, Anderson AS, Bhargava A, et al. Physician-performed point-of-care echocardiography using a laptop platform compared with physical examination in the cardiovascular patient. J Am Coll Cardiol 2001;37:2013–8.

36. Kobal SL, Trento L, Baharami S, et al. Comparison of effectiveness of hand-carried ultrasound to bedside cardiovascular physical examination. Am J Cardiol 2005;96:1002–6.

37. Fedson S, Neithardt G, Thomas P, et al. Unsuspected clinically important findings detected with a small portable ultrasound device in patients admitted to a general medicine service. J Am Soc Echocardiogr 2003;16:901–5.

38. Rich S, Sheikh A, Gallastegui J, et al. Determination of left ventricular ejection fraction by visual estimation during real-time two-dimensional echocardiography. Am Heart J 1982;104:603–6.

39. Hope MD, de la Pena E, Yang PC, et al. A visual approach for the accurate determination of echocardiographic left ventricular ejection fraction by medical students. J Am Soc Echocardiogr 2003;16:824–31.

40. Blume ED, Naftel DC, Bastardi HJ, et al. Outcomes of children bridged to heart transplantation with ventricular assist devices: a multi-institutional study. Circulation 2006;113:2313–9.

41. Fraser CD Jr, Jaquiss RD, Rosenthal DN, et al. Prospective trial of a pediatric ventricular assist device. N Engl J Med 2012;367:532–41.

42. Taeed R, Schwartz SM, Pearl JM, et al. Unrecognized pulmonary venous desaturation early after Norwood palliation confounds Gp:Gs assessment and compromises oxygen delivery. Circulation 2001;103:2699–704.

43. Reddy VM, Liddicoat JR, McElhinney DB, et al. Hemodynamic effects of epinephrine, bicarbonate and calcium in the early postnatal period in a lamb model of single-ventricle physiology created in utero. J Am Coll Cardiol 1996;28:1877–83.

44. Stieh J, Fischer G, Scheewe J, et al. Impact of preoperative treatment strategies on the early perioperative outcome in neonates with hypoplastic left heart syndrome. J Thorac Cardiovasc Surg 2006;131:1122–1129.e2.

45. Tweddell JS, Hoffman GM, Fedderly RT, et al. Phenoxybenzamine improves systemic oxygen delivery after the Norwood procedure. Ann Thorac Surg 1999; 67:161–7 [discussion: 167–8].

46. De Oliveira NC, Ashburn DA, Khalid F, et al. Prevention of early sudden circulatory collapse after the Norwood operation. Circulation 2004;110:II133–8.

47. Hoffman GM, Tweddell JS, Ghanayem NS, et al. Alteration of the critical arteriovenous oxygen saturation relationship by sustained afterload reduction after the Norwood procedure. J Thorac Cardiovasc Surg 2004;127:738–45.

48. Bradley SM, Simsic JM, McQuinn TC, et al. Hemodynamic status after the Norwood procedure: a comparison of right ventricle-to-pulmonary artery connection versus modified Blalock-Taussig shunt. Ann Thorac Surg 2004;78:933–41 [discussion: 933–41].

49. Lai L, Laussen PC, Cua CL, et al. Outcomes after bidirectional Glenn operation: Blalock-Taussig shunt versus right ventricle-to-pulmonary artery conduit. Ann Thorac Surg 2007;83:1768–73.

50. Maher KO, Pizarro C, Gidding SS, et al. Hemodynamic profile after the Norwood procedure with right ventricle to pulmonary artery conduit. Circulation 2003;108: 782–4.

51. Ohye RG, Sleeper LA, Mahony L, et al. Comparison of shunt types in the Norwood procedure for single-ventricle lesions. N Engl J Med 2010;362:1980–92.

# Acute Kidney Injury in Children
## An Update on Diagnosis and Treatment

James D. Fortenberry, MD, MCCM[a,*], Matthew L. Paden, MD[a], Stuart L. Goldstein, MD[b]

## KEYWORDS

- Acute kidney injury • Pediatrics • Continuous renal replacement therapy
- Fluid overload • Septic shock • Extracorporeal therapies

## KEY POINTS

- The definitions and characterization of acute kidney injury (AKI) in children have advanced significantly over the past 2 decades.
- AKI is common in critically ill children and is associated with increased morbidity and mortality.
- AKI in association with sepsis, multiple organ involvement, and fluid overload carries heightened risk.
- Gene probes and urinary biomarkers represent intriguing tools for predicting and monitoring pediatric AKI, as well as potentially guiding treatment intervention.
- Treatment of AKI is problematic, but extracorporeal approaches in AKI and multiple organ system failure continue to grow in use and potential benefit.

*"In the kidneys are seated reasonings, and there dwells in them the faculty of discernment; they distinguish truth from falsehood, and judge what is base and what is noble."*

—*Saint Ephraem (ca 306–373 CE)*[1]

Ancient authors viewed the kidneys to be both the seats of reason and of discernment.[1] The kidneys, later termed "reins" in the English vernacular, were also seen as a source of divine punishment. Job described, among his many maladies, "my reins consume me."[1] Although our scientific understanding of the kidney has markedly evolved, we still find that the kidney does provide both a marker of outcome in critically ill adults and children, and a potential target for improving morbidity and mortality. This review focuses on updates in definition, epidemiology and outcomes, associated

[a] Critical Care Division, Department of Pediatrics, Emory University School of Medicine, Children's Healthcare of Atlanta at Egleston, 1405 Clifton Road North East, Atlanta, GA 30322, USA; [b] Center for Acute Care Nephrology, Cincinnati Children's Hospital Medical Center, Cincinnati, OH, USA
* Corresponding author.
*E-mail address:* james.fortenberry@choa.org

Pediatr Clin N Am 60 (2013) 669–688
http://dx.doi.org/10.1016/j.pcl.2013.02.006
0031-3955/13/$ – see front matter © 2013 Elsevier Inc. All rights reserved.

The KDIGO AKI definition and staging criteria should be used at the current time unless further modifications are warranted by prospective study.

The role of excessive fluid accumulation and its association with poor outcome in critically ill children is discussed later in this article; however, the potential for fluid accumulation to dilute serum creatinine concentration and alter the ascertainment of AKI based on serum creatinine change has been examined recently. In a post hoc analysis of the Fluid and Catheter Treatment trial, Liu and colleagues[14] corrected serum creatinine concentration based on fluid status. In this analysis, patients who fulfilled AKI by serum creatinine–based criteria after, but not before, fluid overload (FO) correction had significantly higher mortality than patients who did not meet AKI criteria before or after FO correction. In a study of infants after arterial switch operation, we found correction of serum creatinine for fluid balance increased the number of patients with severe AKI and strengthened the association of AKI with mortality.[15]

The repeated demonstration of serum creatinine as a late and unmodifiable functional AKI marker has led to a more than decade-long research effort to identify novel urinary AKI biomarkers that reflect kidney injury development and severity earlier than serum creatinine.[16] Numerous biomarkers discovered from animal models of AKI have been validated in humans and include neutrophil gelatinase–associated lipocalin (NGAL), kidney injury molecule-1 (KIM-1), interleukin-18 (IL-18), and liver type fatty acid binding protein, all of which are upregulated in the setting of ischemic kidney injury. Additional biomarkers that leak from tubular cells, such as alpha-glutathione-S-transferase (GST) and pi-GST, are also being investigated.[17] Although it is beyond the scope of this update to review the entire AKI biomarker literature (please see Devarajan[18] for the most recent review), these markers hold promise to identify patients at risk for acute functional kidney decline, much as the troponins have revolutionized identification and directed early management of the acute coronary syndrome to prevent myocardial infarction in adults.[19] In fact, a recent meta-analysis of NGAL across 10 adult and pediatric studies demonstrate similarly poor outcomes for patients with NGAL (+)/serum creatinine (–) and serum creatinine (+)/NGAL (–) AKI.[20] In the future, once these biomarkers have been used widely in clinical practice and linked to clinical outcomes, it is likely that AKI will become defined by biomarker elevations and not by serum creatinine.

## AKI EPIDEMIOLOGY AND INCIDENCE

The epidemiology of AKI has likewise changed over the past 2 decades, transitioning from primary renal disease to a syndrome secondary to other systemic illness or its treatment. Advances in medical management for other organ illnesses, including solid organ and stem cell transplantation, corrective congenital heart surgery, sepsis, and septic shock, have depended on medicinal and mechanical therapeutic interventions that have nephrotoxic side effects. For example, numerous studies demonstrate cardiopulmonary bypass (CPB) to be associated with a 20% to 40% AKI rate.[11,21] Nephrotoxic medications are a commonly reported cause of AKI in critically ill and non–critically ill children,[22] which is independently associated with morbidity and mortality in children.[23,24] Finally, nonrenal disease accounts for 80% of the underlying illnesses associated with the continuous renal replacement therapy provision in children.[25–28] Thus, this epidemiologic shift requires non-nephrologists to be on the lookout for factors that place children at risk for AKI and early signs of AKI to optimize management to prevent or mitigate the effects of AKI. The KDIGO AKI guidelines provide a stage-based management scheme for AKI that incorporates risk assessment in the model.[13]

AKI is quite common in critically ill children, with incidence ranging from 1% to 82% of all ICU or postoperative CPB admissions, as categorized in an excellent review.[29] AKI as defined by AKIN criteria was found in 17.9% of 2106 admissions in a large Canadian pediatric ICU (PICU) cohort[30] and in 10% of 3396 PICU patients by RIFLE criteria.[31] AKI is associated with worsened outcomes in children. AKI in the Canadian study was an independent risk factor for mortality (OR 3.7), increased length of stay, and prolonged mechanical ventilation[31]; ICU length of stay was increased fourfold. Reported mortality in children with AKI receiving continuous renal replacement therapies (CRRTs) has ranged from 32.1% to 58.9% in studies since 2000.[29] AKI synergistically increases morbidity and mortality in children with multiple organ failure, hematopoietic stem cell transplantation, trauma, and extracorporeal membrane oxygenation, independent of severity of illness scoring.[32–35] Effects of AKI are also long lasting in survivors, with chronic renal insufficiency in almost half of patients at 3-year to 5-year follow-up, suggesting permanent alteration of the renal parenchyma.[36]

## AKI AND ASSOCIATED CONDITIONS
### Sepsis-Associated AKI

AKI is a common finding in sepsis, both as a cause and as an effect, and often in association with multiple organ dysfunction.[37] Septic AKI is defined as the simultaneous presence both of RIFLE criteria for AKI and consensus criteria for sepsis, with the absence of other clear and established nonsepsis-related causes of AKI (eg, radiocontrast, other nephrotoxins).[38] Sepsis has been noted as the primary cause of up to 50% of adult AKI.[39] In pediatric AKI series, incidence of sepsis-associated AKI has ranged from 9% to 34%.[7,22,40] Sepsis-associated AKI is also associated with lower survival.[41] The pathogenic mechanisms of AKI in sepsis are complex and multifactorial, but are most likely related to combination of blood flow alterations and cytokine-mediated injury (**Fig. 1**).[42] Resultant injury produces both necrotic and apoptotic renal cell death. Regional or global hypoperfusion has long been thought to be responsible for primary injury, with an associated proinflammatory state adding injury. Likely the answer is more complex. For instance, sepsis-associated AKI can occur even in the face of hyperdynamic renal blood flow.[42] The "peak concentration hypothesis" has been proposed to suggest that elevations and imbalances of both proinflammatory and

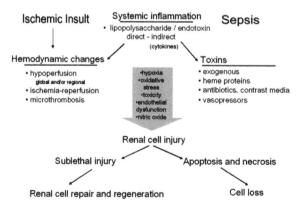

**Fig. 1.** Proposed pathogenic mechanisms of sepsis-induced acute kidney injury. (*From* Loza R, Estremadoyro L, Loza C, et al. Factors associated with mortality in acute renal failure in children. Pediatr Nephrol 2006;21:106–9; with permission.)

anti-inflammatory mediators coupled with endothelial dysfunction and altered coagulation cascade can all function synergistically to induce AKI.[43] The importance of microthrombosis in AKI has been demonstrated by findings that deficiency of ADAMTS-13 (formerly known as von Willebrand factor–cleaving protease), a cardinal finding in thrombotic thrombocytopenic purpura (TTP), is found in septic AKI patients.[44] ADAMTS-13 deficiency in this setting is associated with increased mortality. Specific cytokine gene promoter polymorphisms have also been suggested to predispose some patients with sepsis to develop AKI,[45] and to increase likelihood of mortality in sepsis-associated AKI.[46] Specific gene probes for matrix metalloproteinase-8 and elastase-2 were upregulated in pediatric septic shock–associated AKI with high sensitivity, albeit low specificity,[47] suggesting the potential for serum biomarkers in predicting AKI.

### AKI and Other Organ Involvement

Although AKI manifests itself most commonly as single organ failure, it frequently occurs in concert with other organ failure in critically ill children. Children with multiple organ system failure (MOSF) have decreasing survival with increasing number of organ failures,[48] and AKI is a synergistic contributor to this mortality.[32]

The complex pathophysiologic interaction of heart and kidney dysfunction in children has been increasingly recognized, described as cardiorenal syndrome (CRS).[49] CRS may occur as numerous subtypes, but is primarily caused by acute cardiac disease with secondary acute renal impact (type 1), or vice versa (type 3). Systemic disease can also result in secondary heart and kidney involvement. In children, type 1 CRS is seen most commonly in the perioperative setting with acute decompensated heart failure. AKI was seen in 27% of patients in a postoperative pediatric CPB cohort.[21] Diagnosis of severe AKI after pediatric CPB was also associated with worsened left ventricular function 30 days after CPB.[10] Recent studies have identified several urinary biomarkers, including NGAL, IL-18, and KIM-1,[21] as well as serum biomarkers, such as cystatin C,[50] that can detect AKI children after CPB. They also correlate with AKI severity and outcome. Thus, early diagnosis of CRS and/or AKI through use of biomarkers could help guide use of peritoneal dialysis or ultrafiltration immediately in the postoperative period.[49] Adult studies are ongoing and pediatric trials may be warranted. Excellent pediatric recommendations regarding CRS are found in the review by Jefferies and Goldstein.[49] The interaction of liver and kidney in hepatorenal syndrome is well recognized, although pathophysiologic mechanisms remain elusive.[51]

### AKI and Fluid Overload

Development of AKI would be expected to contribute inherently to FO from decreased renal function and oliguria; however, evidence also suggests that FO itself may contribute to AKI. A number of pediatric and adult studies have supported the association of degree of FO and worsening outcome.[52] Goldstein and colleagues[53] first reported this association. In children receiving continuous venovenous hemofiltration (CVVH) (either alone or with dialysis), percent FO at initiation of hemofiltration was significantly lower in survivors (16.4% ± 13.8%) compared with nonsurvivors (34.0% ± 21.0%), even when controlled for severity of illness. These findings were supported in analysis by Foland and colleagues[28] of a larger population of 113 critically ill children receiving CVVH for a variety of conditions associated with both primary and secondary renal insufficiency. Multiple organ dysfunction syndrome (MODS) was seen in 103 of these patients. Median FO was significantly lower in survivors compared with nonsurvivors (7.8% vs 15.1%, $P = .02$). Percent FO was independently associated with survival in patients with 3 or more organ MODS, adjusting for severity of illness by PRISM III score (**Fig. 2**). Children with high FO (>10%) at CVVH initiation were at 3 times greater risk of mortality ($P$ = .002). Another single-center study[54] also found that pediatric CRRT survival outcomes progressively worsened with increasing percent FO (**Fig. 3**). Subsequently, prospective observation data from the 13 centers of the Prospective Pediatric Continuous Renal Replacement Therapy Registry confirmed the association between FO and outcomes in pediatric patients with AKI selected to receive CRRT.[25,55,56] In these studies, mortality increased with increasing deciles of percent FO, even when adjusted for intergroup differences in severity of illness scores. Children with greater than 20% FO had an adjusted mortality OR of 8.5 times those less than 20%.[56]

Several prospective AKI studies later confirmed pediatric findings more broadly in adolescents and adults with AKI; fluid balance was an independent risk factor for mortality, and early institution of renal replacement therapy was associated with better outcome.[57] The Program to Improve Care in Acute Renal Disease (PICARD), a 618-patient adult AKI observational study,[58] found that FO was associated with mortality and nonrecovery of kidney function (adjusted OR of 2.07 for death associated with FO at time of dialysis initiation), persisting even when adjusted for Acute Physiology and Chronic Health Evaluation (APACHE) and Sequential Organ Failure Assessment (SOFA) severity of illness scores. The data also suggested that aggressive use of diuretics and early initiation of hemofiltration might be associated with improved outcomes. Although adjusting for severity of illness, all these AKI studies do not test the effects of treating FO on outcome and are unable to determine causation. Randomized studies would be important to further evaluate therapeutic benefit in children with AKI.

## TREATMENT OF AKI IN CHILDREN

Although diagnostic classification and characterization of AKI has significantly improved, treatment remains problematic. In part this is a result of the broad etiologies

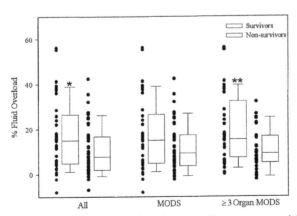

**Fig. 2.** Box plot of the medians, 25th and 75th percentiles, ranges, and individual data values for percentage FO by survival status for all patients, patients with MODS, and patients with ≥3-organ MODS receiving CVVH. Percentage FO was significantly less in overall survivors (*left*) (*$P$ = .02) and survivors with >3-organ MODS (**$P$ = .01) compared with nonsurvivors in each group. (*Reproduced from* Foland JA, Fortenberry JD, Warshaw BL, et al. Fluid overload before continuous hemofiltration and survival in critically ill children: a retrospective analysis. Crit Care Med 2004;32:1771–6; with permission.)

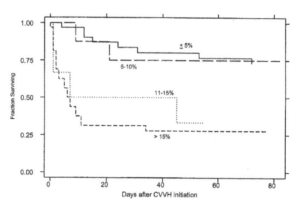

**Fig. 3.** Kaplan-Meier survival estimates over time, by percentage FO category, in children with critical illness and acute kidney injury receiving CVVH. Survival significantly decreased with increasing FO (*P* = .0002). (*From* Gillespie R, Seidel K, Symons J. Effect of fluid overload and dose of replacement fluid on survival in hemofiltration. Pediatr Nephrol 2004;19:1394–9; with permission.)

of AKI and multifactorial causes. Potential therapies, without conclusive data in adults, are even less well defined for use in children.

### Medical Therapies

Numerous medical approaches have been attempted for prevention and treatment of AKI. Trials assessing such AKI treatments are hampered on the reliance of serum creatinine as the marker of AKI. Because, as noted previously, serum creatinine is a late functional marker of AKI, it is unlikely that any treatment is likely to be effective once more than 50% of the functional nephron mass is affected. The most common therapeutic agent used and studied in the setting of AKI has been furosemide, a loop diuretic that causes diuresis, as well as natriuresis and kaliuresis. Bagshaw and colleagues[59] performed a comprehensive meta-analysis of furosemide trials in AKI, and determined that whereas most patients with AKI receive diuretics, they led to no improvement in outcomes.

AKI preventive therapies and AKI prevention trials depend on knowing the precise timing of AKI or detection of an early biomarker of injury to allow for early and optimized directed therapy. The 2 settings most conducive to such study are radiocontrast administration and CPB. Indeed, the CPB setting has been the proving ground for most AKI biomarker studies. Medications tested in this setting have included fluid administration, sodium bicarbonate, diuretics, n-acetylcysteine (NAC),[60] statins, low-dose dopamine, fenoldopam, and theophylline. Although some initial success was seen with NAC in preventing contrast-induced nephropathy, subsequent large randomized trials have yielded negative or equivocal results.[61] Similar disappointing patterns of early success for AKI treatment or prevention followed by lack of substantiation have been observed with almost all the medications listed previously.

Given the potential role of ischemia in AKI, efforts to limit or improve renal blood flow have always been attractive; however, pharmacologic approaches have not proven successful in clinical studies. The classic use of "renal dose" dopamine has been convincingly shown to be ineffective in decreasing need for renal replacement therapy or mortality, and is not recommended.[62] Maintenance of appropriate arterial blood pressure should still be considered essential to optimize renal perfusion.[63]

It is important to note that both low-dose dopamine and loop diuretics may be harmful for AKI prevention, and their use in this context has been largely abandoned. On a positive note, Ricci and colleagues[64] demonstrated that high-dose fenoldopam given during cardiac bypass decreases urinary NGAL and cystatin C levels, as well as serum creatinine–based AKI severity by pRIFLE. This novel trial design, using novel biomarkers as the end point and incorporated in the definition of AKI, should inform future studies going forward.[65]

### Metabolic Control

Efforts to maintain euglycemia have received much attention in light of a seminal randomized trial[66] demonstrating reduced mortality in surgical patients achieving tight glycemic control. The suggested mechanism of benefit of insulin is induction of anti-inflammatory and antiapoptotic effects,[67,68] in line with the suggested mechanisms of septic AKI. Reduction of AKI has accordingly been suggested to benefit from tight control in critical illness hyperglycemia. In the study by van den Berghe and colleagues, severe acute renal failure requiring dialysis or CRRT was reduced (8.2% vs 4.8%; $P = .04$), as well as reduced numbers of patients with elevated creatinine, in patients receiving tight control. Subsequent studies in medical patients have been less encouraging in mortality benefit, although AKI was again reduced, as based on I or F criteria of RIFLE (8.9% vs 5.9%).[69] Subsequent trials in both adults[70] and children[71,72] have not found significant effects on reduction of AKI, or need for dialysis.

### CRRT

CRRT has become recognized as the preferred modality for management of the child with severe AKI with electrolyte abnormalities and FO. Several excellent reviews provide much information on technical details, timing, and dosing.[73,74] Benefits of CRRT over intermittent hemodialysis and peritoneal dialysis remain the technique's ability to provide gradual but constant removal of solutes and independent adjustment of composition and volume of extracellular fluid, minimizing the hemodynamic impact in critically ill patients. An additional theoretical benefit of CRRT has been the potential immunomodulatory effect of inflammatory cytokine removal,[43] related to the classic "peak concentration" hypothesis. Although a multitude of studies have identified decrease in cytokines with CRRT, related both to filtration and adsorption to the membrane,[75] no studies have correlated degree of cytokine removal with outcome in septic patients.

While biologically plausible and intuitively advantageous, randomized trials have unfortunately not demonstrated outcome efficacy of CRRT compared with intermittent hemodialysis therapy in critically ill adults.[76,77] Prospective randomized studies of CRRT compared with standard approaches are lacking in children; however, data from the 13-center Prospective Pediatric Continuous Renal Replacement Therapy (ppCRRT) registry[78] have provided an extensive window into indications for and use of CRRT in children. More than 90% of patients in the registry have received CRRT to treat metabolic or fluid disturbances directly related to AKI.[26] Reports from the ppCRRT registry in patients receiving CRRT for AKI and MOSF[25,55] have supported the association of FO and outcome and the early initiation of CRRT. Anecdotally, mortality in these CRRT series is lower than might be expected from historical series of children with MOSF not treated with CRRT.[25]

Dosing of CRRT has been postulated to accordingly improve outcome. Indeed, an early landmark randomized trial by Ronco and colleagues[79] found significant improvement in survival with high-flow ultrafiltration (35 mL/kg/h) compared with a lower dose (20 mL/kg/h); however, subsequent single-center and multicenter trials found no difference by intensity.[77,80,81] In particular, the Randomized Evaluation of Normal versus Augmented Level Replacement Therapy (RENAL) trial of 1508 adults exclusively receiving continuous venovenous diahemofiltration (CVVDHF) found no difference in survival or renal replacement need at 60 days between the high-intensity ($33.4 \pm 12.8$ mL/kg/h) group and the low-intensity group ($22 \pm 17.8$ mL/kg/h).[81] The cumulative evidence thus leads to the recommendation that provision of an effectively delivered standard dose of renal replacement therapy should be sought over seeking to increase intensity of therapy.[77] Some single-center experience has suggested outcome benefit of convective hemofiltration as a mode compared with diahemofiltration, perhaps because of enhanced cytokine removal in sepsis. However, ppCRRT results did not find comparative benefit in nonrandomized review. Timing of CRRT initiation is also still not well delineated. Although evidence favors earlier initiation to minimize FO,[52,76] no study has been able to successfully assess best-practice cutoff points. Use of urinary biomarkers in combination with FO categories could provide a mechanism for identifying timing; further studies are in progress.

Anticoagulation is a key element of effective CRRT. Although heparin had been a mainstay of therapy, use of sodium citrate anticoagulation with calcium infusion has achieved widespread and majority acceptance because of the ability to provide regional anticoagulation of the circuit, decrease bleeding risk, and minimize heparin exposure.[26,82] The protocol of Bunchman and colleagues[83] is the most commonly used citrate approach. Patients on protocol must be monitored closely for evidence of citrate overload, particularly in patients with impaired hepatic function.

### Plasma Exchange in AKI and MOSF

The use of plasma exchange has markedly improved survival and AKI outcomes of TTP.[84] Findings of a TTP-like subtype of patients, most with sepsis, thrombocytopenia, and multiple organ failure (TAMOF) have led to efforts to use plasma exchange in children.[85] A small randomized trial of pediatric patients with TAMOF found benefit in reduction of organ dysfunction scores.[44] Preliminary results from a more recent multicenter prospective observational trial[86] of children with TAMOF demonstrated reduced ADAMTS-13 levels, a high incidence of AKI, and need for CRRT. Plasma exchange was associated with a more rapid reduction in organ dysfunction scores and with decreased mortality in preliminary studies; further prospective randomized trials are necessary to determine outcome benefit on survival and AKI compared with standard therapies.

### Use of CRRT With Extracorporeal Life Support

Treatment of AKI and multiple organ failure is common in the PICU, and often requires multiple extracorporeal devices, including extracorporeal life support (ECLS) to provide temporary cardiopulmonary support for patients with severe, potentially reversible heart or lung failure when traditional medical managements have failed. Renal findings of oliguria/anuria,[87] FO, transient impairment of renal function,[88,89] and combined renal hypoperfusion and hypoxemia all are manifestations of AKI in this population. AKI rates in patients receiving ECLS include 25% in neonates,[90] 18% to 30% in pediatric patients,[91,92] and 50% in adult patients.[93] Specific subpopulations, such as those receiving CPB for repair of congenital heart disease, have much higher reported AKI rates, up to 71% in one series.[94]

Optimal management of these renal complications in patients receiving ECLS has not been definitively determined. Traditionally, management of FO on ECLS has focused on increasing urine output by using diuretics and restricting fluid intake to achieve a net negative daily fluid balance; however, this approach has recently been called into question. Aggressive management of FO can be performed via high diuretic dosages in critically ill patients with AKI, but is associated with increased risk of death, hearing loss, nonrecovery of renal function,[95] and lowered caloric intake due to fluid restriction with poorer outcome.[96] Although impact on survival is unknown, early intervention with hemofiltration in neonatal and pediatric ECLS has been shown to improve fluid balance, increase caloric intake, and reduce total dose of diuretics.[97]

Much variation currently exists in prevention and management of these ECLS complications. In a recent survey of Extracorporeal Life Support Organization (ELSO) centers providing ECLS, Fleming and colleagues[98] found that 23% of centers did not routinely use any renal supportive therapies (intermittent hemodialysis, sustained low-efficiency dialysis, CRRT, slow continuous ultrafiltration) for their patients receiving ECLS, whereas another 26% included a hemofilter to provide these therapies in every ECLS circuit. The most common indications for use of renal supportive therapies were treatment of FO (43%), acute kidney injury (35%), prevention of FO (16%), and electrolyte disturbances (4%). Of centers using a renal supportive therapy, most used convective therapies (61.4%). Differences between devices used, connection points into the ECLS circuit, and techniques used to provide these therapies were seen as well. Nephrology consultation in the management of these patients varied widely (94.0% consultation rates in the United States compared with 5.6% in all other countries). The survey provided evidence of the variability in the diagnosis and treatment of renal complications in patients receiving ECLS and informs future studies aimed at identifying optimal therapy.

ELSO provides patient care guidelines[99] addressing the management of fluid balance and kidney injury in these patients. Because of edema and FO caused by critical illness and iatrogenic crystalloid infusion worsening lung/heart failure,[100] ELSO recommends a management goal "to return the extracellular fluid volume to normal (dry weight) and maintain it there." To achieve this, guidelines suggest institution of diuretics once the patient is hemodynamically stable and if this effect "is not sufficient to achieve negative fluid balance or if the patient is in overt renal failure, [then] continuous hemofiltration is added to the extracorporeal circuit to maintain fluid and electrolyte balance." ELSO guidelines also address the misperception that use of renal replacement therapies concomitantly with ECLS causes both acute and chronic kidney failure, commenting that renal replacement therapies are "often used" on ECLS, can be useful in helping provide full caloric and protein nutritional support, and do "not cause renal failure." Development of chronic renal failure after concomitant CRRT and ECLS therapy is rare outside of a primary kidney disease and resolution of kidney injury occurs "in >90% of patients."[92,101] Balancing the risks of FO and use of renal replacement therapy in patients receiving ECLS is important because both are associated with death in ELSO registry and individual center patient reviews.[35,92]

Several approaches are currently in use for providing renal replacement therapy on ECLS. A brief review of the 2 most common methods, in-line hemofiltration and connection of a dedicated CRRT device to the ECLS circuit, is provided, with more detailed information available elsewhere.[102,103] No studies have been performed to evaluate comparison devices, although single-center experience has suggested improved outcomes in the time period of dedicated CRRT device use.[35] Of note, no currently available CRRT device approved by the Food and Drug Administration exists to date in the United States for use in neonatal or pediatric populations, nor any device approved for use in conjunction with ECLS. Regardless of technique used, the use of commercially prepared replacement/dialysis fluids and use of standardized protocols are critical to providing safe and effective care.

One common method for CRRT in ECLS used in many institutions is a simplified in-line hemofilter device that does not require addition of a dialysis machine to the circuit. Renal replacement circuit flow is driven by ECLS pump flow rather than requiring an additional blood pump. In this standardized procedure (**Fig. 4**),[102,104] a primed renal replacement circuit is inserted in-line and parallel with the existing ECLS circuit. The renal replacement circuit is constructed using a hemofilter/hemo-dialyzer with CRRT tubing. The filter inlet is connected after the ECLS roller pump, the outlet is connected before the pump, and, where available, to the ECLS bladder. Monitoring of actual delivered flow with an ultrasonic flow probe on the arterial limb after all shunts is recommended to ensure adequate oxygen delivery. The blood path circuit is altered with both inlet and outlet to the renal replacement circuit being post-pump but pre-oxygenator when using a centrifugal pump owing to negative pressures seen on the venous pre-pump limb of the circuit. Regardless of pump type used, the outlet blood should be returned before the oxygenator so that it serves as a trap to avoid sending unanticipated air or clot from the hemofiltration limb to the patient. Existing anticoagulation provided for the ECLS circuit is usually sufficient, and no additional anticoagulation of the renal replacement circuit is needed. Ultrafiltrate from the hemofilter is removed using intravenous (IV) fluid infusion tubing and an IV pump, which is intended to control the hourly fluid removal rate and is measured by a urometer when the device is set up to provide slow continuous ultrafiltration (SCUF). To provide CVVH, a second IV pump is used to deliver replacement fluids to the blood before returning to the ECLS circuit. To provide continuous venovenous hemodialysis mode, the replacement fluids are removed and an appropriate dialysate is connected to the hemofilter. Both convection and diffusive therapies, such as CVVHDF, can also be provided.

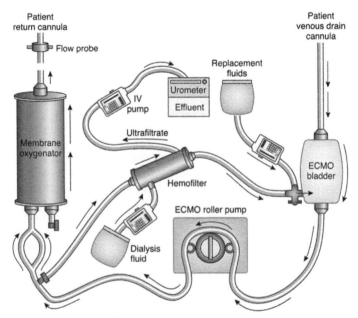

**Fig. 4.** Renal replacement therapy on a roller head ECLS circuit using an in-line hemofilter. (*Reproduced from* Askenazi DJ, Selewski DT, Paden ML, et al. Renal replacement therapy in critically ill patients receiving extracorporeal membrane oxygenation. Clin J Am Soc Nephrol 2012;7:1328–36; with permission.)

Reported advantages to this approach are that it is less costly, easily changed, does not require a dedicated CRRT device, and reduces nursing requirements. However, there are known issues with using this method for providing CRRT on ECLS. The IV pumps used to control ultrafiltration and delivery of replacement fluids have been previously shown to be inaccurate for CRRT and are affected significantly by changing pressure head.[105,106] This represents a significant problem for use of these pumps during ECLS, and, under the pressure and flow conditions seen in ECLS, can produce an error in fluid balance up to 840 mL per day.[107] When using this technique, strong consideration of supplemental monitoring of both ultrafiltrate production and replacement fluid delivery by an alternate means, such as weighing bags or volumetric measurements, is encouraged. When using this technique to provide SCUF, frequent monitoring of electrolytes is recommended to avoid severe abnormalities.

An alternate way to provide CRRT to patients receiving ECLS is to connect a commercially available CRRT device to the ECLS circuit (**Fig. 5**). Connections for the renal replacement therapy blood path are made as described previously for both roller head and centrifugal ECLS setups. However, there is great variation between currently used devices in the inlet and outlet pressures that will trigger an alarm and stop functioning of the device. Trial-and-error alterations of renal replacement circuit inlet and outlet placement are often used in an attempt to reduce alarms and time off of CRRT. However, keeping the return line pre-oxygenator is critically important to reduce the risk of embolism. CRRT devices should also not be placed into the venous pre-pump limb of a centrifugal system because of high risk of cavitation and gases coming out of solution. Other mechanisms of changing pressure, such as external tubing clamps and intentional use of stopcocks designed for much lower flow rates, cannot be recommended because of their increased risk of thrombosis and hemolysis. Again, anticoagulation provided for ECLS is usually adequate for this renal replacement circuit and no additional anticoagulation is necessary.

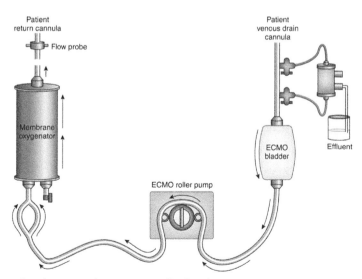

**Fig. 5.** Renal replacement therapy on a roller head ECLS circuit using a commercially available CRRT device. (*Reproduced from* Askenazi DJ, Selewski DT, Paden ML, et al. Renal replacement therapy in critically ill patients receiving extracorporeal membrane oxygenation. Clin J Am Soc Nephrol 2012;7:1328–36; with permission.)

Use of a commercially available CRRT device with ECLS has the potential advantage of using a system that has been designed to provide CRRT, albeit not in this clinical setting. In addition, training requirements for nursing could be reduced because of consistency in CRRT device approaches. A disadvantage is the high initial cost of the commercial CRRT device as compared with the in-line method. Additionally, commercial CRRT pumps use the same peristaltic mechanism as the IV pumps mentioned previously, rendering them vulnerable to suffer from similar inaccuracies. When used with ECLS, commercial CRRT devices have been noted to provide significantly inaccurate fluid balance between ultrafiltrate and replacement fluid volumes and report erroneous values of the fluid removed.[107]

## SUMMARY

The definitions and characterization of AKI in children have advanced significantly over the past 2 decades. AKI is common in critically ill children and is associated with increased morbidity and mortality. AKI in association with sepsis, multiple organ involvement, and FO carries heightened risk. Gene probes and urinary biomarkers represent intriguing tools for predicting and monitoring pediatric AKI, as well as potentially guiding treatment intervention. Treatment of AKI is problematic, but extracorporeal approaches in AKI and MOSF continue to grow in use and potential benefit. The kidney remains a "seat" of reason and discernment, and further studies are needed to guide prevention and treatment of AKI.

## REFERENCES

1. Ekoynan G. The kidneys in the Bible: what happened? J Am Soc Nephrol 2005; 16:3464–71.
2. Kellum JA, Angus DC. Patients are dying of acute renal failure. Crit Care Med 2002;30(2):156–7.
3. Chertow GM, Burdick E, Honour M, et al. Acute kidney injury, mortality, length of stay, and costs in hospitalized patients. J Am Soc Nephrol 2005;16:3365–70.
4. Price JF, Mott AR, Dickerson HA, et al. Worsening renal function in children hospitalized with decompensated heart failure: evidence for a pediatric cardiorenal syndrome? Pediatr Crit Care Med 2008;9:279–84.
5. Bellomo R, Ronco C, Kellum JA, et al. Acute renal failure—definition, outcome measures, animal models, fluid therapy and information technology needs: the Second International Consensus Conference of the Acute Dialysis Quality Initiative (ADQI) Group. Crit Care 2004;8:R204–12.
6. Srisawat N, Hoste EE, Kellum JA. Modern classification of acute kidney injury. Blood Purif 2010;29:300–7.
7. Akcan-Arikan A, Zappitelli M, Loftis LL, et al. Modified RIFLE criteria in critically ill children with acute kidney injury. Kidney Int 2007;71:1028–35.
8. Slater MB, Anand V, Uleryk EM, et al. A systematic review of RIFLE criteria in children, and its application and association with measures of mortality and morbidity. Kidney Int 2012;81:791–8.
9. Mehta RL, Kellum JA, Shah SV, et al. Acute Kidney Injury Network: report of an initiative to improve outcomes in acute kidney injury. Crit Care 2007;11:R31.
10. Blinder JJ, Goldstein SL, Lee VV, et al. Congenital heart surgery in infants: effects of acute kidney injury on outcomes. J Thorac Cardiovasc Surg 2012;143:368–74.
11. Zappitelli M, Bernier PL, Saczkowski RS, et al. A small post-operative rise in serum creatinine predicts acute kidney injury in children undergoing cardiac surgery. Kidney Int 2009;76:885–92.

12. Zappitelli M, Parikh CR, Akcan-Arikan A, et al. Ascertainment and epidemiology of acute kidney injury varies with definition interpretation. Clin J Am Soc Nephrol 2008;3:948–54.

13. Kellum JA, Lamiere N, Aspelin P, et al. Kidney Disease: Improving Global Outcomes (KDIGO) Acute Kidney Injury Work Group. KDIGO clinical practice guideline for acute kidney injury. Kidney Int 2012;2(Suppl):1–138.

14. Liu KD, Thompson BT, Ancukiewicz M, et al. Acute kidney injury in patients with acute lung injury: impact of fluid accumulation on classification of acute kidney injury and associated outcomes. Crit Care Med 2011;39:2665–71.

15. Basu RK, Andrews A, Krawczeski CD, et al. Acute kidney injury based on serum creatinine is associated with increased morbidity in children following the arterial switch operation. Pediatr Crit Care Med, in press.

16. Coca SG, Yalavarthy R, Concato J, et al. Biomarkers for the diagnosis and risk stratification of acute kidney injury: a systematic review. Kidney Int 2008;73: 1008–16.

17. McMahon BA, Koyner JL, Murray PT. Urinary glutathione S-transferases in the pathogenesis and diagnostic evaluation of acute kidney injury following cardiac surgery: a critical review. Curr Opin Crit Care 2010;16(6):550–5.

18. Devarajan P. Biomarkers for the early detection of acute kidney injury. Curr Opin Pediatr 2011;23:194–200.

19. Goldstein SL. Acute kidney injury biomarkers: renal angina and the need for a renal troponin I. BMC Med 2011;9:135.

20. Haase M, Bellomo R, Devarajan P, et al. Accuracy of neutrophil gelatinase-associated lipocalin (NGAL) in diagnosis and prognosis in acute kidney injury: a systematic review and meta-analysis. Am J Kidney Dis 2009;54: 1012–24.

21. Krawczeski CD, Goldstein SL, Woo JG, et al. Temporal relationship and predictive value of urinary acute kidney injury biomarkers after pediatric cardiopulmonary bypass. J Am Coll Cardiol 2011;58:2301–9.

22. Hui-Stickle S, Brewer ED, Goldstein SL. Pediatric ARF epidemiology at a tertiary care center from 1999 to 2001. Am J Kidney Dis 2005;45:96–101.

23. Moffett BS, Goldstein SL. Acute kidney injury and increasing nephrotoxic-medication exposure in noncritically-ill children. Clin J Am Soc Nephrol 2011; 6:856–63.

24. Zappitelli M, Moffett BS, Hyder A, et al. Acute kidney injury in non-critically ill children treated with aminoglycoside antibiotics in a tertiary healthcare centre: a retrospective cohort study. Nephrol Dial Transplant 2011;26:144–50.

25. Goldstein SL, Somers MJ, Baum MA, et al. Pediatric patients with multi-organ dysfunction syndrome receiving continuous renal replacement therapy. Kidney Int 2005;67:653–8, 653–65.

26. Symons JM, Chua AN, Somers MJ, et al. Demographic characteristics of pediatric continuous renal replacement therapy: a report of the prospective pediatric continuous renal replacement therapy registry. Clin J Am Soc Nephrol 2007;2: 732–8.

27. Hayes LW, Oster RA, Tofil NM, et al. Outcomes of critically ill children requiring continuous renal replacement therapy. J Crit Care 2009;24:394–400.

28. Foland JA, Fortenberry JD, Warshaw BL, et al. Fluid overload before continuous hemofiltration and survival in critically ill children: a retrospective analysis. Crit Care Med 2004;32:1771–6.

29. Basu R, Devarajan P, Wong H, et al. An update and review of acute kidney injury in pediatrics. Pediatr Crit Care Med 2011;12:339–47.

30. Alkarandi O, Eddington K, Hyder A, et al. Acute kidney injury is an independent risk factor for pediatric intensive care unit mortality, longer length of stay and prolonged mechanical ventilation in critically ill children: a two-center retrospective cohort study. Crit Care 2011;15:R146.

31. Schneider J, Khemani R, Grushkin C, et al. Serum creatinine as stratified in the RIFLE score for acute kidney injury is associated with mortality and length of stay for children in the pediatric intensive care unit. Crit Care Med 2009;35:2087–95.

32. Zapitelli M. Epidemiology and diagnosis of acute kidney injury. Clin Nephrol 2009;71:602–7.

33. Brophy PD. Renal supportive therapy for pediatric acute kidney injury in the setting of multiorgan dysfunction syndrome/sepsis. Semin Nephrol 2008;28: 457–69.

34. Prodhan P, McCage L, Stroud M, et al. Acute kidney injury is associated with in-hospital mortality in mechanically ventilated children with trauma. J Trauma Acute Care Surg 2012;73:832–7.

35. Askenazi D, Ambalavanan N, Hamilton K, et al. Acute kidney injury and renal replacement therapy independently predict mortality in neonatal and pediatric noncardiac patients on extracorporeal membrane oxygenation. Pediatr Crit Care Med 2011;12:e1–6.

36. Askenazi D, Feig D, Graham N, et al. 3-5 year longitudinal follow-up of pediatric patients after acute renal failure. Kidney Int 2006;69:184–9.

37. Ronco C, Kellum JA, Bellomo R, et al. Potential interventions in sepsis-related acute kidney injury. Clin J Am Soc Nephrol 2008;3:531–44.

38. Wan L, Bagshaw SM, Langenberg C, et al. Pathophysiology of septic acute kidney injury: what do we really know? Crit Care Med 2008;36:S198–203.

39. Bagshaw SM, George C, Bellomo R. Early acute kidney injury and sepsis: a multicentre evaluation. Crit Care 2008;12:R47.

40. Shaheen IS, Watson A, Harvey B. Acute renal failure in children: etiology, treatment and outcome. Saudi J Kidney Dis Transpl 2006;17:153–8.

41. Loza R, Estremadoyro L, Loza C, et al. Factors associated with mortality in acute renal failure in children. Pediatr Nephrol 2006;21:106–9.

42. Bellomo R, Wan L, Langenberg C, et al. Septic acute kidney injury: new concepts. Nephron Exp Nephrol 2008;109:e95–100.

43. Ronco C, Tetta C, Mariano F, et al. Interpreting the mechanisms of continuous renal replacement therapy in sepsis. The peak concentration hypothesis. Artif Organs 2003;27:792–801.

44. Nguyen TC, Han Y, Kiss JE, et al. Intensive plasma exchange increases a disintegrin and metalloprotease with thrombospondin motifs-13 activity and reverses organ dysfunction in children with thrombocytopenia-associated multiple organ failure. Crit Care Med 2008;36:2878–87.

45. Haase-Fielitz A, Haase M, Bellomo R, et al. Genetic polymorphisms in sepsis- and cardiopulmonary bypass-associated acute kidney injury. Contrib Nephrol 2007;156:75–91.

46. Jaber BL, Rao M, Guo D, et al. Cytokine gene polymorphisms and mortality in acute renal failure. Cytokine 2004;25:212–9.

47. Basu RK, Standage S, Cvijanovich N, et al. Identification of candidate serum biomarkers for severe septic shock-associated kidney injury via microarray. Crit Care 2011;15:R273.

48. Watson RS, Carcillo JA, Linde-Zwirble WT, et al. The epidemiology of severe sepsis in children of the United States. Am J Respir Crit Care Med 2003;167: 695–701.

49. Jefferies J, Goldstein S. Cardiorenal syndrome: an emerging problem in pediatric critical care. Pediatr Nephrol 2012. [Epub ahead of print].

50. Hassinger A, Backer C, Lane J, et al. Predictive power of serum cystatin C to detect kidney injury and pediatric-modified RIFLE class in children undergoing cardiac surgery. Pediatr Crit Care Med 2012;13:435–40.

51. Wadei H, Martin M, Ahsan N. Hepatorenal syndrome: pathophysiology and management. Clin J Am Soc Nephrol 2006;1:1066–79.

52. Fortenberry JD. Fluid overload and outcomes in pediatric critical illness. In: Current concepts in pediatric critical care. Chicago: Society of Critical Care Medicine; 2012. p. 71–81.

53. Goldstein S, Brewer E, Currier H, et al. Outcome in children receiving continuous venovenous hemofiltration. Pediatrics 2001;107:1309.

54. Gillespie R, Seidel K, Symons J. Effect of fluid overload and dose of replacement fluid on survival in hemofiltration. Pediatr Nephrol 2004;19:1394–9.

55. Sutherland SM, Zappitelli M, Alexander SR, et al. Fluid overload and mortality in children receiving continuous renal replacement therapy: The prospective pediatric continuous renal replacement therapy registry. Am J Kidney Dis 2010;55: 316–25.

56. Ray K. Fluid overload increases mortality in critically ill children. Nat Rev Nephrol 2010;6:190.

57. Payen D, Cornélie de Pont A, Sakr Y, et al. A positive fluid balance is associated with a worse outcome in patients with acute renal failure. Crit Care 2008; 12:R74.

58. Bouchard J, Soroko SB, Chertow GM, et al. Fluid accumulation, survival and recovery of kidney function in critically ill patients with acute kidney injury. Kidney Int 2009;76:422–7.

59. Bagshaw SM, Delaney A, Haase M, et al. Loop diuretics in the management of acute renal failure: a systematic review and meta-analysis. Crit Care Resusc 2007;9:60–8.

60. Tepel M, van der Giet M, Schwarzfeld C, et al. Prevention of radiographic-contrast-agent-induced reductions in renal function by acetylcysteine. N Engl J Med 2000;343:180–4.

61. ACT Investigators. Acetylcysteine for prevention of renal outcomes in patients undergoing coronary and peripheral vascular angiography: main results from the randomized Acetylcysteine for Contrast-induced nephropathy Trial (ACT). Circulation 2011;124:1250–9.

62. Friedrich JO, Adhikari N, Herridge MS, et al. Meta-analysis: low-dose dopamine increases urine output but does not prevent renal dysfunction or death. Ann Intern Med 2005;142:510–24.

63. Bagshaw SM, Lapinsky S, Dial S, et al. Cooperative Antimicrobial Therapy of Septic Shock (CATSS) Database Research Group. Acute kidney injury in septic shock: clinical outcomes and impact of duration of hypotension prior to initiation of antimicrobial therapy. Intensive Care Med 2009;35:871–81.

64. Ricci Z, Luciano R, Favia I, et al. High-dose fenoldopam reduces postoperative neutrophil gelatinase-associated lipocaline and cystatin C levels in pediatric cardiac surgery. Crit Care 2011;15:R160.

65. Goldstein SL. A novel use for novel acute kidney injury biomarkers: fenoldopam's effect on neutrophil gelatinase-associated lipocalin and cystatin C. Crit Care 2011;15:177.

66. Van den Berghe G, Wouters P, Weekers F, et al. Intensive insulin therapy in critically ill patients. N Engl J Med 2001;345:1359–67.

67. Hansen TK, Thiel S, Wouters PJ, et al. Intensive insulin therapy exerts anti-inflammatory effects in critically ill patients and counteracts the adverse effect of low mannose-binding lectin levels. J Clin Endocrinol Metab 2003;88:1082–8.

68. Allen DA, Harwood S, Varagunam M, et al. High glucose-induced oxidative stress causes apoptosis in proximal tubular epithelial cells and is mediated by multiple caspases. FASEB J 2003;17:908–10.

69. Van den Berghe G, Wilmer A, Hermans G, et al. Intensive insulin therapy in the medical ICU. N Engl J Med 2006;354:449–61.

70. NICE-SUGAR Study Investigators, Finfer S, Chittock DR, et al. Intensive versus conventional glucose control in critically ill patients. N Engl J Med 2009;360:1283–97.

71. Vlasselaers D, Milants I, Desmet L, et al. Intensive insulin therapy for patients in paediatric intensive care: a prospective, randomized controlled study. Lancet 2009;373:547–56.

72. Agus MS, Steil G, Wypij D, et al. Tight glycemic control versus standard care after pediatric cardiac surgery. N Engl J Med 2012;367:1208–19.

73. Sutherland S, Alexander S. Continuous renal replacement therapy in children. Pediatr Nephrol 2012;27:2007–16.

74. Goldstein SL. Advances in pediatric renal replacement therapy for acute kidney injury. Semin Dial 2011;24:187–91.

75. Bellomo R, Tipping P, Boyce N. Continuous veno-venous hemofiltration with dialysis removes cytokines from the circulation of septic patients. Crit Care Med 1993;21:522–6.

76. Murray P, Udani S, Koyner JL. Does renal replacement therapy improve outcome? Controversies in acute kidney injury. Contrib Nephrol 2011;174:212–21.

77. Palevsky P, Zhang J, O'Connor T, et al. Intensity of continuous renal replacement therapy in critically ill patients. N Engl J Med 2008;361:1627–8.

78. Goldstein SL, Somers MJ, Brophy PD, et al. The prospective pediatric continuous renal replacement therapy registry: design, development and data assessed. Int J Artif Organs 2004;27:9–14.

79. Ronco C, Bellomo R, Homel P, et al. Effects of different doses in continuous veno-venous haemofiltration on outcomes of acute renal failure: a prospective randomised trial. Lancet 2000;356:26.

80. Talwani AJ, Campbell RC, Stofan B, et al. Standard versus high-dose CVVHDF for ICU-related acute renal failure. J Am Soc Nephrol 2008;19:1233–8.

81. Bellomo R, Cass A, Cole L, et al. Intensity of continuous renal replacement therapy in critically ill patients. N Engl J Med 2009;361:1627–38.

82. Brophy P, Somers MJ, Baum M, et al. Multi-centre evaluation of anticoagulation in patients receiving continuous renal replacement therapy (CRRT). Nephrol Dial Transplant 2005;20:1416–21.

83. Bunchman T, Maxvold N, Barnett J, et al. Pediatric hemofiltration: normocarb dialysate solution with citrate anticoagulation. Pediatr Nephrol 2002;17:150–4.

84. Rock GA, Shumak K, Buskard N. Comparison of plasma exchange with plasma infusion in the treatment of thrombotic thrombocytopenic purpura. N Engl J Med 1991;325:393–7.

85. Fortenberry JD, Paden M. Extracorporeal therapies in the treatment of sepsis: experience and promise. Semin Pediatr Infect Dis 2006;17:72–9.

86. Fortenberry JD, Nguyen T, Toney R, et al. Organ dysfunction and experience with plasma exchange in children with thrombocytopenia-associated multiple organ failure (TAMOF): findings of the prospective Children's TAMOF Network. Crit Care Med 2010;38:A30.

87. Roy BJ, Cornish JD, Clark RH. Venovenous extracorporeal membrane oxygenation affects renal function. Pediatrics 1995;95:573–8.

88. Heiss KF, Pettit B, Hirschl RB, et al. Renal insufficiency and volume overload in neonatal ECMO managed by continuous ultrafiltration. Trans Am Soc Artif Intern Organs 1987;33:557–9.

89. Sell LL, Cullen ML, Whittlesey GC, et al. Experience with renal failure during extracorporeal membrane oxygenation: treatment with continuous hemofiltration. J Pediatr Surg 1987;22:600–2.

90. Zwischenberger JB, Nguyen TT, Upp JR, et al. Complications of neonatal extracorporeal membrane oxygenation. Collective experience from the Extracorporeal Life Support Organization. J Thorac Cardiovasc Surg 1994;107:838–48.

91. Zahraa JN, Moler FW, Annich GM, et al. Venovenous versus venoarterial extracorporeal life support for pediatric respiratory failure: are there differences in survival and acute complications? Crit Care Med 2000;28:521–5.

92. Paden ML, Warshaw BL, Heard ML, et al. Recovery of renal function and survival after continuous renal replacement therapy during extracorporeal membrane oxygenation. Pediatr Crit Care Med 2011;12:153–8.

93. Yap HJ, Chen YC, Fang JT, et al. Combination of continuous renal replacement therapies (CRRT) and extracorporeal membrane oxygenation for advanced cardiac patients. Ren Fail 2003;25:183–93.

94. Smith AH, Hardison DC, Worden CR, et al. Acute renal failure during extracorporeal support in the pediatric cardiac patient. ASAIO J 2009;55:412–6.

95. Robertson CM, Tyebkhan JM, Peliowski A, et al. Ototoxic drugs and sensorineural hearing loss following severe neonatal respiratory failure. Acta Paediatr 2006;95:214–23.

96. Marik PE, Zaloga GP. Early enteral nutrition in acutely ill patients: a systematic review. Crit Care Med 2001;29:2264–70.

97. Hoover NG, Heard M, Reid C, et al. Enhanced fluid management with continuous venovenous hemofiltration in pediatric respiratory failure patients receiving extracorporeal membrane oxygenation support. Intensive Care Med 2008;34: 2241–7.

98. Fleming FM, Askenazi DJ, Bridges BC, et al. A multicenter international survey of renal supportive therapy during ECMO: The Kidney Intervention During Extracorporeal Membrane Oxygenation (KIDMO) Group. ASAIO J 2012;58:404–14.

99. Extracorporeal Life Support Organization. Guidelines. Available at: http://www. elsonet.org/index.php/resources/guidelines.html. Accessed November 26, 2012.

100. Kelly RE, Phillips JD, Foglia RP, et al. Pulmonary edema and fluid mobilization as determinants of the duration of ECMO support. J Pediatr Surg 1991;26: 1016–22.

101. Meyer RJ, Brophy PD, Bunchman TE, et al. Survival and renal function in pediatric patients following extracorporeal life support with hemofiltration. Pediatr Crit Care Med 2001;2:238–42.

102. Askenazi DJ, Selewski DT, Paden ML, et al. Renal replacement therapy in critically ill patients receiving extracorporeal membrane oxygenation. Clin J Am Soc Nephrol 2012;7:1328–36.

103. Bridges BC, Selewski DT, Paden ML, et al. Acute kidney injury in neonates requiring ECMO. Neoreviews 2012;13:e428–33.

104. Weber TR, Kountzman B. Extracorporeal membrane oxygenation for nonneonatal pulmonary and multiple-organ failure. J Pediatr Surg 1998;33:1605–9.

105. Jenkins R, Harrison H, Chen B, et al. Accuracy of intravenous infusion pumps in continuous renal replacement therapies. ASAIO J 1992;38:808–10.

106. Sucosky P, Dasi LP, Goldman SL, et al. Assessment of current continuous hemo-filtration systems and development of a novel accurate fluid management system for use in extracorporeal membrane oxygenation. J Med Device 2008; 2:35002–10.
107. Santiago MJ, Sánchez A, López-Herce J, et al. The use of continuous renal replacement therapy in series with extracorporeal membrane oxygenation. Kidney Int 2009;76:1289–92.

# Advances in Critical Care of the Pediatric Hematopoietic Stem Cell Transplant Patient

Ranjit S. Chima, MD[a,b,*], Kamal Abulebda, MD[a],
Sonata Jodele, MD[b,c]

## KEYWORDS

- Stem cell transplant • BMT • Pediatrics • Respiratory failure
- Mechanical ventilation • Outcomes

## KEY POINTS

- Despite advances in transplant techniques, recipients of stem cell transplant (SCT) remain a complex cohort of patient, with disproportionately high morbidity and mortality.
- Outcomes for these patients seem to be improving.
- Given the ever-expanding indications and complexity of SCT, it is important for SCT physicians and intensivists to work closely together to ensure the best possible outcomes for critically ill recipients of SCT.

## INTRODUCTION

Recipients of stem cell transplant (SCT) are at risk for a multitude of complications; however, most of these do not require care in an intensive care unit (ICU). The proportion of pediatric recipients of SCT needing admission to an ICU is variable.[1] For example, at Cincinnati Children's Hospital Medical Center, 35% of SCT recipients required ICU admission over a 6-year period.[2] However, those requiring ICU admission are at a disproportionately higher risk of mortality when compared with other SCT patients. Common reasons for ICU admission include life-threatening infections, respiratory failure, shock, fluid overload, acute kidney injury (AKI), bleeding, and seizures. Unlike other patients, the trajectory of illness in SCT recipients is dictated by underlying disease, degree of immune reconstitution, and the presence of

[a] Division of Critical Care Medicine, Cincinnati Children's Hospital Medical Center, 3333 Burnet Avenue, Cincinnati, OH 45229, USA; [b] Department of Pediatrics, University of Cincinnati College of Medicine, Cincinnati, OH, USA; [c] Division of Bone Marrow Transplantation and Immunodeficiency, Cincinnati Children's Hospital Medical Center, 3333 Burnet Avenue, Cincinnati, OH 45229, USA
* Corresponding author. Division of Critical Care Medicine, Cincinnati Children's Hospital Medical Center, 3333 Burnet Avenue, Cincinnati, OH 45229.
E-mail address: ranjit.chima@cchmc.org

Pediatr Clin N Am 60 (2013) 689–707
http://dx.doi.org/10.1016/j.pcl.2013.02.007
0031-3955/13/$ – see front matter © 2013 Elsevier Inc. All rights reserved.

complications such as graft-versus-host disease (GVHD), idiopathic pneumonia syndrome (IPS), veno-occlusive disease (VOD), and transplant-associated thrombotic microangiopathy (TA-TMA).

Historically, pediatric SCT recipients requiring pediatric ICU admission have had high mortality. A recent analysis of retrospective and prospective cohort studies describing ICU mortality for children after SCT[1] reported an overall mortality of 60%. However, most studies in this analysis used data from the 1990s. Recent single-center studies using data from the last decade have reported improved outcomes.[3–5] Data from the largest published cohort of pediatric SCT recipients needing ICU care reported 63% survival to ICU discharge with longer-term survival of 45%.[2]

## OVERVIEW OF SCT

SCT involves the transplantation of hematopoietic progenitor cells from recipients to donors and represents a curative option for patients with malignant and nonmalignant diseases. Therapeutic effects of SCT can be divided into 4 main categories (**Table 1**). The process of SCT is standardized and sequentially involves donor and stem cell selection, recipient conditioning, and infusion of stem cells. After infusion of stem cells, all recipients have a period of immune reconstitution, during which they are at risk for complications and receive prophylaxis against infections and GVHD.

### Donor Selection and Stem Cell Sources

Stem cell donors can be allogeneic (a related or unrelated individual who is HLA-matched with the recipient), syngeneic (genetically identical twin), or autologous (the recipient is the donor). Autologous transplants are almost always performed for malignant disorders not involving hematopoietic cells (eg, solid tumors), whereas allogeneic transplants are performed for disorders that originate from hematopoietic cells (eg, leukemia, marrow failure syndromes such as Fanconi anemia, and immunodeficiencies such as severe combined immune deficiency). Hematopoietic stem cells come from 3 main sources: bone marrow, peripheral blood stem cell (PBSC), or cord blood.[6] The degree of HLA matching, time to engraftment, stem cell dose, and GVHD risk are dependent on the stem cell source.[7] A closer match is needed and quicker engraftment is seen with bone marrow and PBSCs when compared with cord blood. However, the risk of GVHD is lowest with cord blood and highest with PBSCs, and hence the latter are not preferred in children. Unlike bone marrow and PBSCs, a second donation is not possible with cord blood.

**Table 1**
**Therapeutic effect of SCT**

| Effect of SCT | Disorders |
|---|---|
| Correct defects in blood cell function and production | Bone marrow failure syndromes, hemoglobinopathies, immunodeficiencies |
| To replace or rescue bone marrow after ablative therapy | Hematopoietic malignancies, solid tumors |
| To replace underlying enzyme deficiencies | Hurler syndrome |
| To correct immune dysfunction by eliminating autoimmune effector cells or immune modulation by the transplanted cells on existing immune cells | Hemophagocytic syndromes |

Allogeneic donor selection is based on HLA matching between the donor and the recipient. HLA class I (A, B, C) and II (DR, DQ, DP) molecules are important in antigen processing and presentation and are considered major transplant antigens. Typically, donor and recipient are matched at 8 loci (A, B, C, and DR). The ideal donor (a sibling with genetically identical alleles at all 4 loci (8/8 match)) is available to only 15% to 30% of recipients. Most recipients need to find a match from an unrelated donor, and large registries of volunteer adult donors, and banks of frozen cord blood, have been developed for this purpose.

### Conditioning and Infusion of Stem Cells

After donor selection, nearly all recipients receive conditioning therapy, which is then followed by the infusion of stem cells. The goal of conditioning is to make space in the marrow (myeloablation), destroy cancerous marrow, and provide immunosuppression to prevent residual recipient lymphocytes from rejecting the donor stem cells. Myeloablative conditioning regimens are mainly used for malignancies and use high-dose chemotherapy or total body irradiation; these may be associated with significant transplant-related morbidity and mortality related to tissue injury. Patients undergoing autologous SCT for solid tumors such as neuroblastoma or high-risk brain tumors may receive single or multiple high-dose myeloablative chemotherapy courses targeted at their primary tumor. Reduced intensity conditioning (RIC) regimens use medications with significant immunosuppressive properties, but fewer myeloablative effects, and are used in the treatment of immunologic and metabolic disorders or second transplants for leukemias.[8] They cause less immediate organ toxicity, but are associated with a higher incidence of mixed donor chimerism and early and late viral infections. Stem cell infusion is performed through an indwelling central venous catheter. Recipients of autologous and cord blood transplants are at risk for hypertension and bradycardia caused by dimethyl sulfoxide, which is used as a preservative. Late renal injury can also occur, so aggressive hydration is usually administered concomitantly with the infusion. Allogeneic cells are usually collected and infused fresh, but may require processing, including red blood cell depletion if the donor is ABO incompatible with the recipient and T-cell depletion to reduce the risk of GVHD, as is performed for patients with Fanconi anemia.[9,10]

### Infection and GVHD Prophylaxis

Routine prophylaxis for infectious agents has significantly reduced infection-related transplant mortality. Herpes simplex virus (HSV) and cytomegalovirus (CMV) prophylaxis with acyclovir is given to seropositive recipients and those receiving stem cells from seropositive donors. Intravenous immunoglobulin supplementation is used to maintain immunoglobulin G levels within normal limits for age. Pneumocystis jiroveci (formerly Pneumocystis carinii) prophylaxis is provided for approximately 1 year after transplantation using pentamidine or trimethoprim/sulfamethoxazole, the latter being preferred after engraftment because of its myelosuppressive properties. Antifungal prophylaxis is vital after SCT and is directed against yeast (eg, Candida species) and molds (eg, Aspergillus). The most common antifungal medications used are amphotericin B, voriconazole, caspofungin, or micafungin.

GVHD prophylaxis with immunosuppressive agents is standard practice for SCT recipients after allogeneic transplant. The most common prophylactic regimens are calcineurin inhibitors (cyclosporine or tacrolimus), commonly in combination with a second agent such as methotrexate, mycophenolate mofetil (MMF), or corticosteroids. Calcineurin inhibitors are usually started several days before the stem cell infusion to achieve therapeutic levels by the time the new graft is infused. The length of

GVHD prophylaxis varies based on underlying condition and the risk for GVHD and may last from 100 days to 6 to 9 months after transplantation.

## COMPLICATIONS AFTER HEMATOPOIETIC SCT
### Infections

Infections remain a major cause of morbidity and mortality after SCT.[11] All patients after SCT have a prolonged period of immune deficiency, which makes them susceptible to infectious agents. Additional risk factors include underlying disease, indwelling vascular devices, acute GVHD, and use of immunosuppressants. Most organisms infecting SCT recipients are endogenous flora or reactivation of latent infections. The susceptibility to infectious agents is dictated by the phase of immune recovery after transplant.[12] Traditionally, immune recovery after SCT is divided into preengraftment, early engraftment, and late engraftment phases.[13] Specific defects in the immune system and common organisms are presented in **Table 2**. Engraftment does not signify immune reconstitution, and these patients remain immunocompromised up to a year after transplant. In addition, complications such as GVHD are extremely immunosuppressive.

All critically ill SCT patients should be tested for infections. Microbiological tests including blood cultures for bacteria and fungi and polymerase chain reaction (PCR) testing for viruses should be performed. Newer rapid diagnostic tests such as peptide nucleic acid fluorescent in situ hybridization may allow timely identification of bacteria

**Table 2**
**Phases of immune recovery with corresponding immune defect and common infectious agents after SCT**

| | Viral | Bacterial | Fungal/Parasitic |
|---|---|---|---|
| Preengraftment (day 0–30) Neutropenia Mucosal barrier breakdown | HSV Respiratory syncytial virus, parainfluenza, influenza, human metapneumovirus Adenovirus Rotavirus, enterovirus | Gram-positive *Staphylococcus epidermis, Staphylococcus aureus,* viridians streptococci Gram-negative *Escherichia coli, Klebsiella* spp, *Pseudomonas* | *Candida* spp *Aspergillus* spp *Mucor* spp |
| Early engraftment (day 30–100) Impaired cell-mediated immunity GVHD | CMV Adenovirus Respiratory syncytial virus, parainfluenza, influenza, human metapneumovirus Human herpesvirus 6 Adenovirus Epstein-Barr virus Polyoma viruses (BK virus and JC virus) | Gram-positive *Staphylococcus epidermis, Staphylococcus aureus,* viridians streptococci Gram-negative *Escherichia coli, Klebsiella* spp, *Pseudomonas* | *Candida* spp *Aspergillus* spp *Pneumocystis jiroveci* *Toxoplasma gondii* |
| Late engraftment (>100 d) Impaired cell-mediated and humoral immunity Reticuloendothelial dysfunction GVHD | Varicella zoster CMV | *Streptococcus pneumoniae Haemophilus influenzae* | *Toxoplasma gondii* *Pneumocystis jiroveci* *Candida* spp *Aspergillus* spp |

such as *Staphylococcus* spp.[14] If feasible, SCT recipients presenting with respiratory failure and pneumonitis should undergo a bronchoalveolar lavage, with appropriate microbiological studies. Similarly, those presenting with seizures or encephalopathy should undergo neuroimaging and spinal fluid studies.

Given the risk of infections in SCT recipients, prompt initiation of broad-spectrum antimicrobial therapy is warranted. Empirical antibacterial therapy may be tailored to the patient's presentation and the prominent flora in the institution. Particular attention should be paid to drug dosing, given the frequency of underlying kidney dysfunction in these patients. Specific antiviral therapy (**Table 3**) is added after confirmation of a viral infection. Adoptive immunotherapy, in which virus-specific cytotoxic T lymphocytes are used to target affected cells, may be effective for treatment of CMV, Epstein-Barr virus, and adenovirus infections.[15,16] However, this modality is still not available for routine clinical use. Empirical antifungal therapy with amphotericin B is considered in patients who remain febrile or have high suspicion for a fungal infection. Azoles (such as voriconazole) and echinocandins (such as caspofungin) are appropriate treatments of invasive aspergillosis and *Candida* infections, which are the most common opportunistic fungal organisms isolated.[17]

### Acute Lung Injury and Respiratory Failure

Acute lung injury, leading to acute respiratory failure, remains a common reason to require intensive care after SCT. The incidence of acute respiratory failure in children requiring intensive care after SCT remains unclear.[1] However, using mechanical ventilation as a surrogate, up to 30% of children after SCT may require mechanical ventilation.[1] At our center, 20% of SCT recipients required tracheal intubation and mechanical ventilation after SCT.[2] The presence of pretransplant pulmonary complications such as lung damage from chemotherapy (bleomycin, busulfan, and cyclophosphamide), a history of respiratory infections, previous surgical procedures involving the lung, and the use of radiotherapy may affect the course of lung injury after SCT.[18,19]

The cause of acute lung injury after SCT is extensive and encompasses processes that originate in the lung or remote from the lung. From a lung standpoint, injury in the posttransplant setting is divided into infectious and noninfectious categories (**Table 4**).

| Table 3 Viral infections and therapeutic options after SCT | |
|---|---|
| **Viral Pathogen** | **Therapy** |
| CMV | Ganciclovir,[a] foscarnet, cidofovir CMV immune globulin[b] |
| Adenovirus | Cidofovir |
| HSV | Acyclovir, valacyclovir, famciclovir Foscarnet (acyclovir-resistant HSV) Cidofovir (acyclovir/foscarnet resistant HSV) |
| Polyoma virus (BK) | Cidofovir, leflunomide |
| Epstein-Barr virus | Rituximab |
| Human herpesvirus type 6 | Ganciclovir, foscarnet, cidofovir |
| Varicella zoster virus infection | Acyclovir, valacyclovir (low-risk patients) Famciclovir (low-risk patients) |

[a] Myelosuppressive, needs to be used with caution in the early phase after SCT, especially before engraftment.
[b] Along with antiviral medication.

**Table 4**
**Cause of lung injury and respiratory failure after SCT**

| Early (Day 0–100) | Late (Day 100+) |
| --- | --- |
| Noninfectious | Noninfectious |
| Pulmonary edema | Bronchiolitis obliterans |
| Periengraftment respiratory distress syndrome | Bronchiolitis obliterans organizing pneumonia |
| Diffuse alveolar hemorrhage | Delayed pulmonary toxicity syndrome |
| Acute interstitial pneumonitis | Chronic GVHD |
| TA-TMA | |
| TRALI | |
| Infectious | Infectious |
| Bacteria: gram-negative rods and gram-positive cocci | Bacteria: encapsulated bacteria, gram-negative rods and gram-positive cocci |
| Virus: HSV, CMV, adenovirus, HHV6, RSV, influenza, parainfluenza, rhinovirus, human metapneumovirus | Virus: adenovirus, CMV, VZV, Epstein-Barr virus |
| Fungi: *Candida, Aspergillus, Pneumocystis* | Fungi: *Candida, Aspergillus, Pneumocystis* |

*Abbreviations:* HHV, human herpesvirus type 6; RSV, respiratory syncytial virus; TRALI, transfusion-related acute lung injury; VZV, varicella zoster virus.

Both infectious and noninfectious processes follow a temporal profile that parallels immune recovery. Hence, complications occurring within 100 days of SCT are described as occurring early and those after 100 days as late (see **Table 4**). Despite these cutoffs, multiple processes with significant overlap can occur, resulting in lung dysfunction and respiratory failure in these patients.

Most diseases leading to noninfectious lung injury constitute IPS. IPS is a distinct constellation of lung diseases characterized by noninfectious widespread lung injury after SCT, which may affect the pulmonary parenchyma, the vascular endothelium, or the airway epithelium.[20] By definition, this injury cannot be attributable to active infection, cardiogenic causes, or renal failure/fluid overload.[20] The incidence of IPS is variable but may occur in up to a quarter of patients after allogeneic SCT.[19,21–24] The mechanism remains unclear; however, it may occur as a consequence of direct and immune-mediated lung injury during the transplant process. Risk factors for IPS are shown in **Box 1**.[20,25] Extensive work in animal models has suggested a role for tumor necrosis factor $\alpha$ (TNF-$\alpha$).[26,27] The clinical presentations of the entities that constitute IPS are described in **Table 5**.

A variety of other conditions that do not encompass IPS may contribute to lung dysfunction. Transfusion-related acute lung injury should be considered in SCT

**Box 1**
**Risk factors for IPS**

- Myeloablative conditioning
- Allogeneic SCT
- Presence of GVHD
- HLA disparity between donor and recipient
- Pretransplant lung dysfunction
- Older recipient age

**Table 5**
**Diseases constituting IPS**

| | Site of Tissue Injury | Clinical Findings | Time of Onset After SCT | Radiologic Findings |
|---|---|---|---|---|
| Acute interstitial pneumonitis | Pulmonary parenchyma | Fever, cough, dyspnea, hypoxemia | Early, within 3 mo | Bilateral infiltrates |
| Acute respiratory distress syndrome | Pulmonary parenchyma | Fever, cough, dyspnea hypoxemia | Early, within first 3 mo | Bilateral infiltrates |
| Periengraftment respiratory distress syndrome | Pulmonary vascular endothelium | Fever, dyspnea, cough, skin rash, weight gain | Early, 5–7 d after neutrophil engraftment | Bilateral interstitial infiltrates, pleural effusions |
| Diffuse alveolar hemorrhage | Pulmonary vascular endothelium | Cough, dyspnea, bloody lavage, rarely frank hemoptysis | Early, 1–3 mo | Diffuse infiltrates with central appearance initially |
| Bronchiolitis obliterans organizing pneumonia | Airway epithelium | Fever, cough, dyspnea, reduced FVC | Late, 2–12 mo | Ground-glass appearance and patchy airspace disease |
| Bronchiolitis obliterans syndrome | Airway epithelium | Cough, tachypnea, wheeze, reduced $FEV_1$ | Late, 3–24 mo | Chest radiograph: hyperinflation Computed tomography: septal lines, ground-glass appearance, bronchiectasis |

*Data from* Panoskaltsis-Mortari A, Griese M, Madtes DK, et al. An official American Thoracic Society research statement: noninfectious lung injury after hematopoietic stem cell transplantation: idiopathic pneumonia syndrome. Am J Respir Crit Care Med 2011;183:1262–79.

patients in whom respiratory symptoms and an oxygen requirement occur soon after the administration of blood products. We have observed extensive pulmonary vascular disease in a subset of SCT patients with hypoxemic respiratory failure and pulmonary hypertension, who have TA-TMA.[28] Hence, in patients with reassuring imaging studies presenting with unexplained hypoxemia, TA-TMA should be considered. Pulmonary VOD is another rare entity that occurs late after SCT and may present with pulmonary hypertension.[29] Infectious processes may involve the lung, leading to lung injury and respiratory failure. The susceptibility of SCT recipients to specific infectious organisms is dependent on the degree of immune recovery after transplant.

All SCT patients admitted to the ICU for respiratory distress should be assessed clinically for signs and symptoms of infection and fluid overload. Bacterial and fungal cultures as well as viral PCR testing should be performed to identify infectious agents. A bronchoscopy with lavage should be considered early. In addition to a routine chest radiograph, further imaging in the form of a computed tomography scan and echocardiography should be performed. Echocardiography may allow clinicians to document the presence of pulmonary hypertension. A lung biopsy may be considered in patients who have focal processes. In the absence of positive microbiologic studies, a diagnosis of IPS may be considered.

Specific therapeutic options to address lung injury after SCT are limited. Given the paucity of specific therapies to address dysregulated inflammation in the lung, corticosteroids remain the mainstay of therapy. The dose and duration are variable. High-dose (10 mg/kg/d) pulse therapy is used in conditions such as diffuse alveolar hemorrhage; once initiated, corticosteroids should be tapered slowly.[20,23,30,31] Given the role of TNF-α in IPS, etanercept (a soluble TNF-α–binding protein) has been shown to be beneficial when combined with corticosteroids in a small study at a dosage of 0.4 mg/kg (maximum of 25 mg) subcutaneously twice weekly for a maximum of 8 doses.[26,32] Larger clinical trials to assess this therapy are ongoing.

The treatment of lung injury and respiratory failure in the ICU is usually supportive. Aggressive and immediate broad-spectrum antimicrobial coverage, including antiviral and antifungal coverage, should be initiated. Fluid overload should be a consideration in each patient and should be addressed with diuretics or renal replacement therapy. Early renal replacement therapy, especially in patients with AKI, may be beneficial. Small studies in children have suggested both short-term oxygenation and survival benefits; however, the mechanisms by which renal replacement therapy may alter the course of respiratory failure after SCT remain unclear.[33,34] Mechanical ventilation should be considered early; no specific mode of mechanical ventilation or ventilatory strategy has been shown to be of benefit. Noninvasive mechanical ventilation may be considered; however, limitations such as body habitus, skin breakdown, and the presence of mucositis might make this modality not feasible in these patients. In patients with pulmonary hypertension, pulmonary vasodilatory therapies such as inhaled nitric oxide, sildenafil, and bosentan may be considered. Surfactant therapy remains of unproven benefit and is being studied.[35] Extracorporeal membrane oxygenation may be considered; however, most centers exclude SCT patients because of several factors, including reversibility of lung disease.[36,37]

The outcome for SCT recipients with IPS is variable; overall mortality is 60% to 80%, with 95% mortality for patients needing mechanical ventilation.[21–23,32,38] The mortality for children needing ICU admission and mechanical ventilation remains high; however, recent studies suggest an improvement in survival.[3,39] Our recent data showed a 40% survival to ICU discharge for 88 SCT recipients who needed intubation and mechanical ventilation, with a 6-month survival approaching 25%.[2] Similar 6-month survival was noted in another recently published cohort of SCT recipients requiring intensive care.[5]

## AKI

AKI is common after SCT, with up to 50% of SCT recipients having signs of AKI, although 5% to 20% may develop chronic kidney disease.[40–43] AKI in the setting of SCT is likely multifactorial. SCT recipients require significant volumes of fluid, blood products, and medications, which place them at a disproportionate risk for fluid overload in the setting of AKI. Common risk factors for kidney injury in SCT recipients are shown in **Box 2**.

Fluid overload, hypertension, and azotemia are common clinical presentations. Traditionally, the diagnosis of AKI has relied on doubling of serum creatinine and urine output; alternatively, clinical criteria (pRIFLE [pediatric risk, injury, failure and end-stage renal disease]) are used. The latter are sensitive in diagnosing AKI and correlate with mortality.[44,45] Using creatinine and creatinine clearance in SCT recipients to estimate glomerular filtration rate may be unreliable, given the degree of muscle wasting.[46] Cystatin C is not affected by age or muscle mass and has been shown to be a potentially robust marker in assessing GFR.[47,48] Recent data suggest that combining cystatin C and creatinine may afford very high sensitivity and specificity

---

**Box 2**
**Common risk factors for kidney injury in SCT recipients**

- Allogeneic transplant, myeloablative conditioning
- Pretransplant kidney injury
- Drug toxicity (cyclosporine, amphotericin B, cidofovir, foscarnet, cyclophosphamide)
- Sepsis/septic shock
- Sinusoidal obstruction syndrome
- TA-TMA
- BK virus nephropathy

---

in estimating GFR.[48] Hence, cystatin C may be beneficial in monitoring kidney function in SCT recipients.

The approach to AKI in SCT recipients is largely supportive, although prevention is extremely important. Being diligent about limiting risk factors and fluid overload is imperative. Multiple studies have suggested increased mortality and morbidity in patients with fluid overload at the time of initiating renal replacement therapy; similar data are also reported in children with renal failure after SCT.[49–51] Diuretics remain the first choice to address fluid overload, with doses higher than usual needed because of underlying kidney disease; loop diuretics are commonly used as boluses or continuous infusion to achieve desired fluid balance. Early initiation of continuous renal replacement therapy (CRRT) may be beneficial in SCT recipients with renal failure and fluid overload. However, the optimal timing of initiation and dose of CRRT for SCT recipients remains unclear. Outcomes for SCT recipients needing renal replacement therapy remain poor. Single-center data show 33% survival, and data from the prospective pediatric CRRT registry report a 45% survival to ICU discharge for SCT recipients needing CRRT.[52,53]

### Acute GVHD

Acute GVHD is a major SCT-related complication, leading to transplant-related morbidity and mortality. The incidence after SCT is highly variable and dependent on transplant type. The severity of acute GVHD may increase the odds of requiring ICU admission.[5,54] Traditionally, GVHD is divided into acute or chronic if onset is within 100 or after 100 days of SCT. The pathogenesis, histologic features, and clinical presentation of acute and chronic GVHD are distinctly different.[55] Hence, clinical features should be used to distinguish acute from chronic GVHD. However, this distinction may not be clear-cut because there may be overlap. Risk factors for the development of acute GVHD include HLA disparity between donor and recipient, older donor and recipient age, sex mismatch (multiparous female donors for male recipients), infections, and intensity of conditioning regimen.[54] In the intensive care setting, clinicians usually encounter SCT recipients with complications in association with varying severities of acute GVHD.

Acute GVHD typically occurs as a consequence of immune-competent cells in the graft with differing antigens from the recipient. Typically, pathogenesis involves 3 interrelated phases[54]:

- Phase 1: host tissue damage and mucosal barrier disruption related to preparative chemotherapy/radiation

- Phase 2: recipient and donor antigen-presenting cells trigger activation of donor T cell with inflammatory cytokine release and recruitment of more differentiated cells
- Phase 3: damage to host tissue by donor cells

The clinical features of acute GVHD relate to involvement of 3 organ systems: the skin, liver, and gastrointestinal tract.[54] Skin involvement is notable for a maculopapular rash that starts on the sun-exposed areas but involves palms and soles and might progress to erythroderma and bullae. Liver disease is characterized by cholestasis and transaminitis, which may progress to liver failure.[56] Diarrhea is the hallmark of gastrointestinal involvement; secretory diarrhea is common, which may progress and become bloody. Patients usually complain of abdominal pain, nausea, and vomiting. Intensive care is usually needed for management for fluid and electrolyte disturbances related to diarrhea and gastrointestinal bleeding. Ocular involvement and pancreatic insufficiency and sweat impairment may also be seen in recipients with acute GVHD.[57] Acute GVHD and its treatment are profoundly immunosuppressive, making patients as risk for life-threatening infections.

Acute GVHD is diagnosed clinically, with severity being dependent on the degree of skin, liver, and gastrointestinal tract involvement.[58] The grading depends on the combined severity of involvement of the skin, liver, and gastrointestinal tract.[58] Skin and gastrointestinal tract biopsy may be performed to establish a histologic diagnosis of GVHD.[54] The differential diagnosis for acute GVHD is broad and includes skin reactions, conditioning toxicity to the skin, liver or gut, sinusoidal obstruction syndrome, and infection.

Systemic corticosteroids (1–2 mg/kg of prednisone or equivalent) represent first-line therapy for acute GVHD, with the goal of interrupting the cycle of inflammation and tissue injury.[54,59] However, response rates are variable. Failure to respond to corticosteroids is typically defined as any worsening after 3 days of therapy, or the lack of improvement in within 5 to 7 days of therapy. Options for such patients include additional immune-suppressive agents; although some patients may respond, outcomes are generally unsatisfactory.[60] Agents and strategies that have been tried are shown in **Table 6**.[54,60] Because most of these agents are extremely immunosuppressive, the risk of infection remains high. Supportive care for acute GVHD includes diligent antibacterial, antiviral, and antifungal surveillance and prophylaxis, with appropriate escalation of agents with documented or suspected infection; meticulous skin care with topical emollient therapy; wound care is required to prevent against infection. Gut rest and hyperalimentation are needed for gastrointestinal GVHD. Gastrointestinal bleeding may require packed red blood cells and platelet transfusion support, and octreotide may be effective in controlling secretory diarrhea and gastrointestinal bleeding. Pain control can be challenging, and rarely, patients may need intubation

| Table 6 Therapy for steroid refractory acute GVHD | |
|---|---|
| Lymphocyte-targeted drug therapy | Antithymocyte globulin, basiliximab, alemtuzumab, abatacept, alefacept, infliximab, etanercept, MMF, pentostatin, calcineurin inhibitors, sirolimus |
| Phototherapy | Psoralens + UV-A light, extracorporeal photopheresis |
| Cellular therapy | Mesenchymal stem cells |
| Topical/directed therapy | Topical corticosteroids for skin GVHD; oral beclomethasone or budesonide for intestinal GVHD |

for escalating doses of narcotics. Systematic ophthalmologic evaluation for ocular involvement should be performed in patients with GVHD.

The outcomes for acute GVHD are dependent on the severity and grade of disease. Recent data in adults and children showed dismal survival outcomes (5% 5-year survival) for grade 4 GVHD, whereas 5-year survival for grades 1 to 2 was 80% to 85%.[61]

## TA-TMA

Transplant-associated thrombotic microangiopathy (TA-TMA) is a thrombotic micro-angiopathic process that is associated with high morbidity and mortality and may lead to chronic kidney disease in SCT recipients. It usually occurs early (within 100 days) after allogeneic SCT, but also occurs after autologous transplant. The incidence and prevalence remain unclear. The pathogenesis of TA-TMA is unclear.[62] The key to its pathogenesis is likely vascular endothelial damage during the transplant process, which is followed by platelet activation, resulting in microangiopathic hemolytic anemia, microthrombosis, fibrin deposition, and end-organ injury.[62,63] The kidney is most commonly affected; however, involvement of multiple organs, including the lung and the gastrointestinal tract, has been noted.[62,64] Histologic findings of TA-TMA include thickened capillary walls with endothelial cell swelling and separation from the basal membrane, extravasation of fragmented erythrocytes into the tissues, and microvessel occlusion with fibrin thrombi. Multiple triggers like infections (adenovirus, BK virus, CMV, human herpesvirus), high-dose chemotherapy, radiotherapy, calcineurin inhibitors (such as cyclosporine), and GVHD have been associated with TA-TMA.

Current clinical diagnostic criteria for TA-TMA include varying degrees of schistocytosis, de novo thrombocytopenia and anemia, increased lactate dehydrogenase levels, decreased haptoglobin, doubling of serum creatinine, and neurologic symptoms.[65,66] The usefulness of these criteria remains questionable, because the diagnosis of TA-TMA in the transplant setting is challenging, given the numerous conditions that lead to anemia, thrombocytopenia, and kidney injury.[67] Clinical presentation includes polyserositis and multiorgan failure, which may mimic sepsis, sinusoidal obstruction syndrome, and GVHD. Other findings include hypertension and proteinuria, which may allow an earlier diagnosis. Pulmonary arterial hypertension has been observed in patients with prolonged symptoms of TA-TMA, and hence, it should be considered in SCT recipients with new-onset respiratory distress, hypoxemia, and signs of pulmonary hypertension.[28] TA-TMA diagnosis is often delayed using current clinical criteria, and novel diagnostic markers should be evaluated. Renal biopsy, although challenging, may be useful in certain patients.

Lack in understanding of TA-TMA pathogenesis limits specific therapeutic options. Early intervention before irreversible organ damage improves outcomes of TA-TMA.[67] Most commonly used clinical interventions are discontinuing calcineurin inhibitors and treating known triggers like infections and GVHD. Response to rituximab and defibrotide alone or in combination with therapeutic plasma exchange has been reported in small cohorts of patients.[62] Severe TA-TMA with multiorgan failure has high mortality (60%–90%). SCT survivors with a milder but prolonged course of TA-TMA have a high risk of chronic kidney disease and hypertension, affecting long-term outcomes.

### Hepatic VOD

Hepatic VOD or sinusoidal obstruction syndrome is an SCT-related complication, which primarily involves the liver. It occurs early, typically within the first 30 days of transplant, and presents with weight gain, jaundice, hepatomegaly, and ascites. The reported incidence is 8% to 14%, and a higher incidence may be noted in higher-risk patients.[68] Risk factors include high-dose chemotherapy (especially busulfan, melphalan, and cyclophosphamide), total body radiation, preexisting liver disease, unrelated donor, Total parenteral nutrition use, and positive CMV serology in the recipient.[69–72] VOD is believed to occur as a consequence of sinusoidal endothelial damage related to conditioning. Histologically, subendothelial edema, extravasation of red blood cells, and fibrin deposition result in hepatocyte damage and deposition of collagen. Sinusoidal obstruction leads to the development of portal hypertension; with progression, it may result in hepatocyte necrosis and liver failure.[73] Dysregulated coagulation also plays a role in the pathogenesis leading to thrombosis.[74]

Classic presentation is tender hepatomegaly and weight gain (>5% from pretransplant weight) followed by hyperbilirubinemia. Fluid overload with ascites, edema, and pleural effusions is common. Progression of VOD leads to multiorgan failure (specifically, liver and kidney failure). The severity of VOD is classified by prognosis. Mild and moderate disease resolves spontaneously with minimal treatment, whereas severe disease is characterized by multiorgan failure, often resulting in death.[72] Clinical criteria (hyperbilirubinemia, hepatomegaly, ascites, and weight gain) are used for diagnosis; however, these may be nonspecific in the SCT recipient, and hence, a high degree of suspicion is needed.[75,76] Liver dysfunction is suggested by hyperbilirubinemia, transaminitis, thrombocytopenia, and coagulopathy. Thrombocytopenia and reduced levels of antithrombin and protein C may be noted.[74] Doppler evaluation of the liver may show attenuation of hepatic vein flow, slowing or reversal (late finding) of portal vein flow, and an increased resistive index in the hepatic artery.[77] In SCT recipients with suspected VOD, serial ultrasonography might be performed to follow progress of disease. Liver biopsy and transvenous measurement of hepatic venous gradient (increase >10 mm Hg is specific for VOD) may be useful but are rarely performed because of risk of bleeding.[78]

Specific therapies are limited, and hence, prevention may be beneficial. To this end, busulfan dosing guided by pharmacokinetics has been helpful; ursodiol is commonly used as cholestasis prophylaxis.[79,80] Once VOD develops, supportive care remains the cornerstone of treatment, with diligent monitoring and management of fluid overload using diuretics and sodium restriction. There should be a low threshold for instituting renal replacement therapy for fluid retention, especially in patients with worsening renal function. Numerous agents like antithrombin, heparin, and prostaglandin E have been tried without much effect.[81–83] Pulse of high-dose corticosteroids may be beneficial if initiated early in the disease course.[84] Defibrotide, a polydisperse oligonucleotide with antithrombotic and profibrinolytic effects, is the most promising therapy; data from an initial dose escalation study have resulted in multiple studies showing improved outcomes in patients with severe VOD.[85–87] A major risk factor with defibrotide is bleeding, and hence, clinically significant bleeding is a contraindication to it use. As a last resort, liver transplantation may be considered in patients who progress to end-stage liver disease. Outcome from VOD is related to disease severity. Patients with mild to moderate disease have low mortality (up to 20%), whereas mortality is more than 80% with severe disease, especially in the setting of multiorgan failure.[68,71,75,87]

### Neurologic Complications

Neurologic complications may occur in up to 15% of children undergoing SCT and associated with transplant-related morbidity and mortality.[88–90] The spectrum of neurologic complications is broad; however, seizures and acute encephalopathy are

| **Box 3** |
| **Cause of neurologic complications after SCT** |

- Infections:
  - Viral: adenovirus, human herpesvirus 6 and 7, HSV, polyoma viruses (BK and JC virus)
  - Bacterial: *Streptococcus pneumoniae*
  - Fungal: *Aspergillus* spp, *Candida* spp
  - Protozoal: *Toxoplasma gondii*
- Conditioning-related toxicity
  - Chemotherapy: busulfan, ifosafamide, intrathecal methotrexate, cytarabine
  - Radiation
- Drug toxicity
- Stroke
- Intracranial hemorrhage
- Acute disseminated encephalomyelitis
- PRES
- Posttransplant lymphoproliferative disease

common reasons for children to need intensive care after SCT. Risk factors for development of neurologic complications include total body irradiation, GVHD, and hypertension caused by calcineurin inhibitor use for GVHD prophylaxis. Common causes for neurologic complications including infections associated with SCT are presented in **Box 3**.[88,89,91] As with other complications, the risks of infection and bleeding are dictated by engraftment and immune recovery after SCT. The most common complication after allogeneic transplant is drug toxicity related to the use of calcineurin inhibitors (cyclosporine, tacrolimus). Patients on cyclosporine may present with a posterior reversible encephalopathy syndrome (PRES), in which headache, visual changes, seizures, and encephalopathy are associated with classic findings on neuroimaging. This syndrome is often reversible, but recovery may be prolonged.[92–95]

The clinical approach to a patient presenting with neurologic complications, especially with encephalopathy or seizures, includes a detailed history and physical examination, cerebrospinal fluid studies, electroencephalography, and neuroimaging. SCT recipients with PRES show hyperintensity of the subcortical and cortical regions in the parieto-occipital regions on T2-weighted and fluid-attenuated inversion recovery images on magnetic resonance imaging.[91] For patients with PRES, cyclosporine should be discontinued and hypertension should be managed aggressively.[92,96] Other supportive measures include seizure control and correction of thrombocytopenia and coagulopathy.

## SUMMARY

Despite advances in transplant techniques, SCT recipients remain a complex cohort of patients, with disproportionately high morbidity and mortality. Nonetheless, outcomes for these patients seem to be improving. Given the ever-expanding indications and complexity of SCT, it is important for SCT physicians and intensivists to work closely together to ensure the best possible outcomes for critically ill SCT recipients.

## REFERENCES

1. van Gestel JP, Bollen CW, van der Tweel I, et al. Intensive care unit mortality trends in children after hematopoietic stem cell transplantation: a meta-regression analysis. Crit Care Med 2008;36(10):2898–904.
2. Chima RS, Daniels RC, Kim MO, et al. Improved outcomes for stem cell transplant recipients requiring pediatric intensive care. Pediatr Crit Care Med 2012; 13(6):e336–42.
3. van Gestel JP, Bollen CW, Bierings MB, et al. Survival in a recent cohort of mechanically ventilated pediatric allogeneic hematopoietic stem cell transplantation recipients. Biol Blood Marrow Transplant 2008;14(12):1385–93.
4. Cole TS, Johnstone IC, Pearce MS, et al. Outcome of children requiring intensive care following haematopoietic SCT for primary immunodeficiency and other nonmalignant disorders. Bone Marrow Transplant 2012;47(1):40–5.
5. Aspesberro F, Guthrie KA, Woolfrey AE, et al. Outcome of pediatric hematopoietic stem cell transplant recipients requiring mechanical ventilation. J Intensive Care Med 2012. [Epub ahead of print].
6. Haspel RL, Miller KB. Hematopoietic stem cells: source matters. Curr Stem Cell Res Ther 2008;3(4):229–36.
7. Gallardo D, de la Camara R, Nieto JB, et al. Is mobilized peripheral blood comparable with bone marrow as a source of hematopoietic stem cells for allogeneic transplantation from HLA-identical sibling donors? A case-control study. Haematologica 2009;94(9):1282–8.
8. Jacobsohn DA, Duerst R, Tse W, et al. Reduced intensity haemopoietic stem-cell transplantation for treatment of non-malignant diseases in children. Lancet 2004; 364(9429):156–62.
9. Bakken AM. Cryopreserving human peripheral blood progenitor cells. Curr Stem Cell Res Ther 2006;1(1):47–54.
10. Hunt CJ. Cryopreservation of human stem cells for clinical application: a review. Transfus Med Hemother 2011;38(2):107–23.
11. van Burik JA, Weisdorf DJ. Infections in recipients of blood and marrow transplantation. Hematol Oncol Clin North Am 1999;13(5):1065–89, viii.
12. Lujan-Zibermann J. Infections in hematopoietic stem cell transplant recipients. In: Long SL, editor. Principles and practice of pediatric infectious diseases. Philadelphia: Elsevier; 2009. p. 558–62.
13. Storek J, Geddes M, Khan F, et al. Reconstitution of the immune system after hematopoietic stem cell transplantation in humans. Semin Immunopathol 2008; 30(4):425–37.
14. Oliveira K, Brecher SM, Durbin A, et al. Direct identification of Staphylococcus aureus from positive blood culture bottles. J Clin Microbiol 2003; 41(2):889–91.
15. Fujita Y, Rooney CM, Heslop HE. Adoptive cellular immunotherapy for viral diseases. Bone Marrow Transplant 2008;41(2):193–8.
16. Leen AM, Heslop HE. Cytotoxic T lymphocytes as immune-therapy in haematological practice. Br J Haematol 2008;143(2):169–79.
17. Segal BH, Almyroudis NG, Battiwalla M, et al. Prevention and early treatment of invasive fungal infection in patients with cancer and neutropenia and in stem cell transplant recipients in the era of newer broad-spectrum antifungal agents and diagnostic adjuncts. Clin Infect Dis 2007;44(3):402–9.
18. Michelson PH, Goyal R, Kurland G. Pulmonary complications of haematopoietic cell transplantation in children. Paediatr Respir Rev 2007;8(1):46–61.

19. Kaya Z, Weiner DJ, Yilmaz D, et al. Lung function, pulmonary complications, and mortality after allogeneic blood and marrow transplantation in children. Biol Blood Marrow Transplant 2009;15(7):817–26.
20. Panoskaltsis-Mortari A, Griese M, Madtes DK, et al. An official American Thoracic Society research statement: noninfectious lung injury after hematopoietic stem cell transplantation: idiopathic pneumonia syndrome. Am J Respir Crit Care Med 2011;183(9):1262–79.
21. Keates-Baleeiro J, Moore P, Koyama T, et al. Incidence and outcome of idiopathic pneumonia syndrome in pediatric stem cell transplant recipients. Bone Marrow Transplant 2006;38(4):285–9.
22. Kantrow SP, Hackman RC, Boeckh M, et al. Idiopathic pneumonia syndrome: changing spectrum of lung injury after marrow transplantation. Transplantation 1997;63(8):1079–86.
23. Fukuda T, Hackman RC, Guthrie KA, et al. Risks and outcomes of idiopathic pneumonia syndrome after nonmyeloablative and conventional conditioning regimens for allogeneic hematopoietic stem cell transplantation. Blood 2003;102(8):2777–85.
24. Afessa B, Litzow MR, Tefferi A. Bronchiolitis obliterans and other late onset noninfectious pulmonary complications in hematopoietic stem cell transplantation. Bone Marrow Transplant 2001;28(5):425–34.
25. Cooke KR. Acute lung injury after allogeneic stem cell transplantation: from the clinic, to the bench and back again. Pediatr Transplant 2005;9(Suppl 7):25–36.
26. Yanik GA, Ho VT, Levine JE, et al. The impact of soluble tumor necrosis factor receptor etanercept on the treatment of idiopathic pneumonia syndrome after allogeneic hematopoietic stem cell transplantation. Blood 2008;112(8):3073–81.
27. Cooke KR, Hill GR, Gerbitz A, et al. Tumor necrosis factor-alpha neutralization reduces lung injury after experimental allogeneic bone marrow transplantation. Transplantation 2000;70(2):272–9.
28. Jodele S, Hirsch R, Laskin B, et al. Pulmonary arterial hypertension in pediatric patients with hematopoietic stem cell transplant-associated thrombotic microangiopathy. Biol Blood Marrow Transplant 2013;19(2):202–7.
29. Bunte MC, Patnaik MM, Pritzker MR, et al. Pulmonary veno-occlusive disease following hematopoietic stem cell transplantation: a rare model of endothelial dysfunction. Bone Marrow Transplant 2008;41(8):677–86.
30. Heggen J, West C, Olson E, et al. Diffuse alveolar hemorrhage in pediatric hematopoietic cell transplant patients. Pediatrics 2002;109(5):965–71.
31. Afessa B, Tefferi A, Litzow MR, et al. Outcome of diffuse alveolar hemorrhage in hematopoietic stem cell transplant recipients. Am J Respir Crit Care Med 2002;166(10):1364–8.
32. Yanik G, Hellerstedt B, Custer J, et al. Etanercept (Enbrel) administration for idiopathic pneumonia syndrome after allogeneic hematopoietic stem cell transplantation. Biol Blood Marrow Transplant 2002;8(7):395–400.
33. DiCarlo JV, Alexander SR, Agarwal R, et al. Continuous veno-venous hemofiltration may improve survival from acute respiratory distress syndrome after bone marrow transplantation or chemotherapy. J Pediatr Hematol Oncol 2003;25(10):801–5.
34. Elbahlawan L, West NK, Avent Y, et al. Impact of continuous renal replacement therapy on oxygenation in children with acute lung injury after allogeneic hematopoietic stem cell transplantation. Pediatr Blood Cancer 2010;55(3):540–5.
35. Tamburro RF, Thomas NJ, Pon S, et al. Post hoc analysis of calfactant use in immunocompromised children with acute lung injury: impact and feasibility of further clinical trials. Pediatr Crit Care Med 2008;9(5):459–64.

36. Gow KW, Wulkan ML, Heiss KF, et al. Extracorporeal membrane oxygenation for support of children after hematopoietic stem cell transplantation: the Extracorporeal Life Support Organization experience. J Pediatr Surg 2006;41(4):662–7.

37. Morris SH, Haight AE, Kamat P, et al. Successful use of extracorporeal life support in a hematopoietic stem cell transplant patient with diffuse alveolar hemorrhage. Pediatr Crit Care Med 2010;11(1):e4–7.

38. Crawford SW, Hackman RC. Clinical course of idiopathic pneumonia after bone marrow transplantation. Am Rev Respir Dis 1993;147(6 Pt 1):1393–400.

39. Tamburro RF, Barfield RC, Shaffer ML, et al. Changes in outcomes (1996-2004) for pediatric oncology and hematopoietic stem cell transplant patients requiring invasive mechanical ventilation. Pediatr Crit Care Med 2008;9(3):270–7.

40. Gronroos MH, Bolme P, Winiarski J, et al. Long-term renal function following bone marrow transplantation. Bone Marrow Transplant 2007;39(11):717–23.

41. Hazar V, Gungor O, Guven AG, et al. Renal function after hematopoietic stem cell transplantation in children. Pediatr Blood Cancer 2009;53(2):197–202.

42. Kist-van Holthe JE, van Zwet JM, Brand R, et al. Bone marrow transplantation in children: consequences for renal function shortly after and 1 year post-BMT. Bone Marrow Transplant 1998;22(6):559–64.

43. Kist-van Holthe JE, Goedvolk CA, Brand R, et al. Prospective study of renal insufficiency after bone marrow transplantation. Pediatr Nephrol 2002;17(12): 1032–7.

44. Akcan-Arikan A, Zappitelli M, Loftis LL, et al. Modified RIFLE criteria in critically ill children with acute kidney injury. Kidney Int 2007;71(10):1028–35.

45. Plotz FB, Bouma AB, van Wijk JA, et al. Pediatric acute kidney injury in the ICU: an independent evaluation of pRIFLE criteria. Intensive Care Med 2008;34(9): 1713–7.

46. Jacobson P, West N, Hutchinson RJ. Predictive ability of creatinine clearance estimate models in pediatric bone marrow transplant patients. Bone Marrow Transplant 1997;19(5):481–5.

47. Blufpand HN, Tromp J, Abbink FC, et al. Cystatin C more accurately detects mildly impaired renal function than creatinine in children receiving treatment for malignancy. Pediatr Blood Cancer 2011;57(2):262–7.

48. Laskin BL, Nehus E, Goebel J, et al. Cystatin C-estimated glomerular filtration rate in pediatric autologous hematopoietic stem cell transplantation. Biol Blood Marrow Transplant 2012;18(11):1745–52.

49. Foland JA, Fortenberry JD, Warshaw BL, et al. Fluid overload before continuous hemofiltration and survival in critically ill children: a retrospective analysis. Crit Care Med 2004;32(8):1771–6.

50. Hayes LW, Oster RA, Tofil NM, et al. Outcomes of critically ill children requiring continuous renal replacement therapy. J Crit Care 2009;24(3):394–400.

51. Michael M, Kuehnle I, Goldstein SL. Fluid overload and acute renal failure in pediatric stem cell transplant patients. Pediatr Nephrol 2004;19(1):91–5.

52. Sutherland SM, Zappitelli M, Alexander SR, et al. Fluid overload and mortality in children receiving continuous renal replacement therapy: the prospective pediatric continuous renal replacement therapy registry. Am J Kidney Dis 2010; 55(2):316–25.

53. Rajasekaran S, Jones DP, Avent Y, et al. Outcomes of hematopoietic stem cell transplant patients who received continuous renal replacement therapy in a pediatric oncology intensive care unit. Pediatr Crit Care Med 2010;11(6):699–706.

54. Jacobsohn DA. Acute graft-versus-host disease in children. Bone Marrow Transplant 2008;41(2):215–21.

55. Filipovich AH. Diagnosis and manifestations of chronic graft-versus-host disease. Best Pract Res Clin Haematol 2008;21(2):251–7.
56. McDonald GB. Hepatobiliary complications of hematopoietic cell transplantation, 40 years on. Hepatology 2010;51(4):1450–60.
57. Westeneng AC, Hettinga Y, Lokhorst H, et al. Ocular graft-versus-host disease after allogeneic stem cell transplantation. Cornea 2010;29(7):758–63.
58. Przepiorka D, Weisdorf D, Martin P, et al. 1994 Consensus Conference on Acute GVHD Grading. Bone Marrow Transplant 1995;15(6):825–8.
59. Bacigalupo A. Management of acute graft-versus-host disease. Br J Haematol 2007;137(2):87–98.
60. Deeg HJ. How I treat refractory acute GVHD. Blood 2007;109(10):4119–26.
61. Cahn JY, Klein JP, Lee SJ, et al. Prospective evaluation of 2 acute graft-versus-host (GVHD) grading systems: a joint Societé Française de Greffe de Moelle et Thérapie Cellulaire (SFGM-TC), Dana Farber Cancer Institute (DFCI), and International Bone Marrow Transplant Registry (IBMTR) prospective study. Blood 2005; 106(4):1495–500.
62. Laskin BL, Goebel J, Davies SM, et al. Small vessels, big trouble in the kidneys and beyond: hematopoietic stem cell transplantation-associated thrombotic microangiopathy. Blood 2011;118(6):1452–62.
63. Changsirikulchai S, Myerson D, Guthrie KA, et al. Renal thrombotic microangiopathy after hematopoietic cell transplant: role of GVHD in pathogenesis. Clin J Am Soc Nephrol 2009;4(2):345–53.
64. Siami K, Kojouri K, Swisher KK, et al. Thrombotic microangiopathy after allogeneic hematopoietic stem cell transplantation: an autopsy study. Transplantation 2008;85(1):22–8.
65. Ho VT, Cutler C, Carter S, et al. Blood and marrow transplant clinical trials network toxicity committee consensus summary: thrombotic microangiopathy after hematopoietic stem cell transplantation. Biol Blood Marrow Transplant 2005;11(8):571–5.
66. Ruutu T, Barosi G, Benjamin RJ, et al. Diagnostic criteria for hematopoietic stem cell transplant-associated microangiopathy: results of a consensus process by an International Working Group. Haematologica 2007;92(1):95–100.
67. Cho BS, Yahng SA, Lee SE, et al. Validation of recently proposed consensus criteria for thrombotic microangiopathy after allogeneic hematopoietic stem-cell transplantation. Transplantation 2010;90(8):918–26.
68. Carreras E, Diaz-Beya M, Rosinol L, et al. The incidence of veno-occlusive disease following allogeneic hematopoietic stem cell transplantation has diminished and the outcome improved over the last decade. Biol Blood Marrow Transplant 2011;17(11):1713–20.
69. Ozkaynak MF, Weinberg K, Kohn D, et al. Hepatic veno-occlusive disease post-bone marrow transplantation in children conditioned with busulfan and cyclophosphamide: incidence, risk factors, and clinical outcome. Bone Marrow Transplant 1991;7(6):467–74.
70. Barker CC, Butzner JD, Anderson RA, et al. Incidence, survival and risk factors for the development of veno-occlusive disease in pediatric hematopoietic stem cell transplant recipients. Bone Marrow Transplant 2003;32(1):79–87.
71. Coppell JA, Richardson PG, Soiffer R, et al. Hepatic veno-occlusive disease following stem cell transplantation: incidence, clinical course, and outcome. Biol Blood Marrow Transplant 2010;16(2):157–68.
72. Lee SH, Yoo KH, Sung KW, et al. Hepatic veno-occlusive disease in children after hematopoietic stem cell transplantation: incidence, risk factors, and outcome. Bone Marrow Transplant 2010;45(8):1287–93.

73. Rubbia-Brandt L. Sinusoidal obstruction syndrome. Clin Liver Dis 2010;14(4):651–68.
74. Peres E, Kintzel P, Dansey R, et al. Early intervention with antithrombin III therapy to prevent progression of hepatic venoocclusive disease. Blood Coagul Fibrinolysis 2008;19(3):203–7.
75. McDonald GB, Sharma P, Matthews DE, et al. Venocclusive disease of the liver after bone marrow transplantation: diagnosis, incidence, and predisposing factors. Hepatology 1984;4(1):116–22.
76. Jones RJ, Lee KS, Beschorner WE, et al. Venoocclusive disease of the liver following bone marrow transplantation. Transplantation 1987;44(6):778–83.
77. McCarville MB, Hoffer FA, Howard SC, et al. Hepatic veno-occlusive disease in children undergoing bone-marrow transplantation: usefulness of sonographic findings. Pediatr Radiol 2001;31(2):102–5.
78. Kumar S, DeLeve LD, Kamath PS, et al. Hepatic veno-occlusive disease (sinusoidal obstruction syndrome) after hematopoietic stem cell transplantation. Mayo Clin Proc 2003;78(5):589–98.
79. Kashyap A, Wingard J, Cagnoni P, et al. Intravenous versus oral busulfan as part of a busulfan/cyclophosphamide preparative regimen for allogeneic hematopoietic stem cell transplantation: decreased incidence of hepatic venoocclusive disease (HVOD), HVOD-related mortality, and overall 100-day mortality. Biol Blood Marrow Transplant 2002;8(9):493–500.
80. Tay J, Tinmouth A, Fergusson D, et al. Systematic review of controlled clinical trials on the use of ursodeoxycholic acid for the prevention of hepatic veno-occlusive disease in hematopoietic stem cell transplantation. Biol Blood Marrow Transplant 2007;13(2):206–17.
81. Haussmann U, Fischer J, Eber S, et al. Hepatic veno-occlusive disease in pediatric stem cell transplantation: impact of pre-emptive antithrombin III replacement and combined antithrombin III/defibrotide therapy. Haematologica 2006;91(6):795–800.
82. Rosenthal J, Sender L, Secola R, et al. Phase II trial of heparin prophylaxis for veno-occlusive disease of the liver in children undergoing bone marrow transplantation. Bone Marrow Transplant 1996;18(1):185–91.
83. Schlegel PG, Haber HP, Beck J, et al. Hepatic veno-occlusive disease in pediatric stem cell recipients: successful treatment with continuous infusion of prostaglandin E1 and low-dose heparin. Ann Hematol 1998;76(1):37–41.
84. Khoury H, Adkins D, Brown R, et al. Does early treatment with high-dose methylprednisolone alter the course of hepatic regimen-related toxicity? Bone Marrow Transplant 2000;25(7):737–43.
85. Richardson PG, Elias AD, Krishnan A, et al. Treatment of severe veno-occlusive disease with defibrotide: compassionate use results in response without significant toxicity in a high-risk population. Blood 1998;92(3):737–44.
86. Chopra R, Eaton JD, Grassi A, et al. Defibrotide for the treatment of hepatic veno-occlusive disease: results of the European compassionate-use study. Br J Haematol 2000;111(4):1122–9.
87. Richardson PG, Ho VT, Cutler C, et al. Hepatic veno-occlusive disease after hematopoietic stem cell transplantation: novel insights to pathogenesis, current status of treatment, and future directions. Biol Blood Marrow Transplant 2013;19(1 Suppl):S88–90.
88. Faraci M, Lanino E, Dini G, et al. Severe neurologic complications after hematopoietic stem cell transplantation in children. Neurology 2002;59(12):1895–904.

89. Uckan D, Cetin M, Yigitkanli I, et al. Life-threatening neurological complications after bone marrow transplantation in children. Bone Marrow Transplant 2005; 35(1):71–6.

90. Schmidt K, Schulz AS, Debatin KM, et al. CNS complications in children receiving chemotherapy or hematopoietic stem cell transplantation: retrospective analysis and clinical study of survivors. Pediatr Blood Cancer 2008;50(2):331–6.

91. Nishiguchi T, Mochizuki K, Shakudo M, et al. CNS complications of hematopoietic stem cell transplantation. AJR Am J Roentgenol 2009;192(4):1003–11.

92. Saiz A, Graus F. Neurologic complications of hematopoietic cell transplantation. Semin Neurol 2010;30(3):287–95.

93. Wong R, Beguelin GZ, de Lima M, et al. Tacrolimus-associated posterior reversible encephalopathy syndrome after allogeneic haematopoietic stem cell transplantation. Br J Haematol 2003;122(1):128–34.

94. Won SC, Kwon SY, Han JW, et al. Posterior reversible encephalopathy syndrome in childhood with hematologic/oncologic diseases. J Pediatr Hematol Oncol 2009;31(7):505–8.

95. Barba P, Pinana JL, Valcarcel D, et al. Early and late neurological complications after reduced-intensity conditioning allogeneic stem cell transplantation. Biol Blood Marrow Transplant 2009;15(11):1439–46.

96. Heo S, Cho HJ, Jeon IS. A case of posterior reversible encephalopathy syndrome in a child with myelodysplastic syndrome following allogenic bone marrow transplantation. Pediatr Hematol Oncol 2010;27(1):59–64.

# Advances in Pediatric Neurocritical Care

Joshua Cappell, MD, PhD[a,b], Steven G. Kernie, MD[a,c,*]

## KEYWORDS

- Neurocritical care • Advances • Pediatrics • Intensive care units

## KEY POINTS

- Pediatric neurocritical care is focused primarily on 2 sets of problems: (1) injury to the central nervous system and (2) neurogenic respiratory failure.
- A wide range of causes is encompassed, including epileptic, neuromuscular, traumatic, oncologic, immune-mediated, vascular, infectious, and metabolic causes.
- The scope of neurocritical care includes not only medications and surgery for these diseases but neurodiagnostic approaches, neuromonitoring techniques, and neuroprotection strategies as well as clinical and ancillary methods for prognostication.
- The irreversibility of many neurologic injuries implies the necessity of early detection and intervention.
- The role of autoimmune disease in neurocritical illness is greater than previously recognized.
- Although a standardized training route or system for providing neurocritical care does not yet exist, several institutional models are being tried. Better coordination of inpatient and outpatient care is essential for patients who straddle the traditional acute and chronic divide.
- Interinstitutional trials will play an essential role in standardizing and improving care. Several networks have recently formed to facilitate this.

## BACKGROUND AND HISTORY

The concept of specialized neurologic critical care for pediatric patients has existed for nearly a century. In 1928, Philip Drinker and Louis Shaw developed and tested (on themselves) a device that would later come to be known as the iron lung. The

[a] Pediatric Critical Care Medicine, Department of Pediatrics, Morgan Stanley Children's Hospital, Columbia University Medical Center, Columbia University College of Physicians and Surgeons, 3959 Broadway, CHN 10-24, New York, NY 10032, USA; [b] Department of Neurology, Columbia University Medical Center, 630 West 168th Street, New York, NY 10032, USA; [c] Department of Pathology & Cell Biology, Columbia University Medical Center, 630 West 168th Street, New York, NY 10032, USA
* Corresponding author. Pediatric Critical Care Medicine, Columbia University College of Physicians and Surgeons, Morgan Stanley Children's Hospital, 3959 Broadway, CHN 10-24, New York, NY 10032.
E-mail address: sk3516@columbia.edu

Pediatr Clin N Am 60 (2013) 709–724
http://dx.doi.org/10.1016/j.pcl.2013.02.008
0031-3955/13/$ – see front matter © 2013 Elsevier Inc. All rights reserved.

device was first used clinically on an 8-year-old girl with respiratory failure secondary to rapidly advancing poliomyelitis. Although by report she responded remarkably well to this intervention at first, she succumbed to her disease.[1] Although their efforts to save this child failed, their experience set the stage for the emergence and later growth of the modern-day pediatric intensive care unit (PICU). Taking an alternative viewpoint, Drinker and Shaw provided perhaps the first described example of a specialized neurocritical care service for children with neuromuscular diseases.

The advent of modern neurocritical care began in adult intensive care units (ICUs) in the 1980s to provide the necessary infrastructure required to conduct complicated clinical trials testing several emerging neuroprotective strategies for devastating brain injuries, such as ischemic and hemorrhagic stroke, traumatic brain injury (TBI), vasospasm after subarachnoid hemorrhage, and hypoxic-ischemic brain injury after cardiac arrest. These therapies were largely directed toward attenuating the neurotoxicity associated with dying neurons and the concomitant release of excess calcium ions, free radicals, and glutamate, which caused excitotoxic damage. Although the trials themselves uniformly failed to show any benefit to these therapies, the quality of care and outcomes in these diseases nevertheless improved, largely because of the implementation of standardized care pathways, bundles, and uniformity of care.[2] Since that time, numerous studies have shown improved outcomes when neurologically injured patients receive care in specialized neurocritical care units.[3] However, the benefits of these specialized neurocritical care units have been largely championed by key stakeholders in neurology and neurosurgery, such as the United Council of Neurologic Subspecialties, leading others to question the need for separate, specialized, disease-specific or organ system–specific ICUs. The Leapfrog initiative, which was formed in 1998 by a group of large employers to spur greater quality and affordability of purchased health care,[4] has recently supported the concept of specialized, adult neurocritical care units.[2]

In Pediatrics, the establishment of formalized neurocritical care units has been more cautious, because of a variety of factors. Adult critical care encompasses large numbers of patients with few diseases, mostly stroke, TBI, and hypoxic-ischemic injury caused by cardiac arrest. Neurologic causes of disease are more diverse in childhood and include those seen in the adult population as well as primary brain diseases seen more commonly or exclusively in infancy, such as meningitis, encephalitis, and birth asphyxia. At the same time, a variety of both congenital and acquired neuromuscular diseases present, which require different support than is needed for primary brain disease. A recent retrospective review from the Children's Hospital of Pittsburgh, a leader in advancing the neurocritical care of children, suggested that brain injury was the proximate cause of death in two-thirds of pediatric patients at that institution, highlighting the need for better understanding of brain dysfunction from a myriad of causes.[5]

Neonatal ICUs have been at the forefront of pediatric neurocritical care, largely secondary to the infrastructure required to conduct the large hypothermia trials for hypoxic-ischemic birth injuries. Unlike their adult counterparts in the 1980s that investigated antiexcitotoxic therapies for stroke and TBI, the neonatal hypothermia trials have been positive for certain categories and degrees of severity and have thereby resulted in better outcomes, which require improved neurospecific infrastructure.[6] However, despite the success of these trials, neonatal neurocritical care remains largely institution-specific without formalized training pathways. Pediatric neurocritical care is poised to evolve further with select institutions that provide both specialized pediatric neurocritical care services or units and the availability of a few training pathways open to both pediatric neurologists and intensivists.[1,7,8]

## DISEASE CATEGORIES

One of the major challenges in pediatric neurocritical care is the broad number of categories of neurologic disease that are commonly confronted. These categories include central nervous system (CNS)–specific diseases such as brain and spinal cord trauma, status epilepticus from a variety of causes, brain tumors, vascular diseases, metabolic disease, infectious entities, autoimmune diseases, and brain death caused by a variety of both brain-specific and secondary insults. There are also neurogenic respiratory diseases that, because of their severity, are seen almost exclusively in pediatric populations. There are other debilitating neurologic diseases that fail to be placed into any kind of usual categories, all of which require a treatment strategy that is specific or unique to the relevant pathway.

### *TBI Remains Most Common Cause of Death in Children*

TBI occurs commonly in children and is the leading cause of death in children older than 1 year.[9] Treatment of TBI is primarily supportive and has been the subject of numerous attempts at standardized treatment pathways. The first guidelines for the treatment of adult TBI were published in 1993, and since then, treatment has become more uniform, with less use of disproven therapies such as corticosteroids and chronic hyperventilation and more consistent use of therapies directed at intracranial pressure (ICP), which are believed to be beneficial.[10] For pediatric TBI, specific guidelines were first published in 2003 and were recently updated in 2012.[11,12] Although the mainstays of therapy remain supportive, with avoidance of hypotension and hypoxia, there is emerging literature to guide the choice and timing of interventions after severe pediatric TBI, such as hypothermia,[13] decompressive craniectomy (**Fig. 1**), and the use of hypertonic saline (rather than mannitol) for intracranial hypertension.[12]

### *Status Epilepticus Underlies a Vast Assortment of Primary Disorders*

Status epilepticus occurs commonly in the critical care setting as a result of a variety of causes. It is the epitome of the neurocritical illness in that its management requires that neurologic findings and interventions be coordinated with the measurement

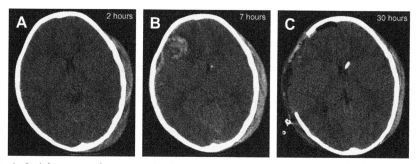

**Fig. 1.** Serial computed tomography (CT) examinations from a 10-year-old with severe TBI who underwent a decompressive craniectomy at 7 hours after injury secondary to evolving hemorrhage and midline shift. (*A*) Initial CT 2 hours after injury shows poor gray-white differentiation and partial cistern effacement. (*B*) Seven hours after injury after placement of external ventricular drain, there is evolving parenchymal hemorrhage in the right frontal area and midline shift, and hemicraniectomy was performed. (*C*) Thirty hours after injury, midline shift resolved and overall less edema. (*Courtesy of* Perot Center for Nerve and Brain Injuries at Children's Medical Center Dallas; with permission.)

and manipulation of systemic vital parameters. The dose-limiting side effects of GABAergic inhibitory medications (chiefly benzodiazepines and barbiturates) are respiratory depression, which can necessitate tracheal intubation, and hypotension, which can necessitate intravenous fluid resuscitation or the use of vasoactive medications. The patient's safety depends on careful titration of antiepileptic drugs and therapies to overcome these adverse effects.

The causes of pediatric status are myriad and include primary epilepsy caused by channelopathy or dysplasia, brain tumors, electrolyte derangements such as hyponatremia or hypoglycemia, disorders of metabolism, meningoencephalitis, TBI, intracranial hemorrhage, child abuse, heat stroke, or a variety of other disorders. Traditionally, status epilepticus was defined by at least 30 minutes of continuous convulsive seizures or intermittent seizures without a return to baseline, a time frame in which neuronal injury becomes evident in some animal models. More recently, it has been recognized that most seizures that stop spontaneously will have done so already in less time, so that when they persist, a deleterious steady-state can already be declared present earlier.[14] The increasing refractoriness of seizures with time and the risk of therapy-related injury increases because control may require more than the initial interventions, which have prompted the view that status epilepticus be redefined to include any seizure lasting longer than 5 minutes.[15] Treatment should occur rapidly and without waiting for transfer to the ICU setting and includes a first-line benzodiazepene, typically 0.1 mg/kg of lorazepam or the equivalent (which can be repeated as needed in the event of incomplete effect) followed by a fosphenytoin load of 20 to 30 mg/kg (measured in phenytoin equivalents [PE]). This treatment can be followed by partial redosing (5–10 mg/kg PE) or the loading of a third-line agent if status has not resolved within 10 minutes. Third-line agents include phenobarbital or levetiracetam. At this point, admission to the PICU is required, often for airway management as well as continuous infusion of midazolam or pentobarbital for unremitting status. Although the single most beneficial protocol has not been established in children, it is clear that initial therapy needs to occur rapidly and should be quickly followed by second-line and third-line agents when initial therapy is ineffective.[15] Propofol is less favored in pediatrics, because of the danger of propofol infusion syndrome, especially in the child who may have an as yet unrecognized mitochondrial cytopathy.[16] Prompt electroencephalography (EEG) is helpful to confirm that seizures have been suppressed not only clinically but electrographically as well and to recognize exceptional circumstances such as atypical absence status, for which different pharmacologic choices are made.

### Nonconvulsive Status Epilepticus is Increasingly Recognized

Although pediatric intensivists have long appreciated the need for prompt attention to convulsive status epilepticus, the identification and treatment of nonconvulsive status epilepticus (NCSE) has emerged as more of a diagnostic and treatment dilemma. The incidence of nonconvulsive status in critically ill children is unknown, although some reports suggest that the incidence is between 7% and 46%.[17] Institutional experience studies report NCSE as a more common finding in pediatric as opposed to adult altered mental status,[18] suggesting that it may be undersuspected and underinvestigated in children. Although it remains unknown how treatment of nonconvulsive status influences outcome in the pediatric ICU, its occurrence and persistence in both neonatal and adult ICUs is associated with poor outcomes.[19] Pediatric patients known to be at risk for nonconvulsive status are a highly heterogeneous group, so the condition should be considered in all patients with encephalopathy that is unexplained or disproportionate to the child's medical state. Because an EEG is needed both to make the diagnosis and confirm effect of treatment, early involvement of a pediatric neurologist is essential.[17]

### *Immune-Mediated Neurologic Disease Occurs Often in Children*

Among the most dramatic shifts in the practice of pediatric neurocritical care is in the ability for early diagnosis and aggressive intervention in antibody-mediated neurologic disease. Traditionally, neurocritical care was focused to a large extent on (1) supportive strategies to compensate for deficit (as with mechanical ventilation for weakness of any kind, or intubation for airway protection in the context of depressed mental status) and (2) prevention of its aggravation (especially in trauma and stroke) rather than the (3) reversal of a disease process. In the past decade, this situation has dramatically changed, as immunomodulation has joined anticonvulsant therapy in the neurointensivist's arsenal of weapons that reverse deleterious processes. Recent identification of putative causative antibodies for a range of neurologic diseases and the availability of treatments directed against antibody-mediated disease, such as intravenous immune globulin (IVIG) transfusion, plasmapheresis, and rituximab, have altered the treatment of central, vascular, and peripheral neurologic conditions. Like seizures, these disorders show that, contrary to stereotype, the differential diagnosis of even the most severe pediatric neurologic presentation is not restricted to inexorably degenerative conditions, but includes recoverable illness. The greater plasticity of the pediatric brain raises the stakes in these conditions, providing both more hope for recovery with rapid recognition and interruption of autoimmune disease but also carrying the threat of maldevelopment as a result of injury of an immature nervous system. The better diagnostic techniques open the possibility and the necessity for head-to-head trials to determine the best therapeutic algorithm for these diseases.

In the CNS, Dalmau syndrome or anti–N-methyl-D-aspartate (NMDA) receptor encephalitis[20] is increasingly recognized to be more common than previously believed in children. Underrecognition prevents accurate incidence estimates, although rate of diagnosis is clearly increasing.[21] Cases may be either paraneoplastic or idiopathic and likely account for much of what in decades past was deemed limbic encephalitis or assumed to be infectious (because of agents that are difficult to culture or not screened for) or postinfectious encephalitis when cerebrospinal fluid (CSF) cultures and viral studies were indeterminate. This disorder can have explosive onset, with rapid loss of cognitive skills and development of movement disorder and seizures coinciding with measurable serum and CSF titers of immunoglobulins against NMDA-type glutamate receptors. ICU admission may be required for multiple reasons, including airway protection, ventilatory support, control of refractory seizures, and severe dysautonomia, including life-threatening arrhythmias. IVIG, plasmapheresis, and, for severe cases, rituximab and cyclophosphamide have been used with apparent success in observational studies.[22] This disorder is probably the most common of what will become recognized as a family of antichannelopathies.[23]

The recognition that Devic disease is caused by antibodies to aquaporin 4[24] allows early diagnosis and intervention for the pediatric patient presenting with transverse myelitis. These patients, who followed a severe progressive course, were previously difficult to distinguish at initial presentation from those with a monophasic demyelinating attack, multiple sclerosis, or even spinal stroke. Consequently, despite the possible benefit of immunotherapy, severe disability was common before the diagnosis was final. Other autoimmune diseases amenable to immunomodulatory therapy require PICU care as well. Database analysis[25] of 25 centers in the United Kingdom found that one-quarter of patients diagnosed with acute disseminated encephalomyelitis were admitted to PICUs, whether for seizures or inability to protect their airway. In this series, all survived to hospital discharge.

Antibody-mediated disease accounts for some cases of pediatric stroke as well. In addition to prothrombotic disorders such as the antiphospholipid antibody syndrome, pediatric stroke may be triggered by antibodies against the von Willebrand factor–cleaving protease known as ADAMTS13.[26,27] Although some children suffer the constellation of complications of thrombotic thrombocytopenic purpura (TTP) because of congenital deficiency of this protein, it is now recognized that children, like adults, are also susceptible to the autoimmune version of this disorder.[26–28] Immunomodulatory therapy can cause the state of hematologic disarray of TTP to remit.[27,29,30] TTP in its acute phase is typically a PICU-requiring condition for many reasons, including renal failure as well as stroke.

### Pediatric Stroke is Unique

Pediatric stroke, although less common than its adult counterpart, is more common than generally appreciated. Its prevalence is comparable with that of childhood brain tumors,[31] which are collectively the most common type of pediatric solid tumors. Adult stroke is to a large extent attributable to a set of common risk factors (influenced by both heredity and lifestyle) including hypertension, hyperlipidemia, and smoking. The causes in childhood are diverse and, although frequently associated with a major other diagnosis such as cardiac disease, sickle cell, or rheumatologic disorder, are probably multifactorial. That stroke is erroneously thought of as an adult disease may contribute to the remarkably late presentation and slow recognition of pediatric stroke. More so than among adults, childhood stroke is an ICU-disease and requires at least initial management and observation in the PICU setting. High rates of tracheal intubation and surgical intervention described among pediatric stroke cases in California[32] strongly suggest that the ICU status did not merely reflect more cautious triaging by pediatricians. A more likely contributing factor, as the investigators point out, was the greater risk of herniation posed by stroke in children because of both their different epidemiology (higher ratio of large vessel to lacunar infarcts) and their anatomy. The pediatric skull has no extra room to accommodate swelling, because the pediatric brain, unlike the adult, fully occupies the cranial vault.

### Primary Metabolic Disease May First Become Manifest in the CNS

Metabolic diseases causing encephalopathy fall largely into 2 categories: (1) those in which the CNS impairment is a consequence of insufficient hepatic (or less often, renal) detoxification (whether because of enzyme deficiency or liver injury) and (2) those in which the biochemical derangement is in the brain itself. Terms such as Reye syndrome or Alpert disease have been used to describe, respectively, acute or chronic conditions in which both factors were present.

Once a regular basis of ICU admissions, Reye syndrome has become increasingly rare. Two major factors likely account for this: (1) the diminished use of salicylates in children with acute febrile illnesses may have reduced the incidence of metabolic crises and (2) the availability of better technology for early specific diagnosis. This factor means that more children with this presentation receive a more precise biochemical (enzyme deficiency) or genetic (DNA mutation) diagnosis rather than the more generic label of Reye syndrome. Diseases that can present in this manner include mitochondrial disorders, including fatty acid oxidation defects, disorders of the urea cycle and adjacent pathways (such as the hyperammonemia, hyperornithinemia, homocitrullinemia syndrome or N-acetylglutamate synthase), disorders of amino acid metabolism including organic acidurias and disorders of gluconeogenesis.[33]

Several fundamental principles guide the management of metabolic crisis. A steady energy source (usually glucose, but in certain conditions, ketone bodies) must be provided, the goal being not merely to provide nutrition, but to exit the catabolic state and restore anabolism. The stressor that triggered the decompensation (often a concomitant infection) must be controlled. Substrates for escape pathways which, depending on the disorder, may include glycine or carnitine, are provided. Those vitamins which are cofactors for impaired enzymes should be provided in pharmacologic quantities. Diagnostic screening tests (such as lactate, pyruvate, ammonia) and metabolic panels (organic acids and acylcarnitines) are often most informative during the crisis to help localize the biochemical defect and identify the symptom-causing metabolite.

### Pediatric-Specific Neuromuscular Disease Requires Innovative Respiratory Support

Neuromuscular diseases causing respiratory failure can be classified by locus in the motor unit, by acuity, and by cause (**Table 1**). In acute or relapsing diseases, it may be the respiratory insufficiency that prompts ICU admission. In the chronic diseases, common reasons for ICU stay include the initial presentation, perioperative state from spinal or gastrostomy surgery, disease progression (which raises the need for higher respiratory support or tracheostomy), or intercurrent respiratory illness.

Most patients with Guillain-Barré syndrome fit the prototype of the best-case scenario PICU patient, for whom critical care need only be a temporary crutch to support vital functions from a previous healthy state until, in most cases, a complete recovery. Historically, the diagnostic challenge was to distinguish it from the chronic devastating weakness of polio, which could present with a similar prodrome of flulike illness. Although a long-recognized disease, several aspects of Guillain-Barré syndrome can make it difficult to recognize at initial presentation. The patient may initially have predominantly sensory ataxia rather than weakness. Also, sensory symptoms may first be noticed by the patient and typically are more subjective paresthesias rather than objective anesthesia. If the weakness is not yet apparent, the patient may seem to have a sensory conversion disorder with the impression of hysterical gait (because they are ataxic with still normal leg strength). However, early recognition is important, because as the progression to respiratory failure inexorably occurs, loss of the ability to protect the airway and development of severe dysautonomia may be rapid. Recent retrospective analysis of cases in the Netherlands[34] shows that preschool children, in whom neurologic testing may be observational rather than formal maximal-effort challenge, are at especially high risk of late diagnosis.

IVIG and plasmapheresis have both been shown to be effective treatments in adults with Guillain-Barré syndrome. The 2 approaches achieved similar times to graduating from ventilatory support, although plasmapheresis has the disadvantage of the risks associated with central lines.[35] The volume and protein load of IVIG, which may be a physiologic burden in the older patient with congestive heart failure or chronic renal insufficiency, is typically well tolerated in most pediatric patients. Recently, a randomized (nonblinded) trial was conducted assigning children to either treatment. Those receiving plasmapheresis had a slightly but significantly shorter mechanical ventilation time and shorter ICU stay.[35] However, the IVIG was given over 5 days, although it generally can be safely administered to children over just 2 days, which may shorten the lag to response. It is not clear whether front-loading IVIG treatment would also accelerate the recovery in this group to equivalence with that seen using plasmapheresis.

The availability of convenient equipment for home mechanical ventilation, whether by tracheostomy or noninvasive ventilation, has revolutionized the care of chronic

**Table 1**
Classic neuromuscular causes of pediatric weakness

| Localization | Disease Class Name | Acute Infectious | Acute Postinfectious/Autoimmune | Autoimmune | Chronic Hereditary/Progressive |
|---|---|---|---|---|---|
| Spinal cord tracts or motoneuron | Myelitis or motoneuronopathy | Polio syndrome (including poliovirus, West Nile virus) | Transverse myelitis Hopkins syndrome | Devic disease, relapsing multiple sclerosis | Spinal muscular atrophy spinocerebellar atrophies, hereditary spastic paraplegias |
| Peripheral nerve (including root) | Neuropathy (radiculopathy) | | Guillain-Barré | Chronic inflammatory demyelinating polyneuropathy | Charcot-Marie-Tooth disease (eg, Dejerine-Sottas disease) |
| Neuromuscular junction (NMJ) | NMJ disorders, myasthenic syndromes | Botulism | | Myasthenia gravis | |
| Muscle | Myopathy and dystrophies | Viral myositis | | Dermatomyositis | Duchenne muscular dystrophy, limb-girdle muscular dystrophy, nemaline and central core myopathy |

neuromuscular disease[36] and altered the natural history of spinal muscular atrophy[37] a major genetic cause of childhood mortality. Similarly the course of advanced Duchenne-type muscular dystrophy has been drastically changed. Although the goals of such technology are to allow the child to not only survive longer but to spend that time at home, inevitably respiratory muscle weakness implies occasional episodes of pneumonia requiring critical care and increased need for PICU beds.[36,38] Optimal respiratory management of this population is challenging because diligent chest physical therapy by suctioning, pressure, or vibratory expectorating modalities and constant vigilance are needed to prevent mucous plugging. Guidelines prepared by the British Thoracic Society[38] can be helpful in training both personnel and parents.

The advent of antisense oligonucleotide medications for spinal muscular atrophy and Duchenne muscular dystrophy[39–41] is hoped to drastically ameliorate the severity of these diseases. Although this treatment may reduce the risk of requiring PICU care (when facing minor respiratory illness) per patient, the overall need for PICU care is likely to remain steady because of the larger population benefiting from improved survival. Already it is the case that these patients are not well served by systems that dichotomize care as acute or chronic. Their needs are chronic temporally but acute in intensity. For example, patients with profound weakness often cannot be moved to floor (non-ICU) care as a step toward discharge home. The level of care that they receive at home may exceed that which a regular hospital floor or rehabilitation facility can provide. These patients show essential factors in the effective delivery of pediatric neurointensive care: (1) the importance, well beyond the standard need in pediatrics, for organized parent education and training, because they are essential caregivers for the medically complex child, and (2) tight integration with outpatient follow-up care, both neurologic and multidisciplinary, for ongoing neurologic and multidisciplinary developmental assessment.

## SYSTEMS AND APPROACHES TO PEDIATRIC NEUROCRITICAL CARE MANAGEMENT
### Physiologic Neuromonitoring Is Largely ICU-Specific

One of the main advantages of the critical care environment is the ability to monitor in real time a variety of physiologic parameters. Recently, several methods for brain monitoring have emerged and become accepted within neurocritical care, although prospective validation of their usefulness is still lacking. The most established neuromonitoring device in pediatrics, after EEG, is the ICP monitor, which exists in several forms. It may be a transducer attached to an intraventricular catheter, which also serves the therapeutic purpose of CSF drainage in settings of intracranial hypertension. Alternatively, it may be purely diagnostic for pressure monitoring in fluid or tissue spaces to guide ICP-directed therapy. Intraparenchymal ICP monitors may also be equipped with probes for extracellular field potential, tissue oximetry, or microdialysis sampling. ICP monitoring is most commonly used in the setting of TBI, but is sometimes also used for other causes of increased ICP, including bacterial meningitis, diabetic-associated cerebral edema, hepatic encephalopathy, obstructive hydrocephalus caused by brain tumors, immune-mediated white matter disease, and encephalitis.[42] The usefulness of ICP monitoring is to establish adequate cerebral perfusion pressure, which in turn is a prerequisite for cerebral oxygenation.

The traditional method for approximating cerebral oxygenation is by measuring jugular venous bulb saturations. This indirect measurement has gradually fallen out of favor in pediatric critical care because of the need for fluoroscopic placement, potential impairment of venous drainage, and questionable usefulness.[42] More recent techniques include direct tissue oxygenation measurements with commercially available systems that measure brain tissue oxygen tension ($PbtO_2$) through a parenchymal monitor. This system provides a direct measurement of tissue oxygenation, which has been shown in small studies to be useful in guiding therapy.[43] The more commonly used indirect measurement of cerebral oxygenation is with near-infrared spectroscopy (NIRS). This noninvasive technology estimates a regional saturation which, under certain assumed tissue conditions, closely approximates regional venous saturations.[44] It has been most extensively used in the setting of congenital heart disease repair, and goal-directed therapy for maintaining normal cerebral saturations may improve neurologic injury associated with repair of congenital heart disease.[44] It remains unclear whether it can be used to guide therapies in other contexts of impaired cerebral perfusion, although it does seem to function well as a noninvasive indicator of changes in cerebral blood flow. Advanced versions of NIRS under development are tomographic, yielding intensity levels across space from an inverse transform of readings across an array of sensors. If validation studies find these NIRS measurements, even if spatially cruder, to correlate with better-understood perfusion-dependent imaging techniques such as functional magnetic resonance imaging (MRI) or positron emission tomography (PET), their greater convenience and temporal resolution would quickly make them essential for any patient whose cerebral perfusion is threatened.

Measurement of electrical brain activity with EEG has long been the gold standard to determine whether a patient is having a seizure. The background organization seen on EEG has been used particularly in the neonatal population to assess brain states and prognosticate outcome.[45] The most valuable information can be obtained when continuous EEG monitoring is accompanied with video to correlate electrical activity with seizures or other abnormal movements. Amplitude-integrated EEG (aEEG) was developed to measure alertness in patients undergoing general anesthesia by personnel less skilled than a pediatric neurologist. It has become popular in neonatal ICUs, where it is used to monitor for seizures as well as to screen infants with hypoxic-ischemic encephalopathy for cooling based on the pattern of activity.[45] However, aEEG has lower spatial resolution than full-montage EEG and so can miss neonatal seizures that are highly focal, because of incomplete myelination and the lesser spatial blurring of the neonatal skull. There is less experience with aEEG technology in the pediatric critical care setting, and its usefulness for monitoring of seizures by nonneurologists or as a surrogate for outcome remains unclear.

### Serum Biomarkers Remain Challenging to Interpret Clinically

Nervous system-specific serum biomarkers have emerged as a largely nonspecific surrogate for the degree of neurologic injury, particularly in the context of TBI and drowning. S100β is a glial-specific marker released presumably by dead and dying astrocytes, which may correlate with outcome after TBI. Neuron-specific enolase is released by neurons, although it seems less useful than S100β as a predictive biomarker, because of nonspecificity to brain injury.[43] Other glial-specific markers such as myelin basic protein found exclusively in white matter and glial fibrillary acidic protein found exclusively in astrocytes are known to be increased after brain injury but remain of uncertain prognostic value.

### Neuroimaging May Be the Most Promising Biomarker

Perhaps the most compelling advances in brain injury detection have occurred with imaging. Although most imaging modalities remain less convenient for critically ill patients than bedside monitors or serum biomarkers, the breadth of information that they can provide about structure, perfusion, and focal abnormalities makes their role in pediatric neurocritical care still expanding. In particular, MRI and spectroscopy have provided the most compelling adjuncts to neurocritical care. Diffusion-weighted imaging, designed to sense the motion of water molecules, detects stroke and differentiates the vasogenic edema altering the extracellular space from the intracellular changes of cytotoxic edema.[43] Diffusion tensor imaging takes advantage of water directionality and has proved to be useful in mapping and quantifying alterations in white matter tracts, which are susceptible to the traumatic shearing effects known as diffuse axonal injury.[46] In addition, PET imaging provides extremely high sensitivity, which, when coupled with computed tomography or MRI, can also provide high spatial resolution, which can quantify glucose uptake and other metabolic derangements associated with a variety of brain injuries.[47] The key limiting factor for these technologies in pediatric neurocritical care is not the resolution of the scans but sufficient image-deficit databases (with image coregistration and morphing to standardized spaces such as Talairach coordinates) on which to base interpretation and inference. Their information richness, which is an advantage, in the interim makes imaging data more complex to simplify to a small set of parameters for study design purposes than the Glasgow Coma Scale or neuron-specific enolase (NSE). Consequently, despite the superiority of the information that they provide over other biomarkers, so far, less guidance is available to the physician from clinical trials for their use in prognostication. The application of the sophisticated image analysis and database tools developed for functional neuroimaging research to clinical lesion-deficit analysis could solve this problem and provide a biomarker capable of telling not only the extent of injury as biomarkers aim to do but, unlike them, also the distribution: to distinguish how much of this injury is in areas that are essential, either in the sense of being required for arousal from coma or in subserving functions that cannot be taken over by surviving brain regions.

### Neuroprotective Strategies Are Still Being Developed

Although the CNS is the most physically shielded organ, it remains especially vulnerable to insults from failure of energy supply, of oxygen delivery, and of electrolyte changes. Two major advances in intraoperative pediatric care show the potential for neuroprotection or neuromonitoring to widen open therapeutic avenues: the use of hypothermia[48] has revolutionized surgery for congenital heart lesions and monitoring of somatosensory evoked potentials, which has reduced morbidity of spine surgery.[49,50] However, the application of neuroprotective and neuromonitoring strategies in the ICU setting, although advancing, has lagged behind what occurs in the operating room and is currently being developed. Whether hypothermia can reduce the neurologic morbidity of cardiac arrest in children as it does in adults is a subject of an ongoing randomized trial (THAPCA [Therapeutic Hypothermia After Pediatric Cardiac Arrest]).[51] Only for a small set of nonsurgical scenarios are neuroprotective strategies standard, such as prophylaxis against busulfan-induced seizures in marrow ablation before stem cell transplant ablative regimens.[52,53] It is hoped that once the indications for cooling or other pharmacologic protocols are better established, these strategies will become an important part of what pediatric neurointensivist physicians and nurses can add to PICU care.

### Neuroprognostication Must Account for Benefits of Protective Techniques

As neuroprotective strategies evolve, better methods will be required to titrate them and assess on an individual patient basis what benefit may be expected with them. The predictive value of several aspects of the clinical picture for comatose patients has been extensively studied in adults, culminating in an American Academy of Neurology practice parameter[54] identifying clinical signs (absent pupils, corneal, or motor reflexes at 72 hours), biochemical markers (NSE >33), and electophysiologic testing (bilateral absent N20 evoked potentials) that are predictive of poor outcome. The relationship of the history and ICP tracings has been more difficult to relate to recovery. Data in children have been useful in replicating some of these findings, such as the prognostic usefulness of N20S.[55] However, the better outcomes in hypothermic adults have altered these prediction rules. Presence and type of limb posturing in particular is less useful in forecasting function.[56–60] Evaluation of the robustness of the coma signs in children is just beginning[60] but already suggests that the meaning of clinical signs is altered in the context of hypothermia. More data on this question are important, because this is a common reason for neurologic consultation in the PICU, and providing families with accurate data on which to base their decisions is among the most profound of medical and ethical responsibilities placed on neurologist intensivists.

### The Delivery of Pediatric Neurocritical Care Is Complex and Multifaceted

The progress of neurointensive care in pediatrics requires not only new physical tools (drugs, imaging equipment) but also new structures (units, training programs, national associations) and even attitudes open to collaborative approaches. The delivery of pediatric neurocritical care is inherently complex, because such a wide range of highly specialized skills is required: to deliver pediatric neurocritical care, it is not only the neurologic or neurosurgical consultant who may be needed but also a pediatric-experienced neuroangiographer, transcranial sonographer, and electromyographer. Few pediatric ICUs have the caseload to allow such services to be provided exclusively by pediatric-specific specialists. Therefore, a key task of the pediatric neurointensivist is to bring a range of non-PICU or nonpediatric services into the therapeutic circle of the PICU.

Several models can be envisioned by which pediatric neurocritical care can be delivered.[1] Most experience has been with a dedicated neurointensivist consult service helping to guide care within a general PICU. Because pediatric neurocritical ICU training is still rare and lacking a defined training route, pediatric neurologists participating in such teams often arrive with a background in EEG epilepsy, with an interest in EEG monitoring, or with subspecialty interest in pediatric stroke. Institutional experiences with a critical care-specific neuroconsult services have been described by both Boston Children's Hospital and Children's National Medical Center.[61] The latter surveys show that as many as a quarter of PICU patients have active neurologic issues among their major problems, more than the number admitted with a neurologic problem as their primary or initial diagnosis. As would be expected, the more complex, higher chronicity and morbidity patients were particularly overrepresented among those who developed neurologic problems requiring consultation and workup.

The development of distinct, cohorted pediatric neurointensive care beds has occurred at fewer institutions. The formation of neurospecific (whether medical or surgical) units in adult hospitals was met with resistance at some institutions; how to best implement this model in pediatrics is yet more complex and controversial.[62] The pediatric patients with only neurologic problems who require ICU observation but no nonneurologic ICU-level interventions may not suffice to populate a unit. The number of pediatric neurologists with primary ICU skills such as intubation or central line placement is smaller than in adult services, in which a generation of neurologists have already been trained to manage ICU patients. The progress of this model requires more dual-trained specialists or jointly managed units.

To achieve their potential, such units need to have curricula for nurse training and a system for neurodevelopmental follow-up. Within adult units, the ability of highly trained nurses to perform neuropsychological batteries more sensitive than the Glasgow Coma Scale has become a key part of vasospasm watch. Analogous systems in neuro-ICUs could help to cut the lag to recognition in pediatric stroke. Neurodevelopmental follow-up would serve to assess the efficacy of PICU interventions for both clinical and research purposes. Such clinics are now a standard expectation of neonatal ICUs.

Although cooperation between institutions has been essential for trials on neuroprotection, it has become recognized that these connections and contacts should be maintained regularly so as to not only implement existing protocols but to foster more proposals even at the conceptual and the design stage. The Pediatric Neurocritical Care Research Group[63] brings together leaders in this emerging filed to share experience and to refine research plans of shared interest. The NeuroNext initiative[64,65] has also, with backing from the National Institutes of Health, made available research tools and expertise to assist with the complexities of designing clinical trials. These networks aim to provide the infrastructure for large multicenter trials. This strategy would allow decision making for common pediatric neurocritical care management to be evidence based and standardized, rather than extrapolated from adult or neonatal data, which may not be applicable. Pediatric neurocritical care services and units, coupled with outpatient multidisciplinary neurodevelopmental follow-up teams, can play a leading, catalyzing role in creating and then implementing this science of developmental intensive care, an approach that saves developmental potential as well as lives.

## REFERENCES

1. Tasker RC. Pediatric neurocritical care: is it time to come of age? Curr Opin Pediatr 2009;21(6):724–30.
2. Markandaya M, Thomas KP, Jahromi B, et al. The role of neurocritical care: a brief report on the survey results of neurosciences and critical care specialists. Neurocrit Care 2012;16(1):72–81.
3. Varelas PN, Abdelhak T, Wellwood J, et al. The appointment of neurointensivists is financially beneficial to the employer. Neurocrit Care 2010;13(2):228–32.
4. Gasperino J. The Leapfrog initiative for intensive care unit physician staffing and its impact on intensive care unit performance: a narrative review. Health Policy 2011;102(2–3):223–8.
5. Au AK, Carcillo JA, Clark RS, et al. Brain injuries and neurological system failure are the most common proximate causes of death in children admitted to a pediatric intensive care unit. Pediatr Crit Care Med 2011;12(5):566–71.
6. Tagin MA, Woolcott CG, Vincer MJ, et al. Hypothermia for neonatal hypoxic ischemic encephalopathy: an updated systematic review and meta-analysis. Arch Pediatr Adolesc Med 2012;166(6):558–66.
7. LaRovere KL, Riviello JJ Jr. Emerging subspecialties in neurology: building a career and a field: pediatric neurocritical care. Neurology 2008;70(22): e89–91.
8. Murphy S. Pediatric neurocritical care. Neurotherapeutics 2012;9(1):3–16.
9. Corrigan JD, Selassie AW, Orman JA. The epidemiology of traumatic brain injury. J Head Trauma Rehabil 2010;25(2):72–80.
10. Marion DW, Spiegel TP. Changes in the management of severe traumatic brain injury: 1991-1997. Crit Care Med 2000;28(1):16–8.

11. Adelson PD, Bratton SL, Carney NA, et al. Guidelines for the acute medical management of severe traumatic brain injury in infants, children, and adolescents. Chapter 19. The role of anti-seizure prophylaxis following severe pediatric traumatic brain injury. Pediatr Crit Care Med 2003;4(Suppl 3):S72–5.

12. Kochanek PM, Carney N, Adelson PD, et al. Guidelines for the acute medical management of severe traumatic brain injury in infants, children, and adolescents–second edition. Pediatr Crit Care Med 2012;13(Suppl 1):S1–82.

13. Hutchison JS, Ward RE, Lacroix J, et al. Hypothermia therapy after traumatic brain injury in children. N Engl J Med 2008;358(23):2447–56.

14. Hirsch LJ. Intramuscular versus intravenous benzodiazepines for prehospital treatment of status epilepticus. N Engl J Med 2012;366(7):659–60.

15. Abend NS, Gutierrez-Colina AM, Dlugos DJ. Medical treatment of pediatric status epilepticus. Semin Pediatr Neurol 2010;17(3):169–75.

16. Wolf A, Weir P, Segar P, et al. Impaired fatty acid oxidation in propofol infusion syndrome. Lancet 2001;357(9256):606–7.

17. Greiner HM, Holland K, Leach JL, et al. Nonconvulsive status epilepticus: the encephalopathic pediatric patient. Pediatrics 2012;129(3):e748–55.

18. Tay SK, Hirsch LJ, Leary L, et al. Nonconvulsive status epilepticus in children: clinical and EEG characteristics. Epilepsia 2006;47(9):1504–9.

19. Shneker BF, Fountain NB. Assessment of acute morbidity and mortality in nonconvulsive status epilepticus. Neurology 2003;61(8):1066–73.

20. Dalmau J, Tuzun E, Wu HY, et al. Paraneoplastic anti-N-methyl-D-aspartate receptor encephalitis associated with ovarian teratoma. Ann Neurol 2007;61(1):25–36.

21. McCoy B, Akiyama T, Widjaja E, et al. Autoimmune limbic encephalitis as an emerging pediatric condition: case report and review of the literature. J Child Neurol 2011;26(2):218–22.

22. Kashyape P, Taylor E, Ng J, et al. Successful treatment of two paediatric cases of anti-NMDA receptor encephalitis with cyclophosphamide: the need for early aggressive immunotherapy in tumour negative paediatric patients. Eur J Paediatr Neurol 2012;16(1):74–8.

23. Lancaster E, Dalmau J. Neuronal autoantigens–pathogenesis, associated disorders and antibody testing. Nat Rev Neurol 2012;8(7):380–90.

24. Lennon VA, Kryzer TJ, Pittock SJ, et al. IgG marker of optic-spinal multiple sclerosis binds to the aquaporin-4 water channel. J Exp Med 2005;202(4):473–7.

25. Absoud M, Parslow RC, Wassmer E, et al. Severe acute disseminated encephalomyelitis: a paediatric intensive care population-based study. Mult Scler 2011;17(10):1258–61.

26. Robson WL, Tsai HM. Thrombotic thrombocytopenic purpura attributable to von Willebrand factor-cleaving protease inhibitor in an 8-year-old boy. Pediatrics 2002;109(2):322–5.

27. Ashida S, Nishimori I, Tanimura M, et al. Effects of von Hippel-Lindau gene mutation and methylation status on expression of transmembrane carbonic anhydrases in renal cell carcinoma. J Cancer Res Clin Oncol 2002;128(10):561–8.

28. Harambat J, Lamireau D, Delmas Y, et al. Successful treatment with rituximab for acute refractory thrombotic thrombocytopenic purpura related to acquired ADAMTS13 deficiency: a pediatric report and literature review. Pediatr Crit Care Med 2011;12(2):e90–3.

29. Albaramki JH, Teo J, Alexander SI. Rituximab therapy in two children with autoimmune thrombotic thrombocytopenic purpura. Pediatr Nephrol 2009;24(9):1749–52.

30. Horton TM, Stone JD, Yee D, et al. Case series of thrombotic thrombocytopenic purpura in children and adolescents. J Pediatr Hematol Oncol 2003;25(4):336–9.

31. Jordan LC, Hillis AE. Challenges in the diagnosis and treatment of pediatric stroke. Nat Rev Neurol 2011;7(4):199–208.

32. Statler KD, Dong L, Nielsen DM, et al. Pediatric stroke: clinical characteristics, acute care utilization patterns, and mortality. Childs Nerv Syst 2011;27(4):565–73.

33. Hoffmann GF, Zschocke J, Nyhan WL. Inherited metabolic diseases: a clinical approach. 2010. p. 386, xiv.

34. Roodbol J, de Wit MC, Walgaard C, et al. Recognizing Guillain-Barre syndrome in preschool children. Neurology 2011;76(9):807–10.

35. El-Bayoumi MA, El-Refaey AM, Abdelkader AM, et al. Comparison of intravenous immunoglobulin and plasma exchange in treatment of mechanically ventilated children with Guillain Barre syndrome: a randomized study. Crit Care 2011; 15(4):R164.

36. Paulides FM, Plotz FB, Verweij-van den Oudenrijn LP, et al. Thirty years of home mechanical ventilation in children: escalating need for pediatric intensive care beds. Intensive Care Med 2012;38(5):847–52.

37. Oskoui M, Levy G, Garland CJ, et al. The changing natural history of spinal muscular atrophy type 1. Neurology 2007;69(20):1931–6.

38. Hull J, Aniapravan R, Chan E, et al. British Thoracic Society guideline for respiratory management of children with neuromuscular weakness. Thorax 2012; 67(Suppl 1):i1–40.

39. Burghes AH, McGovern VL. Antisense oligonucleotides and spinal muscular atrophy: skipping along. Genes Dev 2010;24(15):1574–9.

40. Goemans NM, Tulinius M, van den Akker JT, et al. Systemic administration of PRO051 in Duchenne's muscular dystrophy. N Engl J Med 2011;364(16): 1513–22.

41. Passini MA, Bu J, Richards AM, et al. Antisense oligonucleotides delivered to the mouse CNS ameliorate symptoms of severe spinal muscular atrophy. Sci Transl Med 2011;3(72):72ra18.

42. Wiegand C, Richards P. Measurement of intracranial pressure in children: a critical review of current methods. Dev Med Child Neurol 2007;49(12):935–41.

43. Friess SH, Kilbaugh TJ, Huh JW. Advanced neuromonitoring and imaging in pediatric traumatic brain injury. Crit Care Res Pract 2012;2012:361310.

44. Kasman N, Brady K. Cerebral oximetry for pediatric anesthesia: why do intelligent clinicians disagree? Paediatr Anaesth 2011;21(5):473–8.

45. Bonifacio SL, Glass HC, Peloquin S, et al. A new neurological focus in neonatal intensive care. Nat Rev Neurol 2011;7(9):485–94.

46. Isaacson J, Provenzale J. Diffusion tensor imaging for evaluation of the childhood brain and pediatric white matter disorders. Neuroimaging Clin North Am 2011; 21(1):179–89, ix.

47. Kim S, Salamon N, Jackson HA, et al. PET imaging in pediatric neuroradiology: current and future applications. Pediatr Radiol 2010;40(1):82–96.

48. Barratt-Boyes BG, Simpson M, Neutze JM. Intracardiac surgery in neonates and infants using deep hypothermia with surface cooling and limited cardiopulmonary bypass. Circulation 1971;43(Suppl 5):I25–30.

49. Emerson RG. NIOM for spinal deformity surgery: there's more than one way to skin a cat. J Clin Neurophysiol 2012;29(2):149–50.

50. Nuwer MR, Emerson RG, Galloway G, et al. Evidence-based guideline update: intraoperative spinal monitoring with somatosensory and transcranial electrical motor evoked potentials: report of the Therapeutics and Technology Assessment

Subcommittee of the American Academy of Neurology and the American Clinical Neurophysiology Society. Neurology 2012;78(8):585–9.

51. Moler FW, Donaldson AE, Meert K, et al. Multicenter cohort study of out-of-hospital pediatric cardiac arrest. Crit Care Med 2011;39(1):141–9.

52. Eberly AL, Anderson GD, Bubalo JS, et al. Optimal prevention of seizures induced by high-dose busulfan. Pharmacotherapy 2008;28(12):1502–10.

53. Soni S, Skeens M, Termuhlen AM, et al. Levetiracetam for busulfan-induced seizure prophylaxis in children undergoing hematopoietic stem cell transplantation. Pediatr Blood Cancer 2012;59(4):762–4.

54. Wijdicks EF, Hijdra A, Young GB, et al. Practice parameter: prediction of outcome in comatose survivors after cardiopulmonary resuscitation (an evidence-based review): report of the Quality Standards Subcommittee of the American Academy of Neurology. Neurology 2006;67(2):203–10.

55. Carrai R, Grippo A, Lori S, et al. Prognostic value of somatosensory evoked potentials in comatose children: a systematic literature review. Intensive Care Med 2010;36(7):1112–26.

56. Bouwes A, Binnekade JM, Kuiper MA, et al. Prognosis of coma after therapeutic hypothermia: a prospective cohort study. Ann Neurol 2012;71(2):206–12.

57. Rossetti AO, Carrera E, Oddo M. Early EEG correlates of neuronal injury after brain anoxia. Neurology 2012;78(11):796–802.

58. Samaniego EA, Persoon S, Wijman CA. Prognosis after cardiac arrest and hypothermia: a new paradigm. Curr Neurol Neurosci Rep 2011;11(1):111–9.

59. Al Thenayan E, Savard M, Sharpe M, et al. Predictors of poor neurologic outcome after induced mild hypothermia following cardiac arrest. Neurology 2008;71(19):1535–7.

60. Abend NS, Topjian AA, Kessler SK, et al. Outcome prediction by motor and pupillary responses in children treated with therapeutic hypothermia after cardiac arrest. Pediatr Crit Care Med 2012;13(1):32–8.

61. Bell MJ, Carpenter J, Au AK, et al. Development of a pediatric neurocritical care service. Neurocrit Care 2009;10(1):4–10.

62. Friess SH, Naim MY, Helfaer MA. Is pediatric neurointensive care a legitimate programmatic advancement to benefit our patients and our trainees, or others? Pediatr Crit Care Med 2010;11(6):758–60.

63. Bell MJ, Pineda JA, Vavilala MS, et al. Neurocritical care research networks–pediatric considerations. Neurocrit Care 2012;17:468–9.

64. Heemskerk J, Farkas R, Kaufmann P. Neuroscience networking: linking discovery to drugs. Neuropsychopharmacology 2012;37(1):287–9.

65. The Lancet Neurology. NeuroNEXT: accelerating drug development in neurology. Lancet Neurol 2012;11(2):119.

# End-of-Life Care in Pediatrics
## Ethics, Controversies, and Optimizing the Quality of Death

Rajit K. Basu, MD

## KEYWORDS

- Pediatric end-of-life care • Quality of death

## KEY POINTS

- How care is delivered to the dying child carries remarkable consequence.
- Preparation of a child and family for the end of life is vital.
- The use of pediatric palliative care services can be invaluable for the preparation of a family for a child's death.
- Cultural-specific differences toward dying patients are common.
- A systematic approach to end-of-life care can be created by understanding the critical elements for family and staff and the barriers that need to be overcome.

## INTRODUCTION: UNDERSTANDING THE "WHO"

Although traditionally reported as an "uncommon" occurrence, more than 55,000 children die annually in the United States.[1] An additional estimated 500,000 children confront life-threatening illnesses yearly. Of the children who die, nearly half are outside the neonatal population.[2] For these children, a vast majority are hospitalized at the time of their deaths and most end-of-life (EOL) care occurs in tertiary hospital settings, typically in the intensive care units (ICU) (neonatal, pediatric, and cardiac).[3] This pattern of hospitalization, independent of age stratification, is consistent regardless of the primary etiology of death (**Table 1**). In the ICU, most deaths are "planned," that is, they follow a withdrawal of life-sustaining treatment.[3]

The time trajectory of pediatric death has changed over the past decade. Although the primary etiology of death in children outside the neonatal period continues to be accidental/injury,[2] chronic conditions, such as cancer or cardiovascular disease, account for more than 15,000 deaths per year (~3000 for adolescents and teens).[4]

Conflict of Interest: None.
Disclosures: None.
Division of Critical Care, Department of Pediatrics, University of Cincinnati, Cincinnati Children's Hospital and Medical Center, ML 2005, 3333 Burnet Avenue, MLC 2005, Cincinnati, OH 45229, USA
E-mail address: Rajit.basu@cchmc.org

**Table 1**
**Etiology of pediatric death**

| Rank | Infant <1 y | 1–4 y | 5–14 y | 14–25 y |
|------|-------------|-------|--------|---------|
| 1 | Congenital | Accidents | Accidents | Accidents |
| 2 | Prematurity | Congenital | Malignancy | Homicide |
| 3 | SIDS | Malignancy | Homicide | Suicide |
| 4 | Pregnancy related | Homicide | Congenital | Malignancy |
| 5 | RDS | Cardiac | Cardiac | Cardiac |
| 6 | Placental related | Respiratory | Suicide | Congenital |
| 7 | Accidents | Perinatal injury | Respiratory | Respiratory |
| 8 | Sepsis | Sepsis | Benign oncology | Oncology |

The table lists the most common etiologies of death per age group for pediatrics.
*Abbreviations:* RDS, respiratory distress syndrome; SIDS, sudden infant death syndrome.

Moreover, recent studies suggest an estimated 12,000,000 children living in the United States have special health care needs.[5] Children who previously would not have survived with their chronic conditions or injuries are now living longer (although possibly still not into adulthood) and therefore have a very different death "trajectory" than most children who died in years past (**Fig. 1**). Medical technology has therefore changed the landscape of medicine by widening the distinction between death and dying. The prolonged and variable process of dying ("to disappear or subside gradually"[6]) is typical for many children with chronic conditions who have a slow but inexorable decline toward death, complicating their EOL care.

Death for children is no longer expected. Although this statement seems bizarre in the twenty-first century, at the turn of the nineteenth century, death was commonplace for children younger than 5 years. The decrease in mortality in births from 1915 to 1999 (100 to 7.1/1000 live births) was made possible largely by improvement in general public health and living standards.[2] Common interventions largely taken for granted in 2012 led to the demise of significant numbers of children in 1912 (sanitation, vaccines, antibiotics). Together with other medical advancements, the current reality is that "childhood death is a particular tragedy in developed nations," rather than a common experience.[2] However, although the death rate for children aged 1 to 4 and 5 to 9 has decreased over a decade (2000–2009 decrease from 32.4 and 18.0/100,000 to 26.1 and 13.9/100,000), the population of children in that age group has risen by 5%, meaning more children are currently dying.[2] Recent data suggest that even general pediatricians practicing in the community will care for 3 children per year who die.[2] The numbers are obviously higher for practitioners working in inpatient pediatric settings. In a single-center study in a pediatric academic hospital, the average number of deaths experienced within 1 year for the staff was notable: 4.2 for attending physicians, 6.0 for residents, 19.3 for chaplains, 9.6 for social workers, and 7.7 for respiratory therapists.[7] Despite this exposure, a significant proportion of attending physicians felt inexperienced communicating with dying patients (>50%) or their families (70%), discussing the transition to palliative care (>50%), and discussing resuscitation status (>65%).[7]

The remainder of this article focuses on effects of EOL care on families and providers, the barriers to achieving comfort with EOL care delivery, and the path forward. Because of the high incidence of death in the in-patient pediatric population, it is imperative that caretakers understand the importance of the skill to help dying patients and their families when technology and medicine cannot.

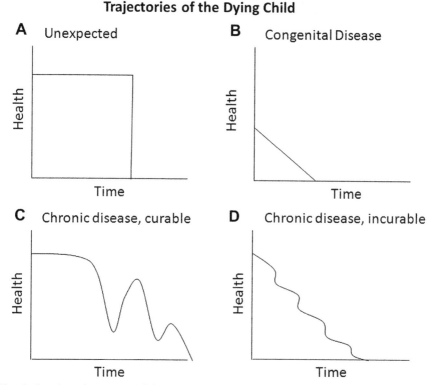

Fig. 1. Death trajectory variability in the ICU. Although death of a child is universally a tragedy, the death can occur after several different trajectories. Depicted are 4 different "death trajectories" frequently encountered in the ICU: (A) sudden, unexpected death, (B) death from a lethal congenital anomaly, (C) death from a potentially curable disease, and (D) death from chronic and terminal disease.

## THE AFTERMATH OF EOL CARE: UNDERSTANDING THE "WHY"

How care is delivered to the dying child carries remarkable consequence. The resultant effects of EOL care on 4 individual "epoch-groups" are illustrative of the cause-effect relationship: (1) Preparation-Family, (2) Active-Family, (3) Recovery-Family, and (4) Recovery-Caretaker. An understanding of the effects on each of these groups is required to understand "why" consistent and compassionate EOL care is vital.

### Preparation-Family

Preparation of a child and family for the end of life is vital. As a child proceeds along the spectrum of illness toward death, care goals generally shift from cure to supportive care to bereavement (Fig. 2). In this care continuum, the manner in which providers transition their focus can be abrupt and difficult to accomplish. A study of 56 families that asked about their experience in the "preparation" period at the end of their children's lives indicated that 28.8% felt inadequately informed about their child's chances for survival, 32.7% were confused about the pros and cons of discontinuing life support, and 51.9% did not know of people they could talk to about questions regarding the process.[8] Alarmingly, 19% of parents believed that the comfort

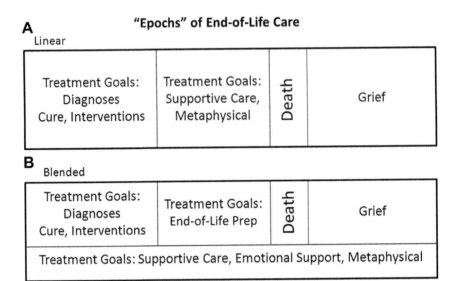

**Fig. 2.** Epochs of EOL care change care delivery. In the ICU, treatment goals do not easily fit a linear construct (*A*) where treatment goals fit into distinct "epochs." A more realistic and appropriate care construct is blended (*B*) where treatment directed at cure and supportive care are intertwined throughout the entire period of a child's dying process.

measures provided were variable and 55% believed they had little to no control over the situation during the final days of their children's lives. Interestingly, most families in this study reported having considered the possibility of withdrawing life support before any discussion was entertained by the hospital staff. Communication "asynchrony" between parents and staff persists in the pediatric EOL literature. A separate, multicenter study of parents of 48 children who died indicated that the most common communication issue was the physician's availability and attentiveness to their informational needs.[9] Communication-related factors playing a significant role in the parents' perceptions of adequate care delivery included honesty and comprehensiveness of information, affect when delivering news, withholding data, provision of false hope, complexity of vocabulary, pace of providing information, contradictory information, and physician's body language. Honesty was cited as extremely important to parents, as an honest prognosis helped parents to make decisions in their child's best interest. Parents noted in numerous instances being "better prepared" with open and honest information, knowing what to expect.[8,10] The withholding of information and provision of false hope were particularly troublesome for families. Adult oncology literature provides evidence that many practitioners do not provide survival estimates to their patients or give *different* (longer) survival estimates to their patients than what they actually believe.[11] Although some parents admitted that it was possible that intentionally withholding prognostic information may have been a way to preserve their optimism and reduce suffering, others felt a sense of betrayal, which eventually led to anger and a lack of trust. Physicians' jargon, pace, and body language were important to parents. Sensitivity and interpersonal skills of the informant were felt to be more important than their professional status. On the whole, families prepared for the EOL by staff who were compassionate, available, and honest felt more comfortable that everything that *could* have been done for their children *was* done.[12] Taken together, parents and families of children carry forward memories of the preparation given to them and their children during the dying process. It is crucial that practitioners be mindful of the method of preparation of families during this time.

The use of pediatric palliative care services can be invaluable for the preparation of a family for a child's death. Published "guidelines" for communication between staff and families for EOL assumes a linear procession from diagnosis, treatment, complications, to death.[13] For children who follow this timeline, palliative care services may be beneficial. The World Health Organization defines palliative care for children as "aiming to improve the quality of life of patients facing life-threatening illnesses and their families through the prevention and relief of suffering by early identification and treatment of pain and other problems, whether physical, psychosocial, or spiritual."[14] Palliative care begins when illness is diagnosed, and continues past the end of life (**Fig. 3**), using a multidisciplinary approach to address psychosocial concerns (including coping mechanisms, previous experiences with death and dying), spiritual needs, advance care planning (including identifying goals of care), and coordination of care (establishing direct communication methods between families and staff, financial needs and limitations, and identifying family preferences of care).[15] Follow-up of 68 family members of 44 deceased children indicated that palliative care services were helpful in remedying inadequate or uncaring communication, preventing procedural oversights, guiding comfort care medications, and coordinating care with multilingual patients.[16] Despite the edict issued by The Institute of Medicine, nearly 10 years ago, to improve the quality and delivery of pediatric palliative care,[2] significant work remains to incorporate this valuable field of service into the standard preparation of a family for the end of life.

## Active-Family

Care for a family when a child's death is imminent carries long-lasting consequence. In this "active" period, many pediatric ICU (PICU) families (approximately 40%–60%) are

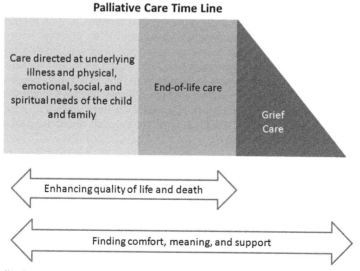

**Palliative Care Time Line**

Care directed at underlying illness and physical, emotional, social, and spiritual needs of the child and family

End-of-life care

Grief Care

Enhancing quality of life and death

Finding comfort, meaning, and support

**Fig. 3.** Palliative care encompasses the entire duration of the dying process. Palliative care services are involved early in a patient's illness providing support via numerous mechanisms. As disease progresses and the focus of medical treatment shifts, palliative care directs support toward comfort and finding a meaning. The care persists after death.

confronted with the decision of withdrawing life-sustaining therapies.[3,17] Exercising autonomy, accepting or refusing medical interventions (even life-sustaining therapy), parents, as the surrogate decision makers for their children, can be influenced heavily by care providers. Intensivists often rely on describing beneficence and nonmalefi-cence (euphemistically stated as "doing things for, rather than to" a child) to lay out options for parents. When asked, parents identified factors, such as quality of life, degree of pain and suffering, and likelihood of improvement, as most important[18]; however, physicians often discuss acute prognosis and neurologic status. Conflicts in these opinions can arise, which, when unresolved, can lead to increased suffering, emotional distress, and high emotional cost.[10] In a study of 14 parents asked about withdrawal of support, the factors that increased comfort with decision making in this active period of death included discussion of past experiences with dying (other family members), honest discussion of the known and unknown regarding prognosis, faith, appreciation of nonmedical influences on care (financial and resource limita-tions), and attention to giving a "time frame" for withdrawal.[18] In a larger, separate study of 70 patients admitted to the PICU for 24 hours to 7 days (not necessarily life-threatening illnesses included), 64% of parents said they would consider with-drawing life-sustaining therapies if their child was suffering, 51% would make a deci-sion based on quality-of-life considerations, and 43% acknowledged the influence of physician-estimated prognosis in their decisions.[19] In this study, faith, financial limita-tions, and reliance on self-intuition were also cited as important. Discussion of resus-citation wishes (code status) is paramount; data suggest that open and honest communication empowers families to dictate what happens at the EOL and the right to tell their own story.[20]

In the "active" period of death, the environment and manner of dying leads to long-lasting effects for parents and families. Environmental and human factors carry poten-tial to reduce stress and improve healing.[21,22] In a follow-up study of 26 parents of children who died in the PICU, factors that exacerbated grief included not being familiar with (or not getting explanations for) the numerous machines, graphs, and noises connected to their children, cramped waiting rooms, restriction of access to their children (eg, during shift change, at night), and facilities to care for themselves (personal hygiene). Parents consistently described how positive environmental memories contributed to comfort during bereavement, whereas negative ones com-pounded an already devastating experience. Other important factors included partic-ipation in their child's care (directly attributed to "space"), being present during invasive procedures and resuscitations, and having easy access to their children. In summary, health care professionals can influence long-term recovery by modulating the environment of a child in the PICU and appreciating the relationship of the child, the family, and their surroundings.

### Recovery-Family

The recovery of a family from grief over a child's death depends on the manner of EOL care. Although a significant proportion of recovery depends on issues outside the scope of PICU staff and care providers, families cite several factors vital to their recovery. Parents consistently report that greater understanding of their child's illness and receiving frequent information from PICU staff were correlated with beneficial short-term and long-term mental and physical health.[12,23,24] Honest and clear infor-mation allows parents to make decisions without a sense of feeling deceived or feel-ings of leaving options on the table. Clinicians previously unknown to the family (as most PICU staff are, vs primary services), are quickly drawn into the family's inner circle of support, thereby becoming an important piece of the support structure[8] and the emotional support of the staff (from empathy to overt expression of sympathy) mattered deeply to parents.[25] Finally, families have indicated a desire to have follow-up with PICU staff to gain information and reassurance and to provide feedback about their experience.[26] Unfortunately, follow-up with families is not commonplace for PICU staff and when done is primarily for study purposes. In the newborn ICU (NICU), however, follow-up with families is more common (NICU follow-up clinics are standard) and studies indicate that discussions of the importance of counseling (marital and sibling), early discussion of autopsy results, and a coordination of the immediate post-death process were vital to parents' grief recovery.[27] Taken together, consistent and compassionate EOL care affects the recovery of a family from a child's death.

### Recovery-Caretakers

Physicians and hospital staff are vulnerable to the effects of EOL care delivery. Several studies suggest that providers who have insufficient training and experience in the delivery of EOL care are susceptible to feelings of "burn-out," inadequacy, and discomfort.[28,29] Other studies indicate that inadequate support for staff members who provide EOL care can lead to depression, emotional withdrawal, and regression at work.[30] House-staff and nurses are especially vulnerable to the effects of posttraumatic stress disorder after the death of patients under their care.[31] Evidence suggests that separate times for staff members to examine intense emotions are beneficial to the long-term health of EOL care providers.[32] During EOL care, from the preparation, to the active dying phase, to the recovery of the family, the personal and professional challenges of providers who repeatedly care for dying children are important to address.[33] A study of 70 critical care physicians from 6 clinical centers indicated that 33% never participated in follow-up meetings with parents, and of the 67% who did, 85% felt the meetings to be beneficial to families and 74% felt the meetings to be beneficial to physicians.[34] Given the widespread lack of follow-up for ICU physicians, this absence of "closure," which can be a part of postmortem meetings, with families may contribute substantially to prolonged grieving and burn-out among staff.

In summary, the resultant effects of EOL care can be felt from both the families of deceased children and the staff who provided care for them in the ICU. EOL literature indicates that consistency, compassion, and constant care were vital to the mental health of all parties involved. Further, the *prospective* delivery of EOL care appears to be affected by the *retrospective* appreciation by staff of the sequelae for each of the 4 "time-groups" of prior EOL care. Put another way, ignoring the past often condemns staff to repeat false steps. To ensure adequate EOL care to dying children, caretakers must understand the factors that are most important to families and to themselves.

## BARRIERS TO CARE: UNDERSTANDING THE "WHAT"

A consistent and compassionate method to deliver EOL care to children faces numerous hurdles. From the metaphysical to the practical, practitioners are confronted with barriers that inhibit optimal care. A proper understanding of these barriers is required to formulate a new working guide to EOL care delivery.

An overarching barrier to the consistent and compassionate care of dying children is *metaphysical*. Simply stated, a child dying does not seem right. Since the days of the ancient Egyptians, the death of a child has been felt to violate the natural order of evolution, where parents outlive their offspring. Existentially, death of children, considered innocent, raises questions about the meaning of life and of morality. Spiritually, noted throughout time in iconography and literature, the death of a child leads to questioning of faith in God and hampers belief in the fairness and balance of the universe. Although the ability to deal with the metaphysical reality of pediatric death is personal and subjective, given the frequency of pediatric death, the issue is more topical than taboo. Appreciation that families also face this intangible hurdle is crucial to delivering compassionate EOL care.

### Infrequency

*Infrequency* is often cited as a barrier as a limitation to consistent EOL care.[33] Although general pediatricians care for approximately 3 children who die per year, PICU physicians and staff care for an obviously high number per year. Although limited experience leads to persistent discomfort and intense emotional responses to death, it also magnifies the feelings of guilt, sadness, and anger a provider may have about their inability to cure.

### Prognostic Uncertainty

*Prognostic uncertainty* is a frequently cited barrier to consistent EOL care. In a study of 240 pediatric health care providers, in 54.6% uncertain prognosis was a barrier to care.[35] In a study of 713 patients (36 deaths), mortality predictions made by physicians of less than 5% or more than 95% were made with significantly more confidence than predictions of more than 5% or less than 95%.[36] The study concluded that the predilection for a "gray area" underscored a difference in therapeutic plan for a patient given a level of confidence. Parents, however, consistently indicate a preference for clear and honest information without delivery of false hope.[9] Many families advocate hearing the "big picture," asking for all the information and the truth, no matter what the truth may be.[25] Complicating the ability to deliver prognostic certainty, however, is the influence of societal and technological expectation. Societal belief that death is avoidable through advanced technology works against physician credibility, a situation magnified in the ICU, where often times trust and a relationship between family and provider has not yet been established. Unfortunately, most physicians prefer to choose the side of overestimating survival when confronted with prognostic uncertainty, one study finding that a more than 3-month gap existed between the time that an oncology provider recognized a child had no chance of survival and the time that the parents recognized the same.[37] The uncertainty barrier is less common in adults than in children, as children (particularly those in the ICU) suffer a diverse range of diseases and congenital conditions. It is imperative, however, that providers overcome prognostic uncertainty by being open and honest with specific details of a child's condition, especially describing the potential for death. The danger of perpetuating uncertainty and not being honest can lead to a confusion of the goals of care (where parents and staff are divergent in the "palliative" vs "cure" goal dichotomy).[35]

A frequently reported barrier to EOL care is the belief that *families are not ready to acknowledge an incurable condition.* Fear of anger or blame from families is compounded by stories of miraculous recoveries sensationalized in mass media, leading people to believe in the endless possibility of medical technology and doctors feeling guilty for this not being reality.[38] The result is the paradox of care providers having an unwillingness or discomfort to eliminate hope while dealing with families who would prefer to *not* receive false hope. Although parents often use denial as a coping mechanism, absence of a consistent and clear message from providers compounds the problem. Using sensitive and caring communication, frank dialogue between parents and staff regarding a child's terminal condition facilitates the preparation for the dying process.[39] Unfortunately, when physicians do not communicate reality, focus is placed on extending the duration of life, as opposed to maximizing the quality of life, driving futile interventions that inhibit optimal comfort care.[33]

Cultural-specific differences toward dying patients are common. A retrospective, descriptive multicenter study of 35 institutions demonstrated significantly less frequent decisions for limitations of care for patients of black race ($P$ = .037) compared with white and Hispanic patients.[40] Whereas white and Hispanic patients were equally represented in cohorts who had care limitations or no limitations, black patients had a nearly 10% higher proportion in the no-limitation cohort. This finding mirrors adult data, which have demonstrated a racial distinction in the receipt of life-prolonging EOL care between white and black patients.[41] Prior work speculated that the reasons for the discordance include characteristics attributable to patients (distrust of the health care system, previous personal experience) and staff (concordance of race).[42] Language also presents a significant barrier to consistent EOL care. A study of Spanish-speaking families reported barriers to care secondary to language and cultural expectations of how physicians should express affection toward pediatric patients.[16] Further, study of death certificates from 1998 to 2003 revealed that non-Hispanic black and Hispanic white children with complex chronic conditions were 40% to 50% less likely to die at home than were white/non-Hispanic children.[43] Native Spanish-speaking families often felt underinformed in EOL or withdrawal situations.[9] Unfortunately, bias, prejudice, and stereotypes often influence patient-clinician engagement during EOL care. Several studies indicate that patients with race-concordant physicians have more positive perceptions of the care they receive.[44] In a survey of 800 respondents from 4 ethnic groups, European Americans emphasized autonomy, Korean Americans expected family members to make EOL decisions, Mexican Americans relied on physician judgments, and African Americans preferred more aggressive treatments.[45] Taken together, to provide consistent EOL care, it is imperative that hospital staff appreciate the cultural and linguistic differences between themselves and their families.

Finally, a significant barrier to proper EOL care is the lack of a formalized education or training for house-staff and nursing staff. A study within a large tertiary pediatric hospital revealed 4 specific topics that staff were uncomfortable discussing: EOL issues with patients, EOL issues with families, transition to palliative care, and resuscitation status.[7] Further, more than 50% of attendings and more than 40% of residents felt inexperienced with pain management in dying patients. A separate study of 49 pediatric residents highlighted a lack of training, experience, knowledge, competence, and comfort in palliative care for children.[46] Another study of 52 fellows and 44 residents at a tertiary pediatric hospital indicated a desire for more formal training in 3 specific areas: discussing prognosis, delivering bad news, and pain control.[47] Finally, a study of 40 pediatric residents with some EOL care experience indicated that fewer than 50% had been formally educated about methodology to hold discussions regarding withdrawal/limitation, death declaration, discussing autopsy, or completing death certificates.[48] The lack of training for EOL situations persists not just in pediatrics but in adult medicine as well, an absence that translates into inconsistent EOL care. At best, this care is disorganized compassion, but conversely can be cold, distant, and chaotic, leaving all involved with long-lasting negative effects.[9,34]

The standardization of an optimal EOL approach for children faces barriers from families and from staff. Parents obviously carry a myriad of wishes for their dying children, some not easily remedied by medical staff. Barriers intrinsic to practitioners (time, language, frequency of death, and education) also complicate the process. Through heightened appreciation of these barriers, however, EOL care can be optimized by creating a clear and concise methodology to enhance a child's quality of death.

## ENHANCING THE QUALITY OF DEATH: UNDERSTANDING THE "HOW"

A systematic approach to EOL care can be created by understanding the critical elements for family and staff and the barriers that need to be overcome. EOL care depends on the following: Questions, Partnership with EOL services, and Designing and Describing the EOL process. Although context always applies, it is possible to create a framework that can be used to provide consistent and compassionate care, enhancing the Quality of Pediatric Death (**Fig. 4**).

Context and situational variability in EOL care can be minimized by asking the proper questions of a patient's family. Amidst uncertainty of prognosis, hospital staff can reach a more personalized understanding of the needs of a family faced with death by asking questions based on the idea of "what would happen if you did NOT win the lottery ticket?"[49] There are 5 principal questions to ask of each patient and family faced with the EOL:

(1) What is your understanding of your prognosis? (2) What fears do you have about what is to come? (3) What are your goals as time grows shorter? (4) How would you prefer your child to live knowing he or she is going to die? (5) What are you willing to go through or put your child through for the possible trade-off of added time?

Robust evidence supports the notion that parents consider withdrawal of care and EOL considerations early, often before being approached by physicians and hospital staff,[8] so the fear of discussing bad news with families is likely overblown. Adherence to parents' priorities is immediately taken care of by having the parents supply the information that is most important to them *before* death is imminent. A frequently cited desire of parents is to preserve the integrity of the parent-child relationship, to feel in control of a situation often seemingly out of their control.[25,50] By asking the questions

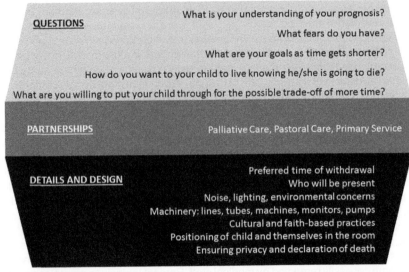

**Quality of Pediatric Death**
*A Framework For Consistency*

**QUESTIONS**
What is your understanding of your prognosis?
What fears do you have?
What are your goals as time gets shorter?
How do you want to your child to live knowing he/she is going to die?
What are you willing to put your child through for the possible trade-off of more time?

**PARTNERSHIPS**
Palliative Care, Pastoral Care, Primary Service

**DETAILS AND DESIGN**
Preferred time of withdrawal
Who will be present
Noise, lighting, environmental concerns
Machinery: lines, tubes, machines, monitors, pumps
Cultural and faith-based practices
Positioning of child and themselves in the room
Ensuring privacy and declaration of death

**Fig. 4.** Quality of Death framework. A logical and consistent approach to EOL care can be facilitated by following this framework: asking crucial questions, partnering with hospital services that specialize with the dying process, and describing/designing the actual procedure of death.

listed previously, providers are better able to understand family-specific context, appreciation that can often define the difference between a positive EOL experience and a negative one. Further, through these questions, staff and family join together to discuss the known and unknown, the limits of care and the understanding of these limits, advance directives, and the ways to balance intervention and prolongation. Perhaps most importantly, the integrity of the parent-child connection is preserved, giving parents a sense of control.[10] It is imperative, obviously, to adhere to standards of communication: meet in private, include all appropriate family members, commit time, do not intimidate, ensure quality interpretation, and affirm nonabandonment.[51] By asking the right questions in the right way and listening to the answers, EOL care providers and family can enhance the quality of a child's death.

Partnership with EOL services is critical to facilitating compassionate and consistent EOL practice. The use of palliative care and hospice services can be particularly beneficial to children with chronic disease. Involvement of these services with families *before* imminent death and through the grieving period (see **Fig. 3**) results in long-lasting satisfaction with the dying process.[14,52] Additionally, palliative care specialists are well equipped to educate and instruct ICU staff, trainees, and attendings alike about specific practices, such as pain management, discussion of organ donation, and discussion of code status. The involvement of pastoral care services facilitates meaningful and respectful dialogue between the ICU staff and families regarding specific culture and faith-based practices and rituals, commonly mentioned by families as important in the EOL process.[25,53] Finally, primary physicians for the child (eg, oncology for patients with malignancy) should be included in the EOL team, as they help build trust between the family and the ICU team. By partnering with other services, the quality of death for a child is enhanced and families are brought closer to the team, forming a cohesive network of individuals dedicated to ensuring the comfort and peace of the child during the dying process.

Designing the dying process in accordance with the family's wishes can optimize the EOL for a child. Because most deaths in the PICU are planned withdrawals,[52] proper design can simultaneously make the process smooth and augment the parents' all-important feeling of control, preserving the sanctity and peace of death. Aside from environmental issues,[54] the following details are important to address:

(1) Preferred time of day to withdraw (if possible); (2) who will be present (family members, staff); (3) what kind of noise and lighting are unacceptable or tolerable (eg, alarms); (4) which lines, tubes, machines, monitors, and pumps to remove (describing in detail how they would be removed and the resultant effect of each removal); (5) what practices they would like to perform before withdrawal (eg, cultural, religious); (6) how they would like to be positioned in the room (eg, positioning of chairs and bed in relation to the door and windows); (7) whether they would prefer laying with the child in bed or holding the child in their arms; (8) any other special requests (eg, having the child's favorite song playing or book being read).

After these questions are answered, the staff should a provide a step-by-step description of how the withdrawal will be performed (from disconnection from monitoring, delivery of analgesia and sedation medication, removal of machinery, to periodicity of checking patient for declaration of death while ensuring privacy of the family). It is imperative that the staff describe to the family what may or may not happen (gasping, agonal breathing, oozing of blood from body cavities) while offering solutions for each of these disconcerting problems. The ability to predict survival time after withdrawal of life-sustaining machinery and medications varies per patient. Giving the family a wider time range, with rationalization of why this range is possible, is an effective way to avoid the feeling of guilt on the part of the family for their decision, and distrust for the medical providers, should a narrow time prediction fail.[51] In aggregate, the proper design and description of the dying process brings the medical providers closer with the family, preserving the peace and decision making of both parties, and ensuring the child's comfort during his or her last hours. When performed in this way, the quality of death for that child is assured.

Optimizing the quality of death is important for both families and practitioners. It is inappropriate and less effective to have the "QOD" discussions in the period of imminent death. Often, both physicians and parents have a sense of the trajectory of death well before these discussions take place. Having these discussions ahead of time enables the family time to process the information and go through the initial stages of grief, identifying the factors most important to them and to their children. Follow-up of parents 6 to 18 months after their child's death indicates that availability and compassion of staff, adequacy of information, and control of the events surrounding the death were associated with their level of grief and overall health.[12,24,55] The Quality of Death framework (see **Fig. 4**) is a simple, comprehensive, and collaborative guide to ensure the greatest compliance of the hospital staff to a child's and family's wishes at the transition period from life to death. A study of the families of 18 children who died in a tertiary pediatric hospital indicates that parents sought meaningful ways to express and assert their parenthood by providing love, comfort, and care; creating security and privacy for themselves; and exercising responsibility for what happens to their children.[56] This Quality of Death framework ensures that these wishes are fulfilled. The guide also will theoretically enable education for trainees, as it systematically addresses the issues of discussing prognosis, formalizing care plans and code status, pain management, and withdrawal procedures. Using this template, family and staff comfort during the dying process can be enhanced, the parent-child relationship can be preserved, and, most importantly, a child's quality of death is improved.

## REFERENCES

1. Burns JP, Rushton CH. End-of-life care in the pediatric intensive care unit: research review and recommendations. Crit Care Clin 2004;20(3):467–85, x.
2. Field MJ, Behrman RE, eds for the Institute of Medicine Committee on Palliative and End-of-Life Care for Children and Their Families. When Children die: improving palliative care and end-of-life care for children and their families. Washington, DC: National Academies Press; 2003.
3. Burns JP, Mitchell C, Outwater KM, et al. End-of-life care in the pediatric intensive care unit after the forgoing of life-sustaining treatment. Crit Care Med 2000;28(8): 3060–6.
4. Feudtner C, Hays RM, Haynes G, et al. Deaths attributed to pediatric complex chronic conditions: national trends and implications for supportive care services. Pediatrics 2001;107(6):E99.
5. Newacheck PW, McManus M, Fox HB, et al. Access to health care for children with special health care needs. Pediatrics 2000;105(4 Pt 1):760–6.
6. Dictionary Merriam Webster On-line: "death" and "dying". 2012.
7. Contro NA, Larson J, Scofield S, et al. Hospital staff and family perspectives regarding quality of pediatric palliative care. Pediatrics 2004;114(5):1248–52.
8. Meyer EC, Burns JP, Griffith JL, et al. Parental perspectives on end-of-life care in the pediatric intensive care unit. Crit Care Med 2002;30(1):226–31.
9. Meert KL, Eggly S, Pollack M, et al. Parents' perspectives on physician-parent communication near the time of a child's death in the pediatric intensive care unit. Pediatr Crit Care Med 2008;9(1):2–7.

10. Sharman M, Meert KL, Sarnaik AP. What influences parents' decisions to limit or withdraw life support? Pediatr Crit Care Med 2005;6(5):513–8.

11. Lamont EB, Christakis NA. Prognostic disclosure to patients with cancer near the end of life. Ann Intern Med 2001;134(12):1096–105.

12. Meert KL, Donaldson AE, Newth CJ, et al. Complicated grief and associated risk factors among parents following a child's death in the pediatric intensive care unit. Arch Pediatr Adolesc Med 2010;164(11):1045–51.

13. Fallowfield L, Jenkins V. Communicating sad, bad, and difficult news in medicine. Lancet 2004;363(9405):312–9.

14. Liben S, Papadatou D, Wolfe J. Paediatric palliative care: challenges and emerging ideas. Lancet 2008;371(9615):852–64.

15. Himelstein BP, Hilden JM, Boldt AM, et al. Pediatric palliative care. N Engl J Med 2004;350(17):1752–62.

16. Contro N, Larson J, Scofield S, et al. Family perspectives on the quality of pediatric palliative care. Arch Pediatr Adolesc Med 2002;156(1):14–9.

17. Garros D, Rosychuk RJ, Cox PN. Circumstances surrounding end of life in a pediatric intensive care unit. Pediatrics 2003;112(5):e371.

18. Meert KL, Thurston CS, Sarnaik AP. End-of-life decision-making and satisfaction with care: parental perspectives. Pediatr Crit Care Med 2000;1(2):179–85.

19. Michelson KN, Koogler T, Sullivan C, et al. Parental views on withdrawing life-sustaining therapies in critically ill children. Arch Pediatr Adolesc Med 2009; 163(11):986–92.

20. Frader J, Kodish E, Lantos JD. Ethics rounds. Symbolic resuscitation, medical futility, and parental rights. Pediatrics 2010;126(4):769–72.

21. Pitts FM, Hamilton DK. Therapeutic environments. The increasingly documented connection between/design and care. Health Facil Manage 2005;18(9):39–42.

22. Ulrich RS. A theory of supportive design for healthcare facilities. J Healthc Des 1997;9:3–7 [discussion: 21–4].

23. Meert KL, Thurston CS, Thomas R. Parental coping and bereavement outcome after the death of a child in the pediatric intensive care unit. Pediatr Crit Care Med 2001;2(4):324–8.

24. Meert KL, Shear K, Newth CJ, et al. Follow-up study of complicated grief among parents eighteen months after a child's death in the pediatric intensive care unit. J Palliat Med 2011;14(2):207–14.

25. Meyer EC, Ritholz MD, Burns JP, et al. Improving the quality of end-of-life care in the pediatric intensive care unit: parents' priorities and recommendations. Pediatrics 2006;117(3):649–57.

26. Meert KL, Eggly S, Pollack M, et al. Parents' perspectives regarding a physician-parent conference after their child's death in the pediatric intensive care unit. J Pediatr 2007;151(1):50–5, 55.e1–2.

27. Williams C, Cairnie J, Fines V, et al. Construction of a parent-derived questionnaire to measure end-of-life care after withdrawal of life-sustaining treatment in the neonatal intensive care unit. Pediatrics 2009;123(1):e87–95.

28. Graham J, Ramirez AJ, Cull A, et al. Job stress and satisfaction among palliative physicians. Palliat Med 1996;10(3):185–94.

29. Ramirez AJ, Graham J, Richards MA, et al. Mental health of hospital consultants: the effects of stress and satisfaction at work. Lancet 1996;347(9003):724–8.

30. Vazirani RM, Slavin SJ, Feldman JD. Longitudinal study of pediatric house officers' attitudes toward death and dying. Crit Care Med 2000;28(11):3740–5.

31. Taubman-Ben-Ari O, Weintroub A. Meaning in life and personal growth among pediatric physicians and nurses. Death Stud 2008;32(7):621–45.

32. Butler R. Support groups address residents' personal development. J Am Osteopath Assoc 1993;93(7):789–91.
33. Sahler OJ, Frager G, Levetown M, et al. Medical education about end-of-life care in the pediatric setting: principles, challenges, and opportunities. Pediatrics 2000;105(3 Pt 1):575–84.
34. Meert KL, Eggly S, Berger J, et al. Physicians' experiences and perspectives regarding follow-up meetings with parents after a child's death in the pediatric intensive care unit. Pediatr Crit Care Med 2011;12(2):e64–8.
35. Davies B, Sehring SA, Partridge JC, et al. Barriers to palliative care for children: perceptions of pediatric health care providers. Pediatrics 2008;121(2):282–8.
36. Marcin JP, Pretzlaff RK, Pollack MM, et al. Certainty and mortality prediction in critically ill children. J Med Ethics 2004;30(3):304–7.
37. Wolfe J, Klar N, Grier HE, et al. Understanding of prognosis among parents of children who died of cancer: impact on treatment goals and integration of palliative care. JAMA 2000;284(19):2469–75.
38. Graham RJ, Robinson WM. Integrating palliative care into chronic care for children with severe neurodevelopmental disabilities. J Dev Behav Pediatr 2005; 26(5):361–5.
39. Mack JW, Hilden JM, Watterson J, et al. Parent and physician perspectives on quality of care at the end of life in children with cancer. J Clin Oncol 2005; 23(36):9155–61.
40. Lee KJ, Tieves K, Scanlon MC. Alterations in end-of-life support in the pediatric intensive care unit. Pediatrics 2010;126(4):e859–64.
41. Mack JW, Paulk ME, Viswanath K, et al. Racial disparities in the outcomes of communication on medical care received near death. Arch Intern Med 2010; 170(17):1533–40.
42. Hopp FP, Duffy SA. Racial variations in end-of-life care. J Am Geriatr Soc 2000; 48(6):658–63.
43. Feudtner C, Feinstein JA, Satchell M, et al. Shifting place of death among children with complex chronic conditions in the United States, 1989-2003. JAMA 2007; 297(24):2725–32.
44. Cooper LA, Roter DL, Johnson RL, et al. Patient-centered communication, ratings of care, and concordance of patient and physician race. Ann Intern Med 2003; 139(11):907–15.
45. Blackhall LJ, Frank G, Murphy ST, et al. Ethnicity and attitudes towards life sustaining technology. Soc Sci Med 1999;48(12):1779–89.
46. Kolarik RC, Walker G, Arnold RM. Pediatric resident education in palliative care: a needs assessment. Pediatrics 2006;117(6):1949–54.
47. Michelson KN, Ryan AD, Jovanovic B, et al. Pediatric residents' and fellows' perspectives on palliative care education. J Palliat Med 2009;12(5):451–7.
48. McCabe ME, Hunt EA, Serwint JR. Pediatric residents' clinical and educational experiences with end-of-life care. Pediatrics 2008;121(4):e731–7.
49. Gawande AA. Letting go, what should medicine do when it can't save your life? The New Yorker 2010;36–48.
50. Truog RD, Meyer EC, Burns JP. Toward interventions to improve end-of-life care in the pediatric intensive care unit. Crit Care Med 2006;34(Suppl 11): S373–9.
51. Spinello IM. End-of-life care in ICU: a practical guide. J Intensive Care Med 2011. [Epub ahead of print].
52. Michelson KN, Steinhorn DM. Pediatric end-of-life issues and palliative care. Clin Pediatr Emerg Med 2007;8(3):212–9.

53. Meert KL, Thurston CS, Briller SH. The spiritual needs of parents at the time of their child's death in the pediatric intensive care unit and during bereavement: a qualitative study. Pediatr Crit Care Med 2005;6(4):420–7.
54. Meert KL, Briller SH, Schim SM, et al. Exploring parents' environmental needs at the time of a child's death in the pediatric intensive care unit. Pediatr Crit Care Med 2008;9(6):623–8.
55. Seecharan GA, Andresen EM, Norris K, et al. Parents' assessment of quality of care and grief following a child's death. Arch Pediatr Adolesc Med 2004; 158(6):515–20.
56. McGraw SA, Truog RD, Solomon MZ, et al. "I was able to still be her mom"—parenting at end of life in the pediatric intensive care unit. Pediatr Crit Care Med 2012;13(6):e350–6.

# Pediatric Delirium
## Monitoring and Management in the Pediatric Intensive Care Unit

Heidi A.B. Smith, MD, MSCI[a],[*], Emily Brink, RN, BSN[b],
Dickey Catherine Fuchs, MD[c], Eugene Wesley Ely, MD, MPH[d],[e],
Pratik P. Pandharipande, MD, MSCI[f]

KEYWORDS

- Delirium • Brain dysfunction • Encephalopathy • Sedation • Agitation • Pain
- Critical care • Pediatric

KEY POINTS

- Pediatric delirium (acute brain dysfunction) can be a complication of critical illness.
- Brain organ dysfunction can manifest as a continuum of psychomotor behaviors that are categorized as hyperactive or hypoactive.
- Delirium can be diagnosed using validated and reliable bedside tools.
- Implementation of delirium monitoring can be enhanced by scheduled in-depth discussions about brain organ dysfunction via multidisciplinary rounds with the medical team.
- Pediatric delirium may be managed with use of nonpharmacologic and, if necessary, pharmacologic interventions thereafter.

Funding Sources: H.A.B. Smith, E. Brink, D.C. Fuchs: Nil. E.W. Ely: VA Clinical Science Research and Development Service and the National Institutes of Health AG027472. P.P. Pandharipande: National Institutes of Health HL 111111-IA and AG027472.
Conflict of Interest: H.A.B. Smith, E. Brink, D.C. Fuchs: Nil. E.W. Ely: Honoraria from Hospira, Inc and Aspect Medical Systems. P.P. Pandharipande: Research grant and honoraria from Hospira, Inc.

[a] Department of Anesthesiology, Division of Pediatric Anesthesiology, Vanderbilt University, 2200 Childrens Way, 3116 VCH, Nashville, TN 37232, USA; [b] Department of Anesthesiology, Vanderbilt University, 1211 21st Avenue South, MAB Room 711, Nashville, TN 37212, USA; [c] Department of Psychiatry, Division of Child and Adolescent Psychiatry, Psychological and Counseling Center, Vanderbilt University, 2015 Terrace Place, Nashville, TN 37203, USA; [d] Division of Allergy/Pulmonary/Critical Care Medicine, Center for Health Services Research, Vanderbilt University, 1215 21st Avenue South, MCE 6100, Nashville, TN 37232, USA; [e] Pulmonary and Critical Care, VA-GRECC, Vanderbilt University, 1310 24th Avenue South, Nashville, TN 37212, USA; [f] Division of Critical Care, Department of Anesthesiology, Vanderbilt University Medical Center, Vanderbilt University, 526 MAB, 1211 21st Avenue South, Nashville, TN 37212, USA
* Corresponding author.
E-mail address: heidi.smith@vanderbilt.edu

Pediatr Clin N Am 60 (2013) 741–760
http://dx.doi.org/10.1016/j.pcl.2013.02.010
0031-3955/13/$ – see front matter © 2013 Elsevier Inc. All rights reserved.

pediatric.theclinics.com

## INTRODUCTION: PEDIATRIC DELIRIUM

Children suffer from delirium during critical illness in a similar manner to adults. The efficient diagnosis of pediatric delirium has recently evolved with the availability of valid and reliable bedside tools,[1-3] although research in this field remains in its infancy. The use of valid delirium-monitoring tools[4,5] and large-scale delirium-monitoring implementation projects have established the prevalence of delirium in critically ill adults to be between 40% and 80%, with a significant association with increase in length of ventilation, length and costs of hospitalization, and greater mortality, after adjusting for severity of illness.[5-12] Furthermore, survivors of critical illness who have suffered from delirium have been predisposed to long-term cognitive impairment (LTCI) and posttraumatic stress disorder (PTSD).[9,13,14] By contrast, pediatric delirium occurs in at least 30% of critically ill children,[1,2] with worse clinical outcomes as described in limited retrospective reports.[15-17] The long-term complications of critical illness and delirium in children remains uncertain, although preliminary studies comparing hospitalized children with those admitted to the pediatric intensive care unit (PICU) demonstrate critical illness to be associated with decreases in spatial and verbal memory and sustained attention.[18] Critically ill children are also more likely to have significantly longer school absences following discharge to home.[19] LTCI following critical illness may impair executive function, an aspect of brain function that is required for purposeful, goal-directed, and problem-solving behavior, such as that required for higher learning.[20] It remains unclear whether the severity of illness associated with critical illness, components of critical illness (eg, diagnosis such as sepsis and cardiac surgery), or its management (eg, delirium, medications administered, metabolic disturbances, hypoxemia) predispose patients to these long-term complications.

Despite the recognition of high prevalence rates of delirium in adults and children, and the associations of adverse outcomes with delirium in adults (some reported cases in children too), there remains a hesitation within the pediatric critical care community to embrace delirium monitoring and therapy, because of ongoing reservations regarding the clinical diagnosis, symptomatology, and pathophysiology. This uncertainty is complicated by a lack of clear treatment options within the pediatric medical literature. For many clinicians, delirium remains an expected and trivial component of illness.[21-24] This article presents a brief overview of pediatric delirium and proposes a model for implementation of delirium monitoring, along with an initial approach to management.

## DEFINITION

Delirium (conceptualized as acute brain dysfunction) is defined in the American Psychiatric Association *Diagnostic and Statistical Manual of Mental Disorders* fourth edition, text revision (DSM-IV-TR) as a disturbance of consciousness and cognition that develops acutely with a fluctuating course of mental status, inattention, and an impaired ability to receive, process, store, or recall information, directly triggered by a general medical condition.[25] Delirium has been described using many terms such as intensive care unit (ICU) psychosis, ICU syndrome, acute confusional state, encephalopathy, and acute brain failure.[22,26-28] A great emphasis therefore needs to be placed on the accurate diagnosis of pediatric delirium within the medical literature and in clinical practice.

## DIAGNOSIS OF DELIRIUM

Historically, diagnosis of delirium has relied on formal evaluation by an expert in psychiatry or neurology using DSM-IV-TR criteria.[17] Unlike other types of organ dysfunction that can be diagnosed by a blood test or monitoring system, diagnosis of delirium currently requires a complete medical examination of the patient, including both careful neurologic evaluation and assessment of mental status. A formal expert consultation is extensive, requiring significant time available to the consultant for a complete physical examination and evaluation of the patient's history and clinical course. Relying on expert consultation alone for delirium monitoring would be impractical for the PICU setting. Pediatric delirium can present with neuropsychiatric symptoms similar to those observed in adults, such as sleep-wake disturbances, disorientation, and inattention. Unique features including purposeless actions, labile affect, inconsolability, and signs of autonomic dysregulation may occur more frequently with pediatric delirium, specifically related to the developmental stage of the child.[15,29] The variation in clinical presentation and cognitive development between children and adults highlights the benefit of pediatric focused diagnostic approaches to delirium.[1,16,30,31]

The Pediatric Confusion Assessment Method for the ICU (pCAM-ICU) was created and successfully validated (specificity 99%, sensitivity 83%) for the diagnosis of delirium against formal neuropsychiatric reference raters in critically ill children older than 5 years, both on and off mechanical ventilation (**Fig. 1**).[1] In the adult population, several screening tools have become standards for delirium monitoring in the hospital and ICU settings, including the Delirium Rating Scale (DRS),[32] Confusion Assessment Method for the ICU (CAM-ICU),[4,33] and the Intensive Care Delirium Screening Checklist (ICDSC).[5] The pCAM-ICU was adapted from the CAM-ICU because of the need for objective and interactive patient assessments focusing on the cardinal features of delirium, including altered or fluctuating mental status and inattention.[1,4,21,33] The hierarchal construction of the pCAM-ICU allows for the evaluation of the most fundamental features of delirium first. If either fluctuation or acute change in mental status (feature 1) or inattention (feature 2) are not present, delirium is absent. Delirium is present when patients demonstrate having both features 1 and 2, followed by either feature 3 or feature 4.[1,4,33] The pCAM-ICU allows for a rapid assessment of delirium, taking less than 2 minutes to complete. The structure of pCAM-ICU algorithm is efficient and is focused on those symptoms most consistent with delirium.

The Corneal Assessment of Pediatric Delirium (CAP-D),[2] a delirium-monitoring tool that has been shown to be valid and reliable for the evaluation of delirium in infants and children, is a modification of the Pediatric Anesthesia Emergence Delirium (PAED) scale.[34] The CAP-D added components to the basic structure of the PAED to increase the likelihood of detecting hypoactive delirium, as the PAED was originally created to recognize emergence delirium, a severe form of hyperactive delirium in the postanesthesia setting. The PAED and CAP-D rely heavily on observation versus patient-caregiver interaction. The developmental and cognitive changes that occur between infancy and childhood are not specifically taken into consideration with either tool. The cardinal features of delirium, such as inattention, are not awarded more weight toward the final score for the diagnosis of delirium in the CAP-D. Rather, all 7 components of the scale have to be completed and have equal value for the determination of delirium.

A limitation for delirium monitoring in pediatric patients is the presence of progressive changes in development and cognition that occurs from infancy to young childhood, and ultimately through adolescence. Tool development must factor in the variable capacity for communication of attention and thought content based on age and stage of development, resulting in the need for more than 1 simple tool for use on all pediatric patients. The pCAM-ICU has been adapted to the PreSchool Confusion Assessment Method for the ICU (psCAM-ICU), which accounts for these unique differences in pediatric patients and is presently being validated at Vanderbilt for use in infants as young as 6 months and children up to 5 years of age. This tool was created

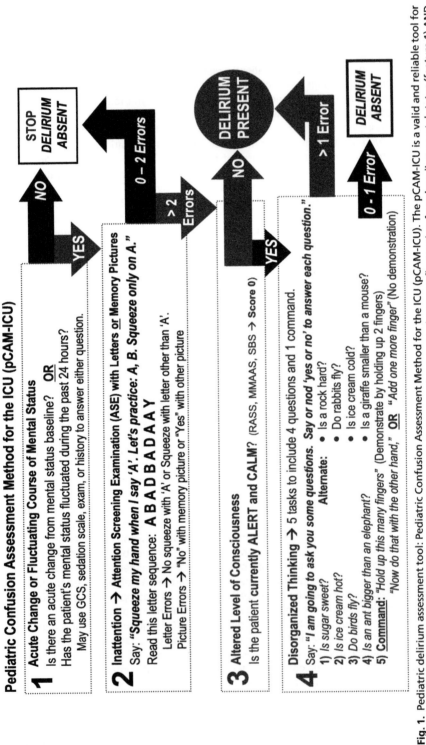

## Pediatric Confusion Assessment Method for the ICU (pCAM-ICU)

**1 Acute Change or Fluctuating Course of Mental Status**

Is there an acute change from mental status baseline?   **OR**

Has the patient's mental status fluctuated during the past 24 hours?

May use GCS, sedation scale, exam, or history to answer either question.

YES → | NO → STOP DELIRIUM ABSENT

**2 Inattention → Attention Screening Examination (ASE) with Letters or Memory Pictures**

Say: *"Squeeze my hand when I say 'A'. Let's practice: A, B. Squeeze only on A."*

Read this letter sequence:   **A B A D B A D A A Y**

Letter Errors → No squeeze with 'A' or Squeeze with letter other than 'A'.

Picture Errors → "No" with memory picture or "Yes" with other picture

> 2 Errors → | 0 – 2 Errors → DELIRIUM PRESENT

**3 Altered Level of Consciousness**

Is the patient currently ALERT and CALM? (RASS, MMAAS, SBS → Score 0)

NO → DELIRIUM PRESENT

YES ↓

**4 Disorganized Thinking → 5 tasks to include 4 questions and 1 command.**

Say: *"I am going to ask you some questions. Say or nod 'yes or no' to answer each question."*       **Alternate:**

1) Is sugar sweet?          • Is a rock hard?
2) Is ice cream hot?        • Do rabbits fly?
3) Do birds fly?            • Is ice cream cold?
4) Is an ant bigger than an elephant?   • Is a giraffe smaller than a mouse?
5) **Command:** *"Hold up this many fingers"* (Demonstrate by holding up 2 fingers)
   *"Now do that with the other hand,"*  **OR**  *"Add one more finger."* (No demonstration)

> 1 Error → DELIRIUM PRESENT | 0 - 1 Error → DELIRIUM ABSENT

**Fig. 1.** Pediatric delirium assessment tool: Pediatric Confusion Assessment Method for the ICU (pCAM-ICU). The pCAM-ICU is a valid and reliable tool for diagnosing delirium in critically ill children at least 5 years old. Patients with an acute change or fluctuation from baseline mental status (feature 1) AND inattention (feature 2) with either an acute alteration in level of consciousness (feature 3) OR disorganized thinking (feature 4) have delirium. (*Courtesy of* Heidi A.B. Smith, MD, MSCI, Nashville, TN; and *From* Smith HA, Boyd J, Fuchs DC, et al. Diagnosing delirium in critically ill children: validity and reliability of the Pediatric Confusion Assessment Method for the Intensive Care Unit. Crit Care Med 2011;39:152, with permission.)

with an expert panel of board-certified pediatric psychologists, neurologists, developmental pediatricians, anesthesiologists, intensivists, and child and adolescent psychiatrists. Furthermore, valid tools to assess pediatric neurocognition,[35,36] pain and behavior,[37,38] and developmental milestones[39,40] were used as a guide to ensure that the cognitive and consciousness assessments within the psCAM-ICU were appropriate for infants and young children. As with the CAM-ICU and pCAM-ICU, the psCAM-ICU places emphasis on the most fundamental features of delirium: acute changes or fluctuations from baseline mental status and inattention.

## ETIOLOGY AND PRESENTATION OF DELIRIUM

Delirium can have a variety of presentations, ranging from an inappropriately sedate, to calm, or agitated patient who does not rest, may resist care, and becomes withdrawn from family or familiar items. Delirium is categorized into subtypes based on these presenting psychomotor behaviors as hypoactive, hyperactive, or a mixed type.[41,42] Normal brain activity depends on a fragile balance of stimulatory and inhibitory neurotransmission that becomes disrupted because of a variety of central nervous system insults occurring during critical illness.[43] Aberrant neurotransmission (delirium) in key areas of the brain is demonstrated as an acute change in mental status, inattention, and altered level of consciousness or cognition, which all forms of delirium (hypoactive, hyperactive, mixed) have in common.[43–47]

The psychomotor responses of patients with delirium are due to an alteration of activity at specific brain receptors within the dopaminergic, cholinergic, and glutamatergic systems (**Fig. 2**).[48–51] Dopamine is a major stimulatory neurotransmitter, whereas acetylcholine and γ-aminobutyric acid (GABA) have inhibitory effects. The balance of both neurotransmitter and receptor action modulate behavior and contribute to the fluctuation of mood, with additional effects on cognitive function.[44,48,52]

Hypoactive delirium may be clinically apparent when patients suffer from a significant deficiency of dopamine or an excess of acetylcholine or $GABA_A$ receptor stimulation.[53] Hypoactive delirium is demonstrated in a patient through apathy, a depressed level of consciousness, and withdrawal from their environment.[47] Unfortunately, these patients rarely arouse concern by the medical team, as they are easily paired and depicted as "good patients,"[30,54] and this mistaken sense of well-being results in a greater likelihood of poorer outcomes.[24,55,56] Patients fluctuating between hypoactive and hyperactive delirium (mixed type) and hypoactive delirium alone are the most commonly observed during critical illness.[41]

Hyperactive delirium may be present when there is an excess of dopaminergic activity and acetylcholine antagonism.[52] The dysfunctional state of hyperactive delirium has been well described in the literature using examples of the anticholinergic toxidrome or dopamine excess, which trigger agitation, restlessness, emotional instability and, ultimately, psychosis.[42,44] Other presentations of delirium have been observed during critical illness, resulting from the scarcity of acetylcholine and commonly used PICU drugs that have anticholinergic properties.[57–60] It remains vital for clinicians to understand the GABAergic system, as many of the most commonly used sedatives in the PICU setting, such as benzodiazepines and propofol, stimulate $GABA_A$ receptors causing sedation, anxiolysis, and even drug-induced delirium and coma.[44,61]

## IMPLEMENTATION OF DELIRIUM MONITORING

There are many obstacles to the institution of a new philosophy, protocol, or monitoring system within the PICU. The bedside nurse is inundated with numerous tasks related to both patient care and hospital protocols/policies. The success of

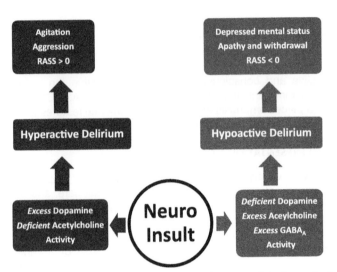

**Fig. 2.** Alteration in neurotransmission leading to psychomotor disturbance in delirium: the psychomotor responses of patients with delirium resulting from aberrant activity at specific brain receptors within the dopaminergic, cholinergic, and glutamatergic systems. Hyperactive delirium may be observed with an excess of dopaminergic activity and acetylcholine antagonism, resulting in agitation, restlessness, emotional instability, and, ultimately, psychosis. Hypoactive delirium may be clinically evident with a significant deficiency of dopamine or an excess of acetylcholine or γ-aminobutyric acid$_A$ (GABA$_A$) receptor activity, demonstrated as patient apathy, depressed level of consciousness, and withdrawal from the environment. RASS, Richmond Agitation-Sedation Scale. (*Data from* Karnik NS, Joshi SV, Paterno C, et al. Subtypes of Pediatric Delirium: A treatment Algorithm. Psychosomatics 2007;48:255.)

implementing delirium monitoring in the PICU depends on the medical team's understanding of the importance, presentation, etiology, and treatment options for delirium, the appreciation of the role of psychiatric or neurology consultation, and the development of confidence that diagnosis of delirium will lead to a change in patient care by the physician. In the early stages of implementation for delirium monitoring at Vanderbilt, in addition to educational in-services and one-on-one training of health care providers, the authors created an opportunity for the education of both physicians and nurses during medical rounds once weekly, with the additional presence of child and adolescent psychiatrist and pediatric anesthesiologists, as well as intensivists with expertise on delirium. The goals for "Brain Rounds" focused on how to redefine the approach to patients within the PICU, recognizing that the overall practice may be deficient in how one diagnoses and manages neurologic, psychiatric, and psychological disease. As an intensivist, the focus of critical care management remains on other vital organ systems (heart, lung, kidneys, and so forth) whereby there is a greater comfort level with diagnosis and treatment. The vast amount of data accumulated on delirium in critically ill adults encourages a transition from the status quo toward a culture change in the PICU for the recognition and management of delirium or brain organ dysfunction in children.

The authors developed Brain Rounds as an opportunity to instruct the medical team on the following: (1) how to identify, describe, and monitor for delirium; (2) how to structure a neuropsychiatric assessment and consider premorbid factors; (3) understand the known risks factors and outcomes for delirium; and (4) how to model interdisciplinary thought regarding management. A case-based approach was used for delirium education grounded in educational theory.[62] Case-based learning is a technique that guides the learner in practical application of new knowledge. Clinical rounds are designed to provide service to the patients, and teaching to the learners on the medical team. The importance of good clinical management of children with delirium was used in the context of challenging trainees and faculty to expand their knowledge base regarding pediatric delirium. Brain Rounds was successful because content experts with knowledge of the presentation, diagnosis, risks, and management of delirium were available to assure consistency in instruction and provide a role model for integrated patient care.

Brain Rounds provides an opportunity to identify specific aspects of delirium education that require further clarification, which are then used as beneficial learning points for new team members. At Vanderbilt, the authors were fortunate to delineate misperceptions held by the medical team that were preliminary obstacles to delirium monitoring and management.

Myth 1: The need for a delirium tool is not necessary.

    Pediatric physicians and nurses take specific care to prevent a child from undergoing further harm in the PICU setting during critical illness. The recent focus on the occurrence of delirium in the authors' PICU challenges the assumption that we already know patients' mental status and cognition well. Delirium tools facilitate the neurologic examination to uncover the key features of delirium that would otherwise potentially be missed.

Myth 2: Delirium monitoring will not lead to a change in patient care.

    Management of delirium requires reassessment of sedation and analgesia practices in the PICU setting, which can be viewed as destabilizing by team members, making intentional and consistent change difficult. This inconsistency leads to ineffective delirium management, contributing to the belief that monitoring of delirium will not lead to a change in patient care. Culture change promoted by the clinical team through intentional changes in patterns of behavior within the PICU is needed for delirium management to be successful.

Myth 3: Delirium management requires the removal of all sedatives, leading to awake and suffering patients.

    Many providers use significant doses of both analgesics and sedatives in critically ill children, hoping to avoid the creation of distressing memories of the PICU experience. The safety of this practice is challenged by literature that identifies not only the development of delirium more often in adults exposed to benzodiazepines during critical illness,[63] but also that children who receive excessive sedation are more likely to have distorted memories of their experience that are associated with the development of PTSD following discharge from the hospital.[64] Medical literature on delirium challenges the caregiver to transition from feeling frustrated over new recommendations for titration of certain drugs, to feeling empowered in having the tools necessary to successfully identify patient needs in regard of pain and anxiety, level of sedation, and delirium. The goal of delirium management is achieved when a child is without significant pain, has adequate anxiolysis via both pharmacologic and nonpharmacologic means using targeted therapy, and responds to treatment of both delirium and the disease state. This approach may result in a child who "experiences" critical illness but without the hurt and fear that we all perceive.

Myth 4: A diagnosis of delirium and psychiatry consultation suggest that the medical team considers the patient "crazy," and management requires "antipsychotics" for an extended period of time.

Delirium differs very little from other types of organ dysfunction in the collaborative approach to monitoring and therapy. As an example, when a child presents with septic shock, the development of acute renal failure is not unexpected. If severe enough, a nephrologist may be consulted to participate in generating strategies for the prevention of worsening kidney function. Aminoglycosides used in the setting of normal renal function requires only monitoring of drug levels; however, with renal insufficiency the kidney is more at risk for further damage, therefore dose or choice of using the drug is reconsidered, often leading to consultation from the specialty service. On discharge from the hospital, renal function usually returns, and ongoing intervention or monitoring by the nephrology service is no longer needed. Similarly, psychiatrists can provide assistance on considering ways to decrease the risk or severity of delirium beyond treatment of the critical disease. This assistance may involve help with the differential diagnosis, identification of risk factors, modifications of ongoing therapy, and in some instances pharmacologic suggestions. In addition, their knowledge regarding the treatment of pain, anxiety, depression, and sleep disturbances can provide an organized and consistent approach to management. The psychiatrist remains a consistent presence for the monitoring of improvement in delirium symptoms and weaning of pharmacotherapy through discharge. The need for the psychiatrist coincides with the acuity and severity of the clinical presentation of delirium.

Brain Rounds offers a tremendous opportunity to discuss real issues and provide key teaching points and procedures to overcome misperceptions that affect the implementation of delirium monitoring in the PICU. A systematic approach to case-based teaching[62] during Brain Rounds including use of consistent information regarding assessment and management, specific patient-based examples, and clinical role modeling has been successful in creating a delirium-monitoring program in the PICU.

## TREATMENT

Delirium management requires a global approach to patient care from the environment we create to the cellular disease process we treat. Through the experiences offered from Brain Rounds, the authors developed a systematic approach to delirium monitoring and management that works in their PICU. The concept of the "Pediatric Road Map" was adapted from the adult delirium group at Vanderbilt to promote the monitoring of pain and anxiety, level of consciousness, and delirium in the PICU, with a guide to a disciplined approach for delirium management.[65] The Pediatric Road Map empowers the nursing staff to observe, report, and discuss the patient's neuropsychological state by creating a "map" using answers to the following questions: (1) Where is my patient now? (2) How did we get here? (3) Where is my patient expected to go? and (4) How do we get them there? To accomplish this, patients are monitored at appropriate intervals for pain using a validated pain scale, for their level of consciousness via the Richmond Agitation-Sedation Scale (RASS)[66,67] or other validated sedation scales, and for delirium using the pCAM-ICU in children older than 5 years. On clinical rounds with the medical team, the nurse or physician in-training presents the current RASS and pCAM-ICU (brain organ assessment) with pain assessment (Where is my patient now?), discusses ongoing therapies and medical conditions that might contribute to that assessment (How did we get here?), then outlines the target RASS and clinical goals for the disease state (Where is my patient expected to go?), followed by creation of a clinical plan of how to successfully titrate therapy that is mutually beneficial for both improvement of critical illness and resolution or prevention of delirium, pain, and anxiety (How do we get them there?).

The Pediatric Road Map uses level of consciousness as a marker to determine the approach for delirium prevention and management. The authors use the RASS (**Fig. 3**) because it provides an objective evaluation of the level of consciousness, separating verbal from physical stimuli via a logical 3-step process: (1) look, (2) talk, and then (3) touch the patient.[66,67] Furthermore, each RASS score depicts a very distinct level of consciousness that can be easily targeted and attained through titration of medications. A change in RASS score may also alert the medical team to an unexpected change in brain function, whether it is a product of a change in sedative/analgesic administration or attributable to a new medical process such as a metabolic derangement. The targeted level of consciousness for patients is set at zero (alert and calm) unless there are factors that warrant a more "sedate" patient. The greatest need for sedation is when patients are on mechanical ventilation, with severe lung disease, and patient-ventilator synchrony is required. The provider should be challenged to determine the minimal level of sedation required to keep the patient comfortable and to tolerate mechanical ventilation, and to maintain adequate oxygenation; no assumption should be made that deep sedation is "necessary." It is easy to use sedation as a mechanism of pharmacologic restraint, and the Pediatric Road Map challenges the medical team to consistently reevaluate the need and target of sedation.

The management of delirium in critically ill children can be generally approached by first assigning patients to one of two groups based on their level of consciousness: (1) comatose or severely obtunded without response to voice (RASS −5, −4), or (2) arousable to voice (RASS −3 to +4). These two groups vastly differ in the degree of altered state of arousal, and the inability to assess the content of consciousness (delirium) in patients whose depressed arousal prevents any response to voice.

The care of comatose or severely obtunded patients can be challenging for the medical team. Evaluation for delirium cannot occur in obtunded or comatose patients, as the neurologic responsiveness required for delirium assessment is lost or minimally present; this does not mean that delirium is absent, only that one cannot clinically diagnose its presence using the pCAM-ICU or any other delirium tool while the patient is comatose. When patients demonstrate a severely depressed level of consciousness, great effort should be exercised in considering possible causes, and therapies that may improve the patient's mental status (**Fig. 4**). This goal may be achieved through the treatment of possible contributing causes (the acronym BRAIN MAPS; see **Fig. 4**), the assessment and targeting of a specific level of consciousness to which psychotropic medications are titrated to reach, and the initiation of preventive measures to decrease the likelihood of ongoing delirium when the patient's sensorium improves. The Pediatric Road Map assists the medical team in consistently reevaluating patients with coma and minimizing risks for the development of delirium while the brain is experiencing an acute state of critical illness.

The care of critically ill patients who are arousable is augmented by the medical team's ability to monitor for pain, anxiety, and delirium. Delirium assessment can be performed accurately using the pCAM-ICU in intubated or nonintubated children 5 years of age and older who are at least arousable to voice (RASS −3 to +4).[1] When delirium is diagnosed, the subtype (hypoactive, hyperactive, mixed) can be determined by the psychomotor behaviors demonstrated by the patient (apathy and

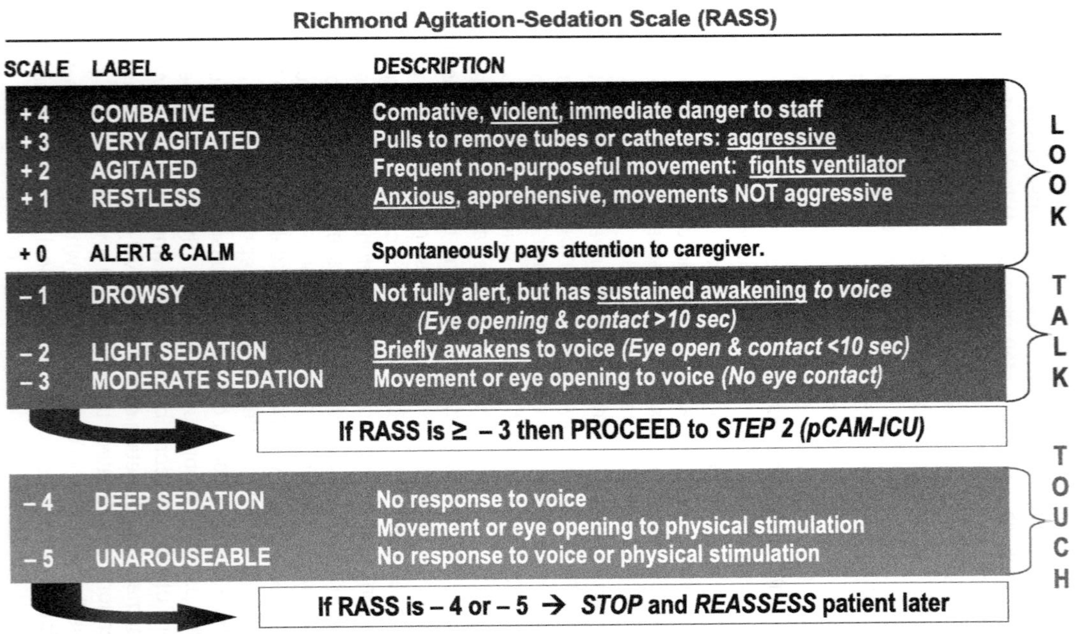

## Richmond Agitation-Sedation Scale (RASS)

| SCALE | LABEL | DESCRIPTION |
|---|---|---|
| +4 | COMBATIVE | Combative, violent, immediate danger to staff |
| +3 | VERY AGITATED | Pulls to remove tubes or catheters: aggressive |
| +2 | AGITATED | Frequent non-purposeful movement:  fights ventilator |
| +1 | RESTLESS | Anxious, apprehensive, movements NOT aggressive |
| 0 | ALERT & CALM | Spontaneously pays attention to caregiver. |
| −1 | DROWSY | Not fully alert, but has sustained awakening to voice (Eye opening & contact >10 sec) |
| −2 | LIGHT SEDATION | Briefly awakens to voice (Eye open & contact <10 sec) |
| −3 | MODERATE SEDATION | Movement or eye opening to voice (No eye contact) |

**LOOK**

**TALK**

If RASS is ≥ − 3 then PROCEED to STEP 2 (pCAM-ICU)

| | | |
|---|---|---|
| −4 | DEEP SEDATION | No response to voice |
| | | Movement or eye opening to physical stimulation |
| −5 | UNAROUSEABLE | No response to voice or physical stimulation |

**TOUCH**

If RASS is − 4 or − 5 → STOP and REASSESS patient later

**Fig. 3.** Targeting the level of consciousness (LOC) using the Richmond Agitation-Sedation Scale (RASS). The RASS is a valid tool for the objective assessment of the level of consciousness. The clinician first observes whether the patient is alert and calm (RASS 0) or demonstrates mild to severe levels of agitation (RASS +1 to +4). If the patient is not alert and calm nor agitated, then the clinician "talks" to the patient to assess mild to moderate levels of depressed consciousness (RASS −1 to −3). If the patient has no response to voice, then the clinician "touches" the patient to elicit either some minimal response (RASS −4) or no response because the patient is comatose (RASS −5). (*Data from* Sessler CN, Gosnell MS, Grap MJ, et al. The Richmond Agitation–Sedation Scale Validity and Reliability in Adult Intensive Care Unit Patients. Am J Respir Crit Care Med 2002;166:1339.)

lethargy, calm, agitation) or the level of consciousness as determined by the RASS, which helps to guide initial management (**Fig. 5**). The approach to delirium management is multimodal, considering untreated pain, disease etiology, and environmental and iatrogenic factors, in addition to pharmacologic treatment of psychomotor symptoms.[15,68–72]

Pain management is a major objective when caring for all critically ill patients. The consistent assessment and treatment of pain in critically ill children may decrease the risk and severity of delirium. This phenomenon may occur partially because of the lessened need for sedatives when a child is already comfortable and calm. A child who is without significant pain is the most likely to maintain a clear sensorium, and often can be comforted by the medical staff and family to relieve anxiety or fear of the strange environment. The goal for an analgesic plan should encourage a multimodal approach[73] with heightened use of acetaminophen and nonsteroidal anti-inflammatory agents[74] when appropriate, and additional use of opioids to treat severe pain. As with any pharmacotherapy in the PICU, the goal remains the aggressive reevaluation of patients' specific needs and titration of therapy as soon as appropriate. Use of opioid infusions that are not patient controlled or titrated based on pain-scale scores should be transitioned to longer-acting, intermittent opioids, which may provide a more stable background and decrease the potential for excessive drug administration and, ultimately, sedation. The longer-acting opioid can be enhanced with the intermittent use of shorter-acting opioids to "rescue" the patient from acute uncontrolled pain caused by procedures or other interventions while critically ill. Patients whose clinical course is rapidly changing may benefit the greatest from continuing opioid infusions that are easily titratable. Regardless of the drug or mode of administration, every patient will benefit from consistent reassessment of pain requirements and titration of analgesia, which allow the patient to continue on the road to recovery.[75]

The PICU environment is unfamiliar and dynamic, frequently demanding the cooperation of patients despite their wishes. The involvement and presence of family, in addition to providing familiar music and filling the room with pictures, toys, and personal items, decreases anxiety and delirium.[15,68] Many of the preventive and interventional approaches used for delirium attempt to keep the healthy brain "awake" and decrease the further dysregulation of neurotransmission in the critical care setting. As pediatricians we support the maintenance of daily and bedtime routines in healthy children, which promote a feeling of safety and well-being for a child. In the PICU setting, these routines are challenging to implement owing to monitoring and therapeutic objectives, with the added perception that the child is too sick. A stable environment and day/night routine may be even more important during critical illness.[47,69] Children are resilient when provided with the tools to deal with stress, anxiety, and grief, which the medical team in concert with Child Life, hospital teachers, and family can supply.

A preliminary step in the management of patients with delirium is to assess their physiologic status, considering the potential medical causes of delirium. This evaluation should be integrated with an assessment of the environment, recognizing that disruption of the environment will exacerbate misperceptions of thought resulting from delirium. Simultaneously the team must assess the safety of the patient and staff. If safety related to behavioral dysregulation is a concern, pharmacologic intervention should be considered. If, however, safety is not an issue, initial efforts should focus on stabilization of the disease state contributing to the delirium. There are some disease states which, although directly contributing to the onset and persistence of delirium, cannot immediately be reversed. When this occurs, the use of pharmacotherapy to

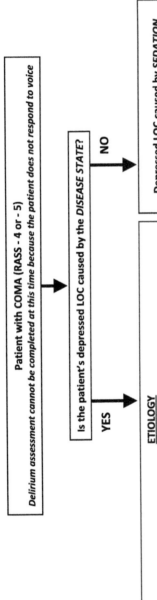

**Patient with COMA (RASS - 4 or - 5)**

*Delirium assessment cannot be completed at this time because the patient does not respond to voice*

**Is the patient's depressed LOC caused by the DISEASE STATE?**

**YES**

**NO**

## Depressed LOC caused by SEDATION

1. *Establish* the **TARGET sedation level**
   - *Set* the TARGET LOC at a **RASS of 0** (alert and calm)
   - If disease intervention requires a 'sedate' patient, *Set* the TARGET LOC at the most 'alert' that will permit needed interventions (e.g., RASS -1, -2, or -3)
   - *Discuss* the specific benefits of sedation in this patient
2. *Provide* titration goals to reach or maintain **TARGET sedation level**
   - *Consider* less deliriogenic sedatives if depressed TARGET LOC required
   - *Titrate* or *discontinue* use of benzodiazepines if not necessary
3. *Follow* a**Pediatric Road Map**

## ETIOLOGY

EVALUATE possible causes of **Acute Brain Dysfunction (Delirium)** → **"BRAIN MAPS"**

B – <u>B</u>ring OXYGEN (hypoxemia, decreased cardiac output, anemia)
R – Remove or <u>R</u>educe deliriogenic drugs like anticholinergics, benzodiazepines
A – <u>A</u>tmosphere (foreign room, lights aglowing, noise loud, restraints, absent family, frequent change of caregivers "strangers," no schedule)
I – Infection, <u>I</u>mmobilization, <u>I</u>nflammation
N – <u>N</u>ew organ dysfunction (CNS, CV, PULM, Hepatic, Renal, Endocrine)
M – <u>M</u>etabolic disturbances (hypo/hypernatremia, hypo/hyperkalemia, hypoglycemia, hypocalcemia, alkalosis, acidosis)
A – <u>A</u>wake (No bedtime routine, Sleep–wake cycle disturbance)
P – <u>P</u>ain (too much and not enough drug OR pain treated and now too much drug)
S – <u>S</u>edation (Assess need and set sedation target)

### PREVENTIVE MEASURES

1. *Maintain* continuity of care, have loved ones present around the child
2. *Create* a calm, reassuring environment (comforting pictures, toys, blankets, music, etc.)
3. *Establish* a day/night routine and periods of uninterrupted rest. Children should be assisted to perform or participate in daily routines of hygiene, mouth care, range of motion exercises, and getting out of bed when awake
4. *Consider* necessity of tubes, lines, restraints (physical or pharmacologic)
5. *Consult* child life specialists and/or hospital teachers when appropriate

manage delirium symptoms is indicated for both safety and support of brain function while efforts continue to address the source of critical illness. Patients with persistent delirium, despite initial treatment of the primary disease state, institution of preventive measures, and initiation of antipsychotics to alleviate unwanted effects of delirium, can be disheartening to the team and family. These patients in particular benefit greatly from case presentation during Brain Rounds, because in this setting ongoing discussion of possible causes (BRAIN MAPS) is encouraged, which may lead to a new culprit for the delirium (**Box 1**). Acute brain dysfunction is not a static process. In the setting of critical illness, aberrant neurotransmission leading to delirium can be cyclic, and caused by new derangements that occur during the patient's medical course. Critical thinking about delirium among the medical team will increase success in developing the most effective management approach for delirium.

**Box 1** summarizes 2 clinical cases highlighted during Brain Rounds in the PICU. Both cases provide examples of how delirium may persist despite pharmacologic treatment of psychomotor symptoms if the source of acute organ dysfunction is not identified and treated. Brain Rounds incorporates the importance of consistently reevaluating possible exacerbating factors for delirium, including new etiologic factors.

It is important to recognize comorbid developmental or psychiatric disorders that may complicate medical management of critically ill children and adolescents. For example, children with autism spectrum disorder have dysregulation when their routine is disrupted. Understanding of the developmental disorder should inform environmental and potentially pharmacologic management of these children. Children with a prior history of trauma may have an increase in dysregulation manifesting as a hyperaroused state (DSM-IV-TR). These children are at risk for increased reactivity in the PICU, which may lead to use of sedatives that complicates the balance of neurotransmitters in the brain. Treatment of their behavioral dysregulation is appropriate; however, the goals of treatment should include understanding of the impact of comorbid disorders on the risk of delirium. Management of the comorbid disorder may result in more beneficial pharmacologic management of delirium.

The management of delirium during critical illness may occasionally require pharmacologic intervention that targets psychomotor behaviors that are harmful to the patient. It must be noted that there is no approval from the Food and Drug Administration for the use of antipsychotics in the treatment of delirium for any age group. Despite this, there is evidence for effective drug therapy in alleviating the symptoms of both adult and pediatric delirium.[15,48,70,76] There remains a misperception that treatment with antipsychotics implies psychiatric disorder and that only patients who are psychotic benefit from these medications. Rather, antipsychotics target

---

**Fig. 4.** Treatment algorithm for the critically ill pediatric comatose patient. This approach to the management of critically ill comatose patients focuses on how to minimize risks for the development or exacerbation of delirium. This method merges the goals for decreasing risk or severity of delirium with those for management of the critical illness. The outcome is a patient care plan that is mutually beneficial. [a] This algorithm incorporates the Pediatric Road Map, a method to consistently evaluate pain and anxiety, level of sedation, and delirium. The Pediatric Road Map helps guide discussion during medical rounds to form a multidisciplinary care plan or "map" by answering the following 4 questions: (1) Where is my patient now? (2) How did we get here? (3) Where is my patient expected to go? and (4) How do we get them there? CNS, central nervous system; CV, cardiovascular; LOC, level of consciousness; PULM, pulmonary; RASS, Richmond Agitation-Sedation Scale.

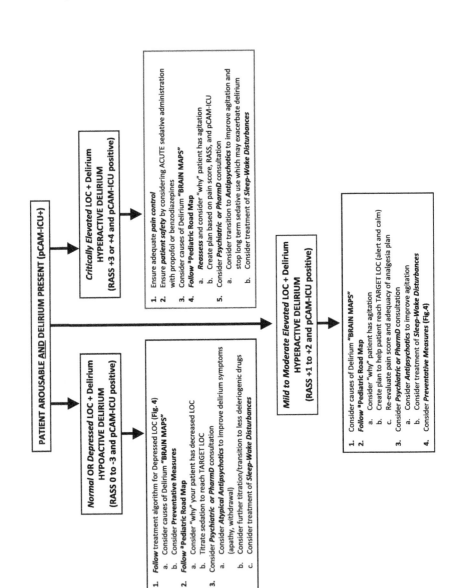

**PATIENT AROUSABLE AND DELIRIUM PRESENT (pCAM-ICU+)**

**Normal OR Depressed LOC + Delirium HYPOACTIVE DELIRIUM (RASS 0 to -3 and pCAM-ICU positive)**

1. *Follow* treatment algorithm for Depressed LOC (Fig. 4)
   a. Consider causes of Delirium "BRAIN MAPS"
   b. Consider Preventative Measures
2. *Follow* ᵃPediatric Road Map
   a. Consider "why" your patient has decreased LOC
   b. Titrate sedation to reach TARGET LOC
3. Consider Psychiatric or PharmD consultation
   a. Consider Atypical Antipsychotics to improve delirium symptoms (apathy, withdrawal)
   b. Consider further titration/transition to less deleriogenic drugs
   c. Consider treatment of Sleep-Wake Disturbances

**Critically Elevated LOC + Delirium HYPERACTIVE DELIRIUM (RASS +3 or +4 and pCAM-ICU positive)**

1. Ensure adequate *pain control*
2. Ensure *patient safety* by considering ACUTE sedative administration with propofol or benzodiazepines
3. Consider causes of Delirium "BRAIN MAPS"
4. *Follow* ᵃPediatric Road Map
   a. *Reassess* and consider "why" patient has agitation
   b. Create plan based on pain score, RASS, and pCAM-ICU
5. Consider Psychiatric or PharmD consultation
   a. Consider transition to Antipsychotics to improve agitation and stop long term sedative use which may exacerbate delirium
   b. Consider treatment of Sleep-Wake Disturbances

**Mild to Moderate Elevated LOC + Delirium HYPERACTIVE DELIRIUM (RASS +1 to +2 and pCAM-ICU positive)**

1. Consider causes of Delirium "BRAIN MAPS"
2. *Follow* ᵃPediatric Road Map
   a. Consider "why" patient has agitation
   b. Create plan to help patient reach TARGET LOC (alert and calm)
   c. Re-evaluate pain score and adequacy of analgesia plan
3. Consider Psychiatric or PharmD consultation
   a. Consider Antipsychotics to improve agitation
   b. Consider treatment of Sleep-Wake Disturbances
4. Consider Preventative Measures (Fig.4)

neurotransmitter dysregulation, which is clinically present in many diseases of the brain. Delirium is one of those syndromes whereby any level of agitation associated with brain dysfunction may benefit from these medications to restore neurotransmission equilibrium and provide anxiolysis and sedation, enhancing the safety of the child. Lack of understanding in regard of these medications may lead to ineffective use or avoidance of this class of drugs. The decision to use antipsychotics requires careful consideration of the risks and benefits, with the ultimate goal of patient safety.

Haloperidol (Haldol) is the most well-known antipsychotic that is supported for use in the treatment of hyperactive delirium in adults.[77,78] Haloperidol blocks primarily dopamine receptors in the brain, offsetting overstimulation of higher cortical pathways, alleviating hallucinations if present, providing anxiolysis or sedation, and restoring attention.[46,61,79] Haloperidol is a reasonable choice for patients who require intravenous medications and demonstrate agitation that fails to respond to nonpharmacologic interventions.

Atypical antipsychotics, namely risperidone (Risperdal), olanzapine (Zyprexa), and ziprasidone (Geodon) among others, are newer-generation drugs that not only have actions on dopamine activity but also more extensive actions on acetylcholine, serotonin, and norepinephrine receptors.[80] Atypical antipsychotics have been shown in adults to be similarly effective in comparison with haloperidol yet with a relatively low burden of side effects,[81] and future studies in children are required. It has been speculated[48] that patients with hypoactive delirium benefit from atypical antipsychotics such as risperidone because of the modulation of dopamine activity through direct antagonism of the dopamine receptor and indirect antagonism via serotonin receptors, leading to small increases in dopamine activity in key areas of the brain. The effect on multiple receptors helps to reduce the side effects that occur when there is more complete dopamine blockade, as in treatment with haloperidol.[48]

Haloperidol and risperidone have been effectively used in children with delirium without causing significant side effects.[15,48,70] Like many other drugs commonly used in the PICU, antipsychotics have side effects that should be considered. Prolonged QTc and extrapyramidal movement disorders, including dystonic reactions, may occur. It is good practice to evaluate and monitor the QTc length in patients who will be receiving haloperidol at baseline and then daily if treatment continues for longer than 24 hours. Dystonic reactions can be easily treated with the use of diphenhydramine and discontinuation of the offending drug. Other cited complications include torsades de pointes, malignant hyperthermia, hypotension, glucose and lipid dysregulation, laryngeal spasm, and anticholinergic effects.[46] As with analgesia or sedation, treatment of delirium also requires reassessment and titration of

**Fig. 5.** Treatment algorithm for the critically ill pediatric patient with delirium. This approach to the management of critically ill patients with delirium focuses on categorizing the subtype of delirium, patient safety when psychomotor symptoms of delirium are extreme, identifying possible causes, and minimizing exacerbating factors for the development of delirium. The initial steps in management are dependent on the psychomotor behaviors demonstrated by the patient (apathy and lethargy, calm, agitation), which determine the subtype of delirium (hypoactive or hyperactive). The management of delirium relies heavily on critical thinking regarding the possible sources of the acute organ dysfunction, followed by decreasing iatrogenic causes related to the environment or clinical practice, preventive measures, and ultimately the use of pharmacologic interventions to modulate the symptoms of delirium. ª This algorithm incorporates the Pediatric Road Map (see explanation in the legend of **Fig. 4**).

---

**Box 1**
**Delirium management: how Brain Rounds can affect patient care in the critical care unit**

*Patient A* is a 10-year-old boy admitted to the pediatric critical care unit with tick-borne septic shock presenting with symptoms of altered mental status, hypoxia, fever, and hypotension. Other complications in the first 24 hours included metabolic abnormalities (hyponatremia, hypocalcemia, metabolic acidosis, and lactic acidosis) and hematologic complications (anemia, consumptive thrombocytopenia, and leukopenia). The patient was diagnosed with delirium in the setting of ehrlichiosis. Neurology was consulted because of concern for seizure activity, and preventive therapy with levetiracetam was initiated. Despite resolution of the metabolic/electrolyte derangements and aggressive treatment of his tick-borne disease, the patient had persistence of his altered level of consciousness, development of dysregulation of sleep, purposeless movements, and psychomotor agitation 72 hours after presentation. His RASS ranged from +1 to −3. An atypical antipsychotic was initiated to address his sleep disturbance and psychomotor agitation. Brain Rounds promoted discussion of persistent delirium and used BRAIN MAPS to review other possible causes. On further presentation of indolent symptoms of mild respiratory insufficiency and oxygen requirement, and a review of chest radiograph revealing mild cardiomegaly and pulmonary edema, an ECHO was obtained, which revealed severe myocardial dysfunction. The treatment plan included the initiation of cardiac-directed therapies in addition to institution of preventive measures with ongoing pharmacotherapy for restoration of his sleep-wake cycle. Within 48 hours, the patient had resolution of his delirium.

*Patient B* is a teenager who suffered a stroke consequent to rupture of a previously undiagnosed arteriovenous malformation. Following intervention to control intracranial hemorrhage and other related acute neurologic events, the patient suffered from extreme agitation and sleep-wake cycle disturbance during his new steady state. He was diagnosed with delirium and initiated on an antipsychotic, owing to his agitation and dysregulation of sleep. Despite improvement in his psychomotor agitation, the patient continued to demonstrate inattention and frustration with verbal communication. Brain Rounds promoted further discussion on possible causes of delirium and a review of the patient's psychiatric premorbid history. In addition, with further description of the patient's agitation there was a realization that he suffered from expressive aphasia, which was likely exacerbating his agitation and sleep disturbance. With the institution of more aggressive occupational therapy and use of creative options for communication, his psychomotor symptoms improved and ultimately the delirium resolved.

---

the amount of drug once clinical status has improved or side effects such as excess daytime sedation occur. In general, all pharmacotherapy for delirium should be discontinued as soon as the acute phase of organ dysfunction has resolved.[70]

## SUMMARY

Monitoring and management of pediatric delirium presents a tremendous opportunity to augment the care of critically ill children. There remain many questions regarding prevalence, risk factors, and outcomes for pediatric delirium, which will be resolved through well-designed prospective pediatric studies. The creation and validation of tools to assist in the diagnosis of delirium among infants and young children will greatly enhance the impact on improving patient care. The lessons learned through the creation and implementation of Brain Rounds, the Pediatric Road Map, and the use of new acronyms for the etiology of delirium (BRAIN MAPS) has provided a consistent mechanism to educate and evaluate the institutional approach to delirium monitoring and management. The reward of the child who survives the PICU and returns to a life of learning, emotional well-being, and future opportunities is worth the considerable effort by the entire medical team in undertaking culture change for delirium monitoring in the PICU.

## REFERENCES

1. Smith HA, Boyd J, Fuchs DC. Diagnosing delirium in critically ill children: validity and reliability of the pediatric confusion assessment method for the intensive care unit. Crit Care Med 2011;39:150–7.
2. Silver G, Traube C, Kearney J. Detecting pediatric delirium: development of a rapid observational assessment tool. Intensive Care Med 2012;38:1025–31.
3. Janssen NJ, Tan EY, Staal M, et al. On the utility of diagnostic instruments for pediatric delirium in critical illness: an evaluation of the Pediatric Anesthesia Emergence Delirium Scale, the Delirium Rating Scale 88, and the Delirium Rating Scale-Revised R-98. Intensive Care Med 2011;37:1331–7.
4. Ely EW, Margolin R, Francis J, et al. Evaluation of delirium in critically ill patients: validation of the Confusion Assessment Method for the Intensive Care Unit (CAM-ICU). Crit Care Med 2001;29:1370–9.
5. Bergeron N, Dubois MJ, Dumont M. Intensive care delirium screening checklist: evaluation of a new screening tool. Intensive Care Med 2001;27:859–64.
6. Pandharipande P, Costabile S, Cotton B. Prevalence of delirium in surgical ICU patients. Crit Care Med 2005;33:A45.
7. Thomason JW, Shintani A, Peterson JF. Intensive care unit delirium is an independent predictor of longer hospital stay: a prospective analysis of 261 non-ventilated patients. Crit Care 2005;9:R375–81.
8. Ely EW, Shintani A, Truman B. Delirium as a predictor of mortality in mechanically ventilated patients in the intensive care unit. JAMA 2004;291:1753–62.
9. Jackson JC, Gordon SM, Hart RP. The association between delirium and cognitive decline: a review of the empirical literature. Neuropsychol Rev 2004;14: 87–98.
10. McNicoll L, Pisani MA, Zhang Y. Delirium in the intensive care unit: occurrence and clinical course in older patients. J Am Geriatr Soc 2003;51:591–8.
11. Ely EW, Gautam S, Margolin R. The impact of delirium in the intensive care unit on hospital length of stay. Intensive Care Med 2001;27:1892–900.
12. Dubois MJ, Bergeron N, Dumont M. Delirium in an intensive care unit: a study of risk factors. Intensive Care Med 2001;27:1297–304.
13. Jackson JC, Gordon SM, Girard TD, et al. Delirium as a risk factor for long term cognitive impairment in mechanically ventilated ICU survivors. Am J Respir Crit Care Med 2007;175:A22.
14. Hopkins RO, Jackson JC. Long-term neurocognitive function after critical illness. Chest 2006;130:869–78.
15. Schieveld JN, Leroy PL, van OJ, et al. Pediatric delirium in critical illness: phenomenology, clinical correlates and treatment response in 40 cases in the pediatric intensive care unit. Intensive Care Med 2007;33:1033–40.
16. Schieveld JN, Leentjens AF. Delirium in severely ill young children in the pediatric intensive care unit (PICU). J Am Acad Child Adolesc Psychiatry 2005;44:392–4.
17. Turkel SB, Tavare CJ. Delirium in children and adolescents. J Neuropsychiatry Clin Neurosci 2003;15:431–5.
18. Fiser DH. Assessing the outcome of pediatric intensive care. J Pediatr 1992;121: 68–74.
19. Rees G, Gledhill J, Garralda ME, et al. Psychiatric outcome following paediatric intensive care unit (PCCU) admission: a cohort study. Intensive Care Med 2004;30:1607–14.
20. Gioia GA, Isquith PK, Guy SC, et al. Behavior rating inventory of executive function. Child Neuropsychol 2000;6:235–8.

21. Smith HA, Fuchs DC, Pandharipande PP, et al. Delirium: an emerging frontier in the management of critically ill children. Crit Care Clin 2009;25:593–614.

22. Ely EW, Siegel MD, Inouye SK. Delirium in the intensive care unit: an under-recognized syndrome of organ dysfunction. Semin Respir Crit Care Med 2001; 22:115–26.

23. Inouye SK. The dilemma of delirium: clinical and research controversies regarding diagnosis and evaluation of delirium in hospitalized elderly medical patients. Am J Med 1994;97:278–88.

24. Francis J, Martin D, Kapoor WN. A prospective study of delirium in hospitalized elderly. JAMA 1990;263:1097–101.

25. Diagnostic and statistical manual of mental disorders. 4th edition. Washington, DC: American Psychiatric Association; 2000. Text Revised (DSM-IV).

26. McGuire BE, Basten CJ, Ryan CJ, et al. Intensive care unit syndrome: a dangerous misnomer. Arch Intern Med 2000;160:906–9.

27. Justic M. Does "ICU psychosis" really exist? Crit Care Nurse 2000;20:28–37.

28. Trzepacz PT, Baker RW. The psychiatric mental status examination. Oxford (England): Oxford University Press; 1993. p. 202.

29. Grover S, Kate N, Malhotra S, et al. Symptom profile of delirium in children and adolescents—does it differ from adults and elderly? Gen Hosp Psychiatry 2012;34:626–32.

30. Turkel SB, Trzepacz PT, Tavare CJ. Comparing symptoms of delirium in adults and children. Psychosomatics 2006;47:320–4.

31. Martini DR. Commentary: the diagnosis of delirium in pediatric patients. J Am Acad Child Adolesc Psychiatry 2005;44:395–8.

32. Trzepacz PT, Mittal D, Torres R, et al. Validation of delirium rating scale: comparison to the delirium rating scale and cognitive test for delirium. J Neuropsychiatry Clin Neurosci 2001;13:229–42.

33. Ely EW, Inouye SK, Bernard GR. Delirium in mechanically ventilated patients: validity and reliability of the confusion assessment method for the intensive care unit (CAM-ICU). JAMA 2001;286:2703–10.

34. Sikich N, Lerman J. Development and psychometric evaluation of the pediatric anesthesia emergence delirium scale. Anesthesiology 2004;100:1138–45.

35. Glascoe FP. The Brigance infant and toddler screen: standardization and validation. J Dev Behav Pediatr 2002;23:145–50.

36. Kube DA, Wilson WM, Petersen MC, et al. CAT/CLAMS: its use in detecting early childhood cognitive impairment. Pediatr Neurol 2000;23:208–15.

37. Malviya S, Voepel-Lewis T, Burke C. The revised FLACC observational pain tool: improved reliability and validity for pain assessment in children with cognitive impairment. Paediatr Anaesth 2006;16:258–65.

38. Freeman BJ, Del'Homme M, Guthrie D, et al. Vineland adaptive behavior scale scores as a function of age and initial IQ in 210 autistic children. J Autism Dev Disord 1999;29:379–84.

39. Feigelman S. The first year. In: Kliegman RM, Stanton B, Behrman RE, et al, editors. Nelson textbook of pediatrics. 19th edition. Philadelphia: Saunders Elsevier; 2007. p. e26–31.

40. Frankenburg WK, Dodds J, Archer P. The Denver II: a major revision and restandardization of the Denver Developmental Screening Test. Pediatrics 1992;89:91–7.

41. Peterson JF, Pun BT, Dittus RS. Delirium and its motoric subtypes: a study of 614 critically ill patients. J Am Geriatr Soc 2006;54:479–84.

42. Meagher DJ, Trzepacz PT. Motoric subtypes of delirium. Semin Clin Neuropsychiatry 2000;5:75–85.

43. Trzepacz PT. Update on the neuropathogenesis of delirium. Dement Geriatr Cogn Disord 1999;10:330–4.

44. Gunther ML, Morandi A, Ely EW. Pathophysiology of delirium in the intensive care unit. Crit Care Clin 2008;24:45–65.

45. Meagher DJ, Moran M, Raju B, et al. Phenomenology of delirium. Assessment of 100 adult cases using standardized measures. Br J Psychiatry 2007;190:135–41.

46. Pandharipande P, Jackson J, Ely EW. Delirium: acute cognitive dysfunction in the critically ill. Curr Opin Crit Care 2005;11:360–8.

47. Trzepacz PT. Delirium. Advances in diagnosis, pathophysiology, and treatment. Psychiatr Clin North Am 1996;19:429–48.

48. Karnik NS, Joshi SV, Paterno C, et al. Subtypes of pediatric delirium: a treatment algorithm. Psychosomatics 2007;48:253–7.

49. Pavlov VA, Wang H, Czura CJ, et al. The cholinergic anti-inflammatory pathway: a missing link in neuroimmunomodulation. Mol Med 2003;9:125–34.

50. Crippen D. Treatment of agitation and its comorbidities in the intensive care unit. In: Hill NS, Levy MM, editors. Ventilator Management Strategies for Critical Care. New York: Marcel Dekker Inc; 2001. p. 243–84.

51. Webb JM, Carlton EF, Geeham DM. Delirium in the intensive care unit: are we helping the patient? Crit Care Nurs Q 2000;2:247–60.

52. Bloom FE, Kupfer DJ, Bunney BS, et al. Amines. In: Psychopharmacology: the fourth generation of progress. An official publication of the American College of Neuropsychopharmacology. New York: Raven Press; 1995. p. 1287–359.

53. Bloom FE, Kupfer DJ, Bunney BS, et al. Transmitter Systems. In: Psychopharmacology: the fourth generation of progress. An official publication of the American College of Neuropsychopharmacology. New York, NY: Raven Press; 1995. p. 1287–359.

54. Pandharipande P, Ely EW. Scoring and managing delirium in the PICU. In: Zimmerman JJ, Shanley TP, editors. Current concepts in pediatric critical care—Society of Critical Care Medicine. Mount Prospect (IL): 2008. p. 69–77.

55. Inouye SK, Schlesinger MJ, Lydon TJ. Delirium: a symptom of how hospital care is failing older persons and a window to improve quality of hospital care. Am J Med 1999;106:565–73.

56. O'Keefe ST, Chonchubhair AN. Postoperative delirium in the elderly. Br J Anaesth 1994;73:673–87.

57. Han L, McCusker J, Cole M, et al. Use of medications with anticholinergic effect predicts clinical severity of delirium symptoms in older medical inpatients. Arch Intern Med 2001;161:1099–105.

58. Tune LE, Egeli S. Acetylcholine and delirium. Dement Geriatr Cogn Disord 1999; 10:342–4.

59. Flacker JM, Cummings V, Mach JR Jr, et al. The association of serum anticholinergic activity with delirium in elderly medical patients. Am J Geriatr Psychiatry 1998;6:31–41.

60. Tune LE, Strauss ME, Lew MF, et al. Serum levels of anticholinergic drugs and impaired recent memory in chronic schizophrenic patients. Am J Psychiatry 1982;139:1460–2.

61. Maldonado JR. Delirium in the acute care setting: characteristics, diagnosis and treatment. Crit Care Clin 2008;24:657–722.

62. Irby D. What clinical teachers in medicine need to know. Acad Med 1994;69: 333–42.

63. Pandharipande PP, Pun BT, Herr DL. Effect of sedation with dexmedetomidine vs lorazepam on acute brain dysfunction in mechanically ventilated patients: the MENDS randomized controlled trial. JAMA 2007;298:2644–53.

64. Colville G, Kerry S, Pierce C. Children's factual and delusional memories of intensive care. Am J Respir Crit Care Med 2008;177:976–82.
65. Ely EW. ICU delirium and cognitive impairment study group. 2009. Available at: www.icudelirium.org. Accessed October 1, 2012.
66. Ely EW, Truman B, Shintani A. Monitoring sedation status over time in ICU patients: reliability and validity of the Richmond Agitation-Sedation Scale (RASS). JAMA 2003;289:2983–91.
67. Sessler CN, Gosnell MS, Grap MJ, et al. The Richmond Agitation-Sedation Scale: validity and reliability in adult intensive care unit patients. Am J Respir Crit Care Med 2002;166:1338–44.
68. Association American Psychiatric. Practice guideline for the treatment of patients with delirium. Arlington (TX): American Psychiatric Pub; 2006.
69. Hipp DM, Ely EW. Pharmacological and nonpharmacological management of delirium in critically ill patients. Neurotherapeutics 2012;9:158–75.
70. Turkel SB, Jacobson J, Munzig E, et al. Atypical antipsychotic medications to control symptoms of delirium in children and adolescents. J Child Adolesc Psychopharmacol 2012;22:126–30.
71. Schieveld JN, Valk JA, Smeets I, et al. Diagnostic considerations regarding pediatric delirium: a review and a proposal for an algorithm for pediatric intensive care units. Intensive Care Med 2009;35:1843–9.
72. Esseveld MM, Leroy PL, Leue C, et al. Catatonia and refractory agitation in an updated flow chart for the evaluation of emotional-behavioral disturbances in severely ill children. Intensive Care Med 2012. http://dx.doi.org/10.1007/s00134-012-2763-1.
73. Deshpande JK, Tobias JD. The pediatric pain handbook. St Louis (MO): Mosby; 1996.
74. Carney DE, Nicolette LA, Ratner MH, et al. Ketorlac reduces postoperative narcotic requirement. J Pediatr Surg 2001;36:76–9.
75. Tobias JD, Deshpande JK. Pediatric pain management for primary care. 2nd edition. Elk Grove Village (IL): American Academy of Pediatrics; 2005.
76. Silver GH, Kearney JA, Kutko MC, et al. Infant delirium in pediatric critical care settings. Am J Psychiatry 2010;167:1172–7.
77. Ely EW, Stephens RK, Jackson JC, et al. Current opinions regarding the importance, diagnosis, and management of delirium in the intensive care unit: a survey of 912 healthcare professionals. Crit Care Med 2004;32:106–12.
78. Jacobi J, Fraser GL, Coursin DB, et al, Task Force of the American College of Critical Care Medicine (ACCM) of the Society of Critical Care Medicine (SCCM), American Society of Health-System Pharmacists (ASHP), American College of Chest Physicians. Clinical practice guidelines. Crit Care Med 2002;30:119–41.
79. Lavid N, Budner LJ. Review of the pharmacological treatment of delirium in the pediatric population with accompanying protocol. Jefferson J Psych 2000;15:25–33.
80. Skrobik YK, Bergeron N, Dumont M, et al. Olanzapine vs haloperidol: treating delirium in a critical care setting. Intensive Care Med 2004;30:444–9.
81. Boettger S, Breitbart W. Atypical antipsychotics in the management of delirium: a review of the empirical literature. Palliat Support Care 2005;3:227–37.

# Family-Centered Care in the Pediatric Intensive Care Unit

Kathleen L. Meert, MD[a],*, Jeff Clark, MD[a], Susan Eggly, PhD[b]

## KEYWORDS

- Family • Parent • Sibling • Visitation • Rounding • Conferences
- Invasive procedures

## KEY POINTS

- Patient-centered and family-centered care (PFCC) is care that is respectful and responsive to the preferences, needs, and values of patients and families.
- Efforts to implement PFCC in pediatric intensive care units (PICUs) include open visitation, family-centered rounding, family presence during invasive procedures, and family conferences.
- Research on PFCC programs in PICUs generally suggests benefits to patients, families, and staff.
- Further development of PFCC programs requires continued input from patients, families, and staff.

## INTRODUCTION

Patient-centered and family-centered care (PFCC) as an approach to care in adult and pediatric settings has been endorsed by major professional organizations, including the Institute of Medicine (IOM), the American College of Critical Care Medicine (ACCM), and the American Academy of Pediatrics (AAP).[1–3] In 2001, the IOM[1] made recommendations for changes to the health care system that emphasized the need for patient-centered care and the ongoing and open exchange of information between health care providers and patients. Patient-centered care was defined as care that is respectful of and responsive to individual patient preferences, needs, and values. In 2007, the ACCM[2] strongly endorsed patient-centered care as defined by the 2001 IOM report, suggesting that patient and family involvement can profoundly influence clinical decisions and patient outcomes in intensive care units. This endorsement was based on the recognition that critically ill patients are often unable to participate

a Department of Pediatrics, Critical Care Medicine, Children's Hospital of Michigan, 3901 Beaubien Boulevard, Detroit, MI 48201, USA; b Department of Internal Medicine, Karmanos Cancer Institute, Wayne State University, 4100 John R MMO3CB, Detroit, MI 48201, USA
* Corresponding author.
E-mail address: kmeert@med.wayne.edu

Pediatr Clin N Am 60 (2013) 761–772
http://dx.doi.org/10.1016/j.pcl.2013.02.011
0031-3955/13/$ – see front matter © 2013 Elsevier Inc. All rights reserved.

in health care decisions and the expressed concerns of families and other surrogates that they are often poorly informed and excluded from decision making and day-to-day care of their loved ones.

With regard to the pediatric context, the AAP defines PFCC as "an innovative approach to the planning, delivery, and evaluation of health care that is grounded in a mutually beneficial partnership among patients, families, and providers that recognizes the importance of the family in the patient's life."[3] The AAP policy is based on the concept of collaboration among patients, families, physicians, nurses, and other professionals. These collaborative relationships are guided by 6 principles of PFCC (**Box 1**). The AAP policy grows out of recent evidence that PFCC can improve outcomes for patients, families, and health care providers, decrease health care costs, and lead to more effective use of health care resources.

In this article, some of the ways that PFCC has been operationalized in pediatric intensive care units (PICUs) are discussed. Although PFCC is intended to permeate all aspects of health care, 4 areas of pediatric critical care practice have been emphasized in the literature. These areas include (1) family visitation; (2) family-centered rounding; (3) family presence during invasive procedures and cardiopulmonary resuscitation (CPR); and (4) family conferences.

## FAMILY VISITATION

Historically, PICUs have had restrictive visiting policies, allowing only brief visits by parents and disallowing visits by siblings or multiple family members (please see accompanying article elsewhere in this issue).[4] Concerns underlying these restrictive policies included the potential for spread of infection; breach of privacy and confidentiality, emotional trauma to patients, parents and siblings; and lack of space and staff to accommodate family. However, research on the needs of families of critically ill patients has consistently shown that families desire information, assurance from staff, and proximity to their loved ones.[5,6] Parents are the natural caregivers for their children. During their child's critical illness, much of the caregiving role of parents is transferred to health professionals, because of the complex care required. This alteration of parental role has been identified as the greatest source of stress among parents in PICUs.[7–10] Parents want to be recognized as important to their child's recovery and participate in their child's care. In response to an increasing awareness of parents' needs, many PICUs have adopted 24-hour open visiting policies. Open visitation has been viewed as a first step in promoting family presence and involvement in care.

---

**Box 1**
**AAP core principles of PFCC**

1. Listening to and respecting each child and their family
2. Ensuring flexibility in organizational policies, procedures, and practices
3. Sharing complete, honest, and unbiased information with patients and families
4. Providing and ensuring formal and informal support for the child and family
5. Collaborating with patients and families at all levels of health care
6. Recognizing and building on the strengths of individual children and families

*Data from* American Academy of Pediatrics, Committee on Hospital Care and Institute for Patient- and Family-Centered Care. Patient- and family-centered care and the pediatrician's role. Pediatrics 2012;129:394–404.

PICU environments may pose many challenges to open visitation. Environmental needs identified by parents include privacy, proximity, adequate space, control of sensory stimuli (eg, noise, lighting, smell), cleanliness, safety, facilities to care for self and others, access to their child, and the presence of people who provide professional and personal support.[11] Having a place to sleep in the hospital or PICU has been identified by parents as an important yet frequently unmet need.[12] In a study conducted before and after renovation of 2 PICUs, Smith and colleagues[8] explored the impact of providing bed space for parents in the PICU on parents' stress levels. Parents experiencing PICUs with parent bed space had less total stress and less stress related to parental role alteration than those experiencing PICUs without bed spaces. In addition to sleeping arrangements, other provisions such as meal vouchers, transportation, and daily amenities may be helpful in supporting family presence in the PICU.

Siblings of critically ill children may also experience stress during their brother's or sister's hospitalization related to parental absence, substitute caregiver arrangements, changes in daily routine, and lack of information.[13] Presence at the bedside may help siblings cope with these changes. Suggestions for facilitating visits by children in pediatric and adult intensive care units include educating nurses on developmental stages and goals, preparing parents for their well child's questions and reactions, preparing siblings for what they might see and hear through age-appropriate books and other materials, screening for infection, maintaining a child-friendly atmosphere, keeping visits brief, using appropriate language, encouraging questions, debriefing after visits, and respecting decisions not to visit.[13,14] Child life specialists are a valuable resource for assisting with sibling visitation.

Based on the available evidence, the ACCM[2] recommends that parents be allowed to visit in PICUs 24 hours per day. Siblings should be able to visit with parental approval after previsit education, and siblings of immune-compromised patients should be allowed to visit with physician approval.[2] Despite these recommendations, a recent ethnographic study[10] conducted in 1 North American PICU with a long-standing 24-hour open visitation policy found that parents are still often forced to relinquish their parental role because of staff attitudes and practices that diverge from the goal of family-centeredness. A survey of Italian PICUs[15] showed that only 12% had unrestricted visiting policies, 59% did not allow continuous presence of a parent, 76% did not allow child visitors, and 32% had no waiting room. However, 48% of these units were in the process of revising their visiting policies, suggesting a readiness for change.

## FAMILY-CENTERED ROUNDS

The ACCM and the AAP recommend that attending physician rounds, case presentations, and discussions take place at the bedside of critically ill children in the presence of parents.[2,3] During rounds, parents should be given the opportunity to ask questions, clarify information, and participate in decision making. Recent studies[16–24] exploring parents' and health professionals' perceptions, attitudes, and preferences regarding parental presence on rounds, and the impact of parental presence on parent and health professional satisfaction, patient privacy, resident teaching, nursing practice, and length of rounds are generally supportive.

Potential benefits of family-centered rounds include increased opportunity for parents to give and receive information and to improve their understanding of their child's condition and treatment plan.[16–24] Other benefits for parents include support of their parental role, increased capacity to advocate for their child and participate in clinical decisions, increased transparency and trust of health professionals, and increased feelings of respect. Attending physicians have an increased opportunity to educate parents, role model communication skills to residents, and observe resident competencies. Residents have increased opportunity to gain understanding of family perspectives. Parental presence on rounds may also reduce the need for nurses to mediate physician-parent communication. Potential risks of family-centered rounds include increased parental anxiety and confusion because of misinterpretation of topics discussed on rounds, breaches in privacy and confidentiality, inhibition of difficult discussions that are medically relevant (eg, poor home care, medical errors, poor prognoses), increased duration of rounds, reduced teaching related to resident discomfort when making presentations and asking questions, and attending limitation of discussions to avoid exposing gaps in resident knowledge.

Most studies of parental presence during rounds are descriptive, consisting of direct observation of rounds and surveys or qualitative interviews with parents and staff. Most studies lack adequate controls, including only parents who are present during rounds, or comparing parents who self-select whether or not to be present during rounds.[17-20] In general, these studies suggest that families prefer to be present on rounds, residents perceive decreased teaching when families are present, and no change in length of rounds or time spent teaching.

Using a predesign and postdesign, Kleiber and colleagues[22] surveyed parents, nurses, and physicians at 1 PICU before implementation of a policy inviting parental presence on rounds and again 6 months after implementation of the policy. Parents were more likely to report daily physician contact with the new policy; nurses were less likely to feel caught in the middle between parents and physicians; all physicians perceived benefit to parents and enhanced trust. There was no increase in the length of rounds under the new policy.

Landry and colleagues[23] conducted a randomized trial comparing bedside versus conference room case presentations in a PICU. Patients who had 2 consecutive morning rounds in the presence of the same resident, attending, and parent were randomized to bedside or conference room rounds on the first study day. On the second day, the alternative was performed. Parents were more satisfied with bedside presentations, felt a greater sense of confidentiality and intimacy, and more often reported being well informed about medical tests. Residents reported no difference in satisfaction or comfort level between bedside and conference room presentations, although they reported more comfort asking and being asked questions in the conference room.

Most studies of family-centered rounding have been conducted in Western societies, and some have cautioned that the findings may not be directly applicable to all cultures.[25] In a nonrandomized prestudy and poststudy conducted in a private hospital in Pakistan, Ladak and colleagues[21] found that parents preferred family-centered rounds over traditional rounds and that patient length of stay was reduced during the family-centered rounding period. In contrast to studies of family-centered rounding from the West, in which most parent participants are mothers, most parents in Ladak and colleagues' study were fathers. These investigators point out that in Pakistani culture, mothers are the primary care providers, whereas male family members are the decision makers; hence, family-centered rounds may be experienced differently based on cultural beliefs and practices.

Educating staff about the underlying principles of PFCC and reconciling these principles with staff needs and expectations is an important step toward successful implementation of family-centered rounding.[18] In addition to educating staff, educating parents about rounding procedures in the PICU has been recognized as a way to maximize benefits and reduce risks.[17,18,20] For example, Aronson and colleagues[17] found that parents present for rounds on the first day of PICU admission, compared with those present for rounds later in the PICU stay, were less likely to understand the plan, to feel comfortable asking questions, to want bad news delivered during rounds, and more likely to have privacy concerns and to want 1 person to convey the plan after rounds. These investigators suggest that parents may need special attention on the first PICU day, such as educational tools about the purpose and process of rounds and the option of family participation.

## FAMILY PRESENCE DURING CPR AND INVASIVE PROCEDURES

In 2000, the American Heart Association became the first national organization to recommend the option of family presence during CPR and other invasive procedures.[26] These guidelines prompted several studies exploring health professionals' views on family presence during CPR and invasive procedures for adult and pediatric patients in emergency departments and intensive care units.[27–33] Health professionals supporting family presence believe that witnessing CPR increases family understanding and sense of control over the situation, allows the family to see that everything was done, and increases family rapport with physicians and nurses. These health professionals also believe that when patients die during CPR, family presence facilitates grieving. Health professionals opposing family presence during CPR caution that family presence may lead to increased anxiety and fear among family members, misunderstanding of events, interference with procedures or decisions to stop CPR, violations of patient privacy, performance anxiety and distraction among health providers, increased malpractice law suits, and the need for more resources such as additional staff, space, and time.

Several factors are associated with health professionals' support or opposition to family presence during CPR and invasive procedures.[28,30,34] In general, nurses are more supportive of family presence than physicians, attending physicians more than physicians in training, and pediatricians more than physicians who care for adults. Health professionals experienced with family presence, with previous education on the topic, or who work in units with formal policies in favor of family presence are also more supportive. Some health professionals believe that family presence should be considered only for less invasive procedures. Regional differences in health professionals' attitudes have been documented across the United States, with Midwesterners more likely to favor family-witnessed CPR than professionals in other areas.[27] Differences in experience and attitudes also exist between countries. Studies from the United States, United Kingdom, and Australia suggest a growing acceptance of family presence during CPR and invasive procedures. However, a recent study from Greece reported that most physicians and nurses working in the neonatal and pediatric departments or intensive care units of 3 hospitals were not familiar with, were not educated about, did not agree with, and had no written policies on family presence.[33]

The views of parents and families regarding presence during CPR and invasive procedures are overwhelmingly supportive.[35–38] Most parents believe that their presence during their child's CPR or invasive procedure helped their child and helped them. In a nonrandomized study comparing parents who were present during their child's PICU procedure with those who were not present, Powers and Rubenstein[38] found that being present reduced parents' anxiety about the procedure but not their anxiety related to the child's condition. In a randomized study comparing relatives (including some parents) who witnessed CPR on a family member in the emergency room with those who did not, Robinson and colleagues[39] found that those who witnessed CPR had a tendency for lower degrees of intrusive thoughts, posttraumatic avoidance behavior, and symptoms of grief 3 months later. In interview studies with parents whose children have undergone CPR,[35,36] parents recommend being present during the event. Parents report that feelings of fear or anxiety are not related to witnessing the CPR but rather to the possibility that their child may not survive. Health professionals have suggested that parental presence during CPR might be most beneficial for parents of children with chronic illnesses[28]; however, parents more often prefer to be present for children who were previously healthy.[35]

Few studies have attempted to measure direct effects on the child of parental presence during invasive procedures. In a randomized crossover trial, Johnston and colleagues[40] evaluated a *Touch and Talk* intervention designed for use by mothers as a means of distracting their infant or toddler during PICU procedures. The intervention did not affect the child's physiologic stability as measured by heart rate, heart rate variability, or oxygen saturation during the procedure but did lead to shorter recovery times by a mean of 24 seconds. A qualitative study exploring how parents experienced the *Touch and Talk* intervention identified an overarching theme about the importance that mothers place on being able to comfort their child and concluded that the option of parental presence during invasive procedures supports the parental role during the PICU stay.[37]

In 2006, representatives from 18 national organizations published consensus recommendations regarding family presence during pediatric procedures and CPR (**Box 2**).[41] The recommendations advise that policies for family presence during procedures and CPR should include definitions of family member, what procedures are covered, who facilitates, how to prepare the family, how to escort the family, how to handle disagreements, and how to support staff. Several investigators contend that the presence of a facilitator (eg, chaplain, social worker, nurse) is essential to maximize the benefits of family presence during procedures and CPR and to maintain safety.[30,42] The facilitator invites the family to be present, stays with the family during the procedure or CPR, provides explanations and emotional support, and occasionally removes those who obstruct care.

Staff education is also a key component of family presence during invasive procedures and CPR. Pye and colleagues[43] described a simulation program in which

---

**Box 2**
**Consensus recommendations on family presence during pediatric procedures and CPR**

1. Consider family presence as an option during procedures and CPR

2. Offer the option after assessing factors that could have an adverse effect

3. If not offered, document reasons why

4. Consider the health care team's safety at all times

5. Develop written policies for family presence

6. Obtain legal review of policies

7. Educate health care professionals about family presence

8. Promote research on family presence

*Data from* Henderson DP, Knapp JF. Report of the National Consensus Conference on family presence during pediatric cardiopulmonary resuscitation and procedures. J Emerg Nurs 2006;32:23–9.

standardized persons acting as parents and grandparents were present in the resuscitation room as CPR skills were practiced on manikins. One of the goals of the simulation was hands-on training in the support of the family during CPR. Staff comfort with parental presence increased from before to immediately after training and at 1 year after training.

## FAMILY CONFERENCES

Family conferences are planned meetings between family members and the interdisciplinary team of professionals caring for the patient.[2,44,45] Family conferences are considered an essential forum for shared decision making in the intensive care setting. Many critically ill patients are unable to communicate with health professionals or participate in decisions about their own care because of severity of illness, use of sedation and endotracheal intubation, and in the case of children, young age and developmental state. Relatives of critically ill adults are asked to provide information about the patients' preferences for care based on the principle of substituted judgment. Parents of critically ill children are asked to consider what would be best for the child based on the best interest standard. Shared decision making, whether guided by the principle of substituted judgment or the best interest standard, requires mutual understanding of the patient's diagnosis, treatment options, prognosis, preferences, values, and wishes. Such mutual understanding can potentially be achieved through family conferences.

Most research on family conferences has been conducted with relatives of critically ill adults in the context of end-of-life decision making.[45–50] These studies have identified several attributes of family conferences associated with increased satisfaction and better psychological outcomes among family members. These attributes include conducting conferences within 72 hours of intensive care admission, having a private place for meeting, providing consistent communication from all team members, allowing adequate time for families to express their concerns, expressing empathy, and providing assurance. Types of empathic statements associated with increased family satisfaction during conferences include those acknowledging the difficulty of having a critically ill loved one, of surrogate decision making, and of confronting death.[49] Types of assurances associated with increased family satisfaction include those that confirm that the patient is not abandoned and does not suffer, and explicit support for the family's end-of-life decisions.[50]

In a randomized controlled trial conducted across 22 adult intensive care units in France, Lautrette and colleagues[51] evaluated the effect of a proactive family end-of-life conference and bereavement brochure on psychological outcomes of family members. The intervention had 5 objectives for health professionals summarized by the mnemonic VALUE (**Box 3**). Family members in the intervention group had less posttraumatic stress, depression, and anxiety 3 months after their relative's death compared with those randomized to standard end-of-life conferences.

Michelson and colleagues[52] interviewed PICU clinicians and parents whose children died in the PICU to explore their experiences with family conferences in the context of end-of-life decision making. Clinicians indicated that family conferences provide a means for communication between clinicians and parents, communication between clinicians, and support of families. Components of the interaction considered most important by staff included providing parents with information and emotional support, and allowing parents to express their needs and concerns. Recommendations from parents included regularly scheduled conferences and use of a private room. In a survey study examining the circumstances surrounding end

---

**Box 3**
**The VALUE mnemonic for use by health providers during family conferences**

1. Value family statements

2. Acknowledge family emotions

3. Listen to family

4. Understand the patient as a person

5. Elicit family questions

*Data from* Curtis JR, White DB. Practical guidance for evidence-based family conferences. Chest 2008;134:835–43; and Lautrette A, Darmon M, Megarbane B, et al. A communication strategy and brochure for relatives dying in the ICU. N Engl J Med 2007;156:469–78.

---

of life in a PICU, Garros and colleagues[53] found that more than 1 family conference was required to reach consensus about forgoing life support for about half the patients.

In addition to family conferences during a child's PICU stay, family meetings after a child's discharge or death may be beneficial to some parents. Colville and colleagues[54] conducted an exploratory randomized controlled trial to evaluate the effect of follow-up meetings on parents' psychological health after their child's PICU discharge. Although no significant differences were found between groups overall, parents who reported higher levels of stress during the PICU stay had lower rates of posttraumatic stress and depression 5 months later when offered a follow-up meeting compared with those not offered a meeting. In a series of qualitative studies conducted among parents bereaved in the PICU and pediatric intensivists,[55–57] the Eunice Kennedy Shriver National Institute of Child Health and Human Development Collaborative Pediatric Critical Care Research Network described parents' and physicians' experiences and perspectives on follow-up meetings after a child's death. From these studies, a framework for follow-up meetings was developed, which focuses on providing information, reassurance, and an opportunity for parental feedback.[58]

## SUMMARY

PFCC as an approach to care is strongly endorsed by many professional organizations. Preliminary research on the implementation of programs related to PFCC in the PICU setting generally suggests benefits to patients, families, and staff. However, more research is needed using experimental designs to further define both the benefits and risks of these practices. The development of PFCC policies and their implementation in clinical practice should reflect the needs of specific patient populations and settings, and thus requires continued input from patients, families, and staff. To reduce the possibility of creating additional stress or other adverse effects, implementation also require careful education and training.

Patient-centered communication is the ideal process through which PFCC is implemented in daily practice. As applied to pediatric critical care, the key components of patient-centered communication are: addressing the patient's and family's perspective; understanding patients and families within their psychosocial context; involving patients and families in care to the extent they desire; reaching a shared understanding of the problem and agreeing on a treatment plan; and making decisions that are based on the best clinical evidence, consistent with patient and family values, and that are feasible.[2,59,60] The PICU setting presents unique challenges to communicating effectively and providing PFCC, but research-based and practical guidance is available to enable effective communication in this and other pediatric settings.[61] Thus, the growing evidence base regarding patient-centered communication and PFCC will provide guidance for future policy and practice, potentially leading to better patient and family outcomes.

## REFERENCES

1. Institute of Medicine. Crossing the quality chasm. A new health system for the 21st century. Washington, DC: National Academy Press; 2001.
2. Davidson JE, Powers K, Hedayat KM, et al. Clinical practice guidelines for support of the family in the patient-centered intensive care unit: American College of Critical Care Medicine Task Force 2004-2005. Crit Care Med 2007; 35:605–22.
3. American Academy of Pediatrics, Committee on Hospital Care and Institute for Patient- and Family-Centered Care. Patient- and family-centered care and the pediatrician's role. Pediatrics 2012;129:394–404.
4. Frazier A, Frazier H, Warren NA. A discussion of family-centered care within the pediatric intensive care unit. Crit Care Nurs Q 2010;33:82–6.
5. Scott DL. Perceived needs of parents of critically ill children. J Soc Pediatr Nurs 1998;3:4–12.
6. Meert KL, Schim SM, Briller SH. Parental bereavement needs in the pediatric intensive care unit: review of available measures. J Palliat Med 2011;14:951–64.
7. Kirschbaum MS. Needs of parents of critically ill children. Dimens Crit Care Nurs 1990;9:344–52.
8. Smith AB, Hefley GC, Anand KJ. Parent bed spaces in the PICU: effect on parental stress. Pediatr Nurs 2007;33:215–21.
9. Board R, Ryan-Wenger N. Long-term effects of pediatric intensive care unit hospitalization on families with young children. Heart Lung 2002;31:53–66.
10. MacDonald ME, Lien S, Carnival FA, et al. An office or a bedroom? Challenges for family-centered care in the pediatric intensive care unit. J Child Health Care 2012;16(3):237–49.
11. Meert KL, Briller SH, Schim SM, et al. Exploring parents' environmental needs at the time of a child's death in the pediatric intensive care unit. Pediatr Crit Care Med 2008;9:623–8.
12. Meert KL, Templin TN, Michelson KN, et al. The bereaved parent needs assessment: a new instrument to assess the needs of parents whose children died in the pediatric intensive care unit. Crit Care Med 2012;40(11):3050–7.
13. Rozdilsky JR. Enabling sibling presence in pediatric ICU. Crit Care Nurs Clin North Am 2005;17:451–61.
14. Hanley JB, Piazza J. A visit to the intensive care unit. A family-centered culture change to facilitate pediatric visitation in an adult intensive care unit. Crit Care Nurs Q 2012;35:113–22.
15. Giannini A, Miccinesi G. Parental presence and visiting policies in Italian pediatric intensive care units: a national survey. Pediatr Crit Care Med 2011;12:e46–50.
16. Cypress BS. Family presence on rounds. A systematic review of the literature. Dimens Crit Care Nurs 2012;31(1):53–64.
17. Aronson PL, Yau J, Helfaer MA, et al. Impact of family presence during pediatric intensive care unit rounds on the family and medical team. Pediatrics 2009;124: 1119–25.

18. McPherson G, Jefferson R, Kissoon N, et al. Toward the inclusion of parents on pediatric critical care unit rounds. Pediatr Crit Care Med 2011;12:e255–61.
19. Phipps LM, Bartke CN, Spear DA, et al. Assessment of parental presence during bedside pediatric intensive care unit rounds: effect on duration, teaching and privacy. Pediatr Crit Care Med 2007;8:220–4.
20. Cameron MA, Schleien CL, Morris MC. Parental presence on pediatric intensive care unit rounds. J Pediatr 2009;155:522–8.
21. Ladak LA, Premji SS, Amanullah MM, et al. Family-centered rounds in Pakistani pediatric intensive care settings: non-randomized pre- and post-study design. Int J Nurs Stud 2012. [Epub ahead of print]. http://dx.doi.org/10.1016/j.ijnurstu.2012.05.009.
22. Kleiber C, Davenport T, Freyenberger B. Open bedside rounds for families with children in pediatric intensive care units. Am J Crit Care 2006;15:492–6.
23. Landry MA, Lafrenaye S, Roy MC, et al. A randomized controlled trial of bedside versus conference- room case presentation in a pediatric intensive care unit. Pediatrics 2007;120:275–80.
24. Eggly S, Meert KL. Parental inclusion in pediatric intensive care unit rounds: how does it fit with patient- and family-centered care. Pediatr Crit Care Med 2011;12: 684–5.
25. Kalloghlian A. Parental presence during bedside pediatric intensive care unit rounds. Pediatr Crit Care Med 2007;8:291–2.
26. Guidelines 2000 for Cardiopulmonary Resuscitation and Emergency Cardiovascular Care. Part 2: ethical aspects of CPR and ECC. Circulation 2000;102 (8 suppl):I12–21.
27. McClenathan BM, Torrington KG, Uyehara FT. Family member presence during cardiopulmonary resuscitation. Chest 2002;122:2204–11.
28. Gold KJ, Gorenflo DW, Schwenk TL, et al. Physician experience with family presence during cardiopulmonary resuscitation in children. Pediatr Crit Care Med 2006;7:428–33.
29. Kuzin JK, Yborra JG, Taylor MD, et al. Family-member presence during interventions in the intensive care unit: perceptions of pediatric cardiac intensive care providers. Pediatrics 2007;120:e895–901.
30. Dingeman RS, Mitchell EA, Meyer EC, et al. Parent presence during complex invasive procedures and cardiopulmonary resuscitation: a systemic review of the literature. Pediatrics 2007;120:842–54.
31. Fulbrook P, Latour JM, Albarran JW. Paediatric critical care nurses' attitudes and experiences of parental presence during cardiopulmonary resuscitation: a European survey. Int J Nurs Stud 2007;44:1238–49.
32. Jones BL, Parker-Raley J, Maxson T, et al. Understanding health care professionals' views of family presence during pediatric resuscitation. Am J Crit Care 2011;20:199–208.
33. Vavarouta A, Xanthos T, Papadimitriou L, et al. Family presence during resuscitation and invasive procedures: physicians' and nurses' attitudes working in pediatric departments in Greece. Resuscitation 2011;82:713–6.
34. MacLean SL, Guzzetta CE, White C, et al. Family presence during cardiopulmonary resuscitation and invasive procedures: practices of critical care and emergency nurses. J Emerg Nurs 2003;29:208–21.
35. Tinsley C, Hill B, Shah J, et al. Experience of families during cardiopulmonary resuscitation in a pediatric intensive care unit. Pediatrics 2008;122:e799–804.
36. Maxton FJ. Parental presence during resuscitation in the PICU: the parents' experience. Sharing and surviving the resuscitation: a phenomenological study. J Clin Nurs 2008;17:3168–76.

37. Rennick JE, Lambert S, Childerhose J, et al. Mothers' experiences of a Touch and Talk nursing intervention to optimize pain management in the PICU: a qualitative descriptive study. Intensive Crit Care Nurs 2011;27:151–7.

38. Powers KS, Rubenstein JS. Family presence during invasive procedures in the pediatric intensive care unit. Arch Pediatr Adolesc Med 1999;153:955–8.

39. Robinson SM, Mackenzie-Ross S, Campbell Hewson GL, et al. Psychological effect of witnessed resuscitation on bereaved relatives. Lancet 1998;352:614–7.

40. Johnston CC, Rennick JE, Filion F, et al. Maternal touch and talk for invasive procedures in infants and toddlers in the pediatric intensive care unit. J Pediatr Nurs 2012;27:144–53.

41. Henderson DP, Knapp JF. Report of the National Consensus Conference on family presence during pediatric cardiopulmonary resuscitation and procedures. J Emerg Nurs 2006;32:23–9.

42. Nibert L, Ondrejka D. Family presence during pediatric resuscitation: an integrative review for evidence-based practice. J Pediatr Nurs 2005;20:145–7.

43. Pye S, Kane J, Jones A. Parental presence during pediatric resuscitation: the use of simulation training for cardiac intensive care nurses. J Spec Pediatr Nurs 2010;15:172–5.

44. Cypress BS. Family conference in the intensive care unit. A systematic review. Dimens Crit Care Nurs 2011;30:246–55.

45. Curtis JR, White DB. Practical guidance for evidence-based family conferences. Chest 2008;134:835–43.

46. Lilly CM, De Meo DL, Sonna LA, et al. An intensive communication intervention for the critically ill. Am J Med 2000;109:469–75.

47. Pochard F, Azoulay E, Chevret S, et al. Symptoms of anxiety and depression in family members of intensive care unit patients: ethical hypothesis regarding decision-making capacity. Crit Care Med 2001;29:1893–7.

48. McDonagh JR, Elliott TB, Engelberg RA, et al. Family satisfaction with family conferences about end-of-life care in the intensive care unit: increased proportion of family speech is associated with increased satisfaction. Crit Care Med 2004;32:1484–8.

49. Selph RB, Shiang J, Engelberg R, et al. Empathy and life support decisions in intensive care units. J Gen Intern Med 2008;23:1311–7.

50. Stapleton RD, Engelberg RA, Wenrich MD, et al. Clinician statements and family satisfaction with family conferences in the intensive care unit. Crit Care Med 2006; 34:1679–85.

51. Lautrette A, Darmon M, Megarbane B, et al. A communication strategy and brochure for relatives dying in the ICU. N Engl J Med 2007;156:469–78.

52. Michelson KN, Emanuel L, Carter A, et al. Pediatric intensive care unit family conferences: one mode of communication for discussing end-of-life decisions. Pediatr Crit Care Med 2011;12:e336–43.

53. Garros D, Rosychuk RJ, Cox PN. Circumstances surrounding end of life care in a pediatric intensive care unit. Pediatrics 2003;112:e371–9.

54. Colville GA, Cream PR, Kerry SM. Do parents benefit from the offer of a follow-up appointment after their child's admission to intensive care?: an exploratory randomized controlled trial. Intensive Crit Care Nurs 2010;26:146–53.

55. Meert KL, Eggly S, Pollack M, et al. Parents' perspectives regarding a physician-parent conference after their child's death in the pediatric intensive care unit. J Pediatr 2007;151:50–5.

56. Meert KL, Eggly S, Pollack M, et al. Parents' perspectives regarding physician-parent communication near the time of a child's death in the pediatric intensive care unit. Pediatr Crit Care Med 2008;9:2–7.

57. Meert KL, Eggly S, Berger J, et al. Physicians' experiences and perspectives regarding follow-up meetings with parents after a child's death in the pediatric intensive care unit. Pediatr Crit Care Med 2011;12:e64–8.

58. Eggly S, Meert KL, Berger J, et al. A framework for conducting follow-up meetings with parents after a child's death in the pediatric intensive care unit. Pediatr Crit Care Med 2011;12:147–52.

59. McCormack LA, Treiman K, Rupert D, et al. Measuring patient-centered communication in cancer care: a literature review and the development of a systematic approach. Soc Sci Med 2011;72:1085–95.

60. Epstein RM, Street RL Jr. Patient-centered communication in cancer care: promoting healing and reducing suffering. Bethesda (MD): National Cancer Institute; 2007 (NCI Document No. 07–6225).

61. Levetown M, the American Academy of Pediatrics Committee on Bioethics. Communicating with children and families: from everyday interactions to skill in conveying distressing information. Pediatrics 2008;121:e1441–60.

# A Parents' Perspective on the Pediatric Intensive Care Unit
## Our Family's Journey

Lynne Merk*, Rick Merk

## KEYWORDS

- Parent perspective • PICU • Pediatric intensive care unit • Patient-centered care
- Family-centered care

## KEY POINTS

- Family time is important to the overall medical care of patients in the PICU.
- In addition to providing excellent medical care, it is also important for PICU teams to focus upon compassion and the patient's unique life situation.
- Improved communication (between staff and with patients/families) is key in providing good patient- and family-centered care.
- Due to the intensity of the emotional experience for patients/families in a critical care setting, patients/families may need access to PICU staff for reassurance and clarification long after leaving the PICU.
- When a patient dies, it is important for PICU staff to learn from that patient and to take steps to make the learning long-term.

## EDITOR'S NOTE

*I first had the pleasure of meeting the Merk family during Tony's second admission to our PICU. Although I never really got to know Tony outside of the confines of our hospital, it was clear from multiple discussions with his family and some of his other health care providers that he was truly a special child. I was privileged to care for Tony and his family again during his final admission to our PICU. Unfortunately, we were not good enough to save Tony's life. Even more disturbing for me, some of our words and actions made an incredibly difficult and sad time for his family even worse. Caring for critically ill children and their families is a unique and special privilege. We owe it to our patients to learn from each and every one of them so that we will be better for our next patient. Our PICU has come a long way over the past 10 years in becoming more patient- and family-centered, but as you will learn from Rick and Lynne Merk's experience, we still have a long way to go. Tony has left our PICU staff with these*

The Pray~Hope~Believe Foundation, PO Box 53236, Cincinnati, OH 45253, USA
* Corresponding author.
*E-mail address:* info@PrayHopeBelieve.org

Pediatr Clin N Am 60 (2013) 773–780
http://dx.doi.org/10.1016/j.pcl.2013.02.012
0031-3955/13/$ – see front matter © 2013 Elsevier Inc. All rights reserved.

*lessons. I want to thank Rick and Lynne for sharing this very difficult and personal story with us, so that all of us may learn from their family's experience.*

### The Beginning

"Intensive care unit." Wow, those are scary words for parents to hear! Before our unwanted entry into the world of serious childhood illness in October, 2008, we viewed the intensive care unit as a place people went when their medical situation was desperate or where they were likely to die. Our first exposure to the pediatric intensive care unit (PICU) began when our then-3-year-old son, Tony, was treated there following intensive brain surgery, just 2 days after a brain tumor was discovered in the base of his skull. As we entered the PICU for the first time, we were greeted by the sweet sound of Tony crying down the hallway. We were told this was a good sign that Tony was waking up and alert. We could not wait to see him after dropping him off 10 long hours earlier for his surgery. Seeing our sweet boy with his head bandaged and all of those tubes, wires, and machines attached to him was scary. Honestly, it was an image we had never seen before. Television shows and movies do not show pictures of children who have just had brain surgery. Our biggest concern in that moment, however, was to reassure Tony that we were there and he was OK. Thankfully, he was able to communicate with us so we knew he was not in pain; he was just scared and uncomfortable. It was important that we, his parents, could take care of him in any way possible. There was so much we could not do for him and we felt helpless, but we appreciate the PICU staff letting us do what we could: touch him, kiss him, talk to him, give him a popsicle. We also appreciated them doing what they could to prevent pain and promote healing (**Fig. 1**).

We came to understand that because of the seriousness of Tony's surgery, he would need to be in the PICU for intensive observation. We quickly learned how

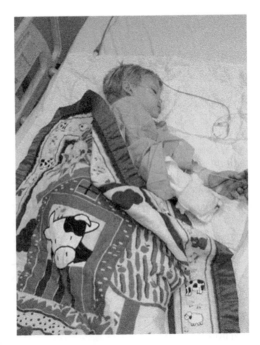

**Fig. 1.** Tony Merk.

parents place total trust in the doctors and nurses of the PICU. Parents are scared and rely on the expertise of the medical professionals to get their children back to health; this was especially true for us during our first trip to the PICU when we were in total shock about our sweet, beautiful 3-year-old son receiving such a difficult diagnosis.

We were comforted by the intensity of care at the time because we were so new to the medical world. We were also struck by the strictness of rules. It felt a bit like a prison, and at that time we did not fully understand the reasons for the strictness regarding who could enter the PICU, where we could eat, and so forth. Tony was allowed numerous visitors while on the neurology floor the couple of days before his surgery, so when we were told Tony's brothers could not visit with him after surgery in the PICU, we were shocked and saddened. Thankfully, Tony's brothers were permitted a very brief visit, just so they could be reassured Tony was OK. It was a necessary visit during a time full of fear and uncertainty.

While there, we met one mother in the kitchen whose child had been in and out of the PICU for his whole young life of less than 2 years. We began to get a picture of how fragile life can be, a thought that rarely occurs when one is around children. This PICU stay only lasted a couple of days, because Tony progressed very quickly to the point at which he no longer required intensive care. Leaving the PICU that day felt good, because we knew it meant Tony was on the road to recovery from his surgery. That was our primary focus at the time. The future battle was before us, but we could not focus on that just yet. At that time, we did not have a complete understanding of Tony's condition, but we knew metastases were found throughout his spine and in another spot of the brain. We were terrified about the future, but our primary focus was in the moment—comforting Tony toward healing while also supporting his older 3 brothers. As we left the PICU, we thanked the staff and told them we hoped to never see them again, at least not in the PICU.

## The Middle

Tony's second visit to the PICU was not planned, and occurred because of emergency circumstances, which is the more common scenario for entry to the PICU. We were sent to the PICU via the emergency department when seizure activity was suspected and Tony would not wake up. It was eventually confirmed Tony was, in fact, experiencing cluster seizures that could not be stopped by ordinary means. Tony had to be placed in a medically induced coma, which required intubation. Tony had already undergone 31 craniospinal radiation treatments and intensive high-dose chemotherapy followed by an autologous stem cell transplant. He had clean scans for almost a year, but experienced a relapse in June 2010. We were told that no treatment existed for relapsed medulloblastoma. None of the treatments we had tried were working, but we were awaiting a new treatment when the seizures started. We were not only terrified by the seizures but also unable to do anything about Tony's brain cancer because of the seizures.

At this point, we were no longer new to the medical world. We had now lived more than 2 years as a family with a seriously ill child. During this stay, Tony remained in the PICU for almost 12 days, which was a long time in the PICU world. The time spent with PICU staff was intense and emotional. This visit was the first time we had an immediate concern about Tony's life. Compared with our first PICU visit, we were now much more aware of what was happening around us. During Tony's journey, we had come to know many other children with cancer or blood disorders, and we knew of way too many who had lost their lives in the PICU. It was a hard place to be, not just because of our own ordeal, but also because we knew everyone on the unit with us was facing a potentially life-threatening situation with a child or teen.

We would sometimes talk with parents in the kitchen or just meet their eyes as we passed in the hallway. The fear, helplessness, and hope were so evident. We remember a night when individuals were being brought to the room next to us, a few at a time, seemingly to say their final goodbye to the sick child or teen being cared for there. We never had this confirmed by the PICU staff, because they do a great job maintaining confidentiality and calm on the floor, but it struck us then that life and death sometimes hang in the balance in the PICU.

### Prescription: family time

During this scary stay in the PICU, we were thankful to Child Life staff who helped us prepare our older sons for what they would see when they visited Tony, given that Tony was in a medically induced coma, on a ventilator, and had been unresponsive for days. We recall Tony's attending physician entering the room during the family visit and commenting, "this is better for Tony than anything I can do for him." We so appreciated that, even with the strict PICU rules, family interaction was recognized as an important part of Tony's healing.

During this PICU stay, we continued to experience the patient- and family-centered care that is part of the hospital environment. We were invited to join both morning and evening rounds. We had an almost constant flow of professionals entering Tony's room, so we appreciated it when they introduced themselves to us. At this point, we had experience on the oncology and bone marrow transplant units, but life on the other medical specialty floors is quite different from life in the PICU.

### The End

Tony had another brief visit in the PICU when his oxygen dropped during a seizure, but his final visit to the PICU began almost 2 weeks before his death. Tony developed a side effect from his chemotherapy and/or tumor growth that required him to receive an intravenous medication that could only be administered in the PICU. We were sent to the PICU not because Tony's physical condition warranted it, but because of the medication he needed. We were not aware that his death was imminent, nor were his treatment providers. We have since had discussions with Tony's doctors about how difficult it is to predict death (**Fig. 2**).

### Missed opportunity: family time

Although most of our experience with the PICU staff was positive, we did have one major problem situation while Tony was there—one that bothers us even more now

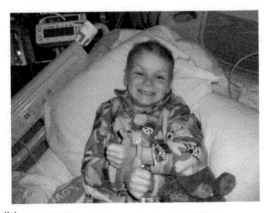

**Fig. 2.** Tony's condition worsens.

that Tony is gone. The issue involved 4 members of the nursing staff denying visitation to our 10-year-old son, Max, just 10 days before Tony's death. On this evening, Lynne brought 2 of Tony's brothers for a visit. Tony's 14-year-old brother, Ben, met the age criteria for visitation, but the 10-year-old did not. We informed the day nurse of the upcoming visit and were under the impression that it would be no problem for Max to visit. However, when we arrived, we were told Max could not visit because Child Life staff were not available to "approve" his visit.

We were confused and frustrated on hearing this. The nursing staff told us Child Life needed to approve all visits for siblings younger than 14 years (we later learned the actual visitation policy says sibling visits can also be approved by the charge nurse). The nursing staff agreed that Max did not pose a medical risk to Tony, but they needed to be sure Max was emotionally prepared to handle what he might see in the PICU. We understand the importance of this preparation in some situations (eg, child severely injured in a car accident), but there was no need for this type of screening in this situation. Did they have any knowledge of Tony's medical history at all? We of course shared with them that Max had been previously cleared by Child Life and had visited with Tony when Tony was in a pentobarbital-induced coma and intubated seven months earlier; Tony's current condition would not be remotely upsetting for Max, given other things Max had seen regarding Tony's treatment. We were told they have 30 families, and if the rules were bent for us, they would have to bend the rules for anyone. (We went through the proper channels to arrange this visit; PICU staff dropped the ball somewhere). Furthermore, because Max was denied visitation, one parent was in Tony's room while the other parent had to stay with Max in the waiting room. Therefore, we were not able to address this issue together with the nurses. Rather, we each took turns going to Tony's room to discuss the issue with the nurses. We spoke with Tony's night nurse, the charge nurse, nurse manager, and manager of patient services. We were continually told the PICU is different from other floors. We reminded them that we were aware of the difference, considering this was our fourth trip to the PICU with Tony in the almost 3 years since his diagnosis, and reminded them of the particularly difficult hospitalization he had 7 months prior when he was intubated and in a coma. In the end, we were told by the Manager of Patient Services that she was "the ultimate authority in the hospital" that night. Talk about feeling helpless! We were already fearful about Tony's condition, because his medical condition precluded him from getting chemotherapy during the past 7 weeks for his growing brain cancer.

For a hospital that prides itself on being patient- and family-centered, this was not at all a patient- or family-centered experience for us. We were honestly shocked at the rigidity and lack of compassion these individuals showed, because this had not been our typical experience at this hospital or in the PICU. The staff was wrong to respond in the way they did. In the end, it felt like a power struggle where they were determined to win, to the detriment of our sons and family. Tony had been in the hospital most of the time during the prior 2 months, which meant our family had very little time together, especially Tony and his brothers. Every moment together was precious. As a family full of helpless feelings, we tried to maximize time spent as a family; that was something we could control, at least until it was denied us. On this particular evening, Tony was awake and interactive, which was a rarity because he was often tired and not feeling well when his brothers visited. It was a missed opportunity, and an important one.

In trying to make sense of this situation, we thought about how it happened in the first place, especially in a hospital that stresses patient- and family-centered care.

Following are some of our guesses, which we hope will elicit discussion among Critical Care teams.

**Chronic versus acute illness/injury.** It is our belief that part of the problem with the visitation denial rested in our family being treated as if we were new to the hospital setting and policies when, in fact, we were quite knowledgeable in these after almost 3 years of coping with our son's life-threatening condition. It felt very much to us like these staff members had no idea about our son's history or even his current status or prognosis. We wish these nurses would have recognized that, as parents of a chronically ill child battling cancer, we truly understood the importance of safety and health. Of course, no safety or health issues were present in this situation. We wish it would have occurred to them that Tony's brothers had witnessed many upsetting situations in the prior 2.5 years and that, with Tony's prognosis, spending time together was a priority. Separation was more upsetting than witnessing Tony's current health status. We wish they would have realized that Tony spent most of the prior 2 months in the hospital, thus making family time extremely difficult and precious. We wish their focus would have been in line with that of families like ours, to "treasure every moment," which became (and remains) one of our family's primary themes. We wish we could get those precious minutes back so our boys could have that time together.

**Day shift versus night shift.** Typically, we interacted less with night shift than with day shift staff, simply because, it was our hope, much of the night shift would involve sleep time. We wonder if night shift staff have sufficient time to get to know their patients. Also, how well did the day and night shift nurses communicate with one another? The day nurse led us to believe that all had been arranged for Max's visit, but the night nurse did not comply.

**Frequent change in nursing staff.** Nursing staff usually changed on a daily basis (or perhaps every other day), but the team of doctors changed weekly. Therefore, although we spent more time with nurses, we had greater consistency in our relationship with the doctors (at least that was our experience in the PICU). We also had the same team of doctors during Tony's hospitalization 7 months prior, so the physician team knew us well and what we had been through. They not only knew Tony and us (his parents) but even recalled the strength of Tony's brothers. We had never had any interaction with this particular night nurse, the charge nurse, or the nurse managers. We wonder also how removed the nurse manager and manager of patient services might be from direct patient care. Have they forgotten the compassion needed for day-to-day interaction with patients and families?

**Dynamics between physicians and nurses.** To us as parents, the visitation denial felt like an opportunity for these particular members of the nursing staff to exert their power. In these situations, when focusing on enforcement of rules, it is important that the individual patient's/family's situation is considered. This would seem to be especially true in a critical care unit where some patients truly are fighting for their lives. Those in the PICU (and elsewhere in the hospital) who knew us and the details of our story would have readily approved this short visit that evening. We chose not to involve the attending physician in the discussion about visitation, because we knew he was tending to a critically ill patient and we did not want to bother him with our situation. We talked briefly with a Fellow about the issue, but were told by the nurses involved that this was a "nursing issue" and therefore it would not be appropriate to involve the doctors. We tried to be respectful of the nurse/doctor dynamic that we imagined might exist, and did not involve the physicians that evening. We witnessed how hard nurses work and how vital they are to health care. We were respectful of their role and did not want to usurp their authority by going "above them" to the physicians.

**An opportunity for learning.** As the family of a child with a life-threatening illness, we had been through so much in the prior 2.5 years and often had to cope with the reality that there was only so much the hospital staff could do to help our son. However, this was a situation in which the hospital staff could have easily done something to help Tony and our family. They simply chose not to, seemingly just because they had the power to do so. On top of our other stress from that day and the prior few months, this situation added significant stress to our family. We all had great difficulty falling asleep that night because we were so upset with how we were treated. We were frustrated by the missed opportunity for Tony and Max to interact (even briefly) when Tony was actually awake. We were sad about the shift in our feelings toward the hospital staff, because we had typically felt that we were treated with the utmost compassion. Added stress was certainly not what we needed at this time in our lives, and I am sure that is the case for any family in the PICU. It seems that anyone working in the PICU would have a greater appreciation for the preciousness of every moment a family has with their loved one; they certainly should.

Weeks later, we eventually brought this matter to the attention of the hospital's Director of Nursing because we wanted to do what we could to prevent other families from having a similar experience. Even though it appeared to us this issue might have been circumscribed to this small group of nurses, these particular nurses were among the management team within the PICU. It concerned us greatly that these individuals might be teaching newer staff these practices. Many doctors and other nurses apologized to us for the visitation denial, but none of the 4 nurses involved in the denial did so. Did they ever conclude that what they did was wrong? Would they do the same thing to another family? Thankfully, the senior nursing administrators of the hospital were appropriately apologetic and made no excuses for the behavior of their nurses on that evening. We have been told changes have since taken place within the PICU such that compassion and an individual patient's unique circumstances are hallmarks of important decision making. In the end, we understand people make mistakes and we are thankful our concerns were taken seriously by the senior nursing administration. We sincerely hope the staff will continue to be reminded of our story in order to maintain the changes they are making.

**A return to family-centered care.** Our story ends on a note of truly family-centered care. On July 3rd, 2011, Tony's status changed. We made a last ditch effort to relieve pressure on his brain. The PICU staff coordinated with all of Tony's treatment providers—over a holiday weekend, no less—to help us make the hardest decisions of our lives. In the end, there was nothing more that could be done to preserve Tony's life, but there was much that could be done to help our family. The PICU staff knew of our large family and how important they are to us. They also knew of our strong faith. Our very large family was permitted to visit with Tony in his final days. They joined in when the priest gave Tony his last rites. We were now that family bringing in family members, a few at a time, to say their final goodbyes. The staff answered our many questions and assured us that whatever decisions we made would be the right ones. They provided the reassurance we needed to hear that we were making loving choices for Tony. As we, Tony's 3 brothers, and Tony's grandparents watched Tony take his last breath, the PICU staff remained professional but were also full of compassion and love. They exemplified the family-centered care we had come to know as the "norm" within the hospital. We continue to be grateful (**Fig. 3**).

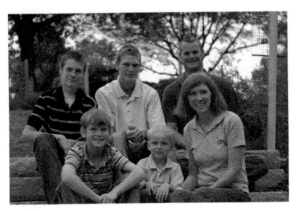

**Fig. 3.** The Merk family.

### Beyond

We imagine many health care providers see the death of a patient as an end to the relationship. However, in our case, after an almost 3-year battle that included a lot of time to become attached, saying goodbye to Tony's caregivers was an added burden to that of grieving the loss of Tony. We had a great deal of emotional investment in Tony's caregivers, that they would be able to find a way to make Tony feel better and, ultimately, save his life. We saw firsthand how hard they tried and how difficult it was for them when Tony passed away. Many of Tony's caregivers offered us the opportunity to talk with them after Tony's death at any time if we needed it. We have taken several of these caregivers up on their offers. We have needed some continued reassurance that we did all we could for Tony. Tony's PICU caregivers shared with us that they learn from every patient. They demonstrated an ability to appreciate the specialness of every patient. Thankfully, they shared with us the ways our son and family touched them. We feel great comfort knowing this. As we continue to relive Tony's final moments, we also feel comfort in knowing we can continue to reach out to the PICU caregivers if we need more reassurance in the future. After all, even though the patient is no longer in need of help, his family members might still be in need, and they matter too!

In conclusion, we want to thank those who are reading our story right now. Thank you for your interest and for considering our experience when treating your patients in critical care situations. Although our story is not representative of all families, there are likely many similarities. Our ultimate hope in sharing our experience is that all staff working within Critical Care medicine will recognize that although excellent medical care is the most important aspect of treatment, there is an important place for compassion. Consideration of the individual patient's situation and that of the family is also paramount; this is what children and families need and deserve, whether they spend a few hours, days, or weeks in your care.

# Index

*Note:* Page numbers of article titles are in **boldface** type.

Printed and bound by CPI Group (UK) Ltd, Croydon, CR0 4YY

03/10/2024

01040441-0008